HANDBOOK OF
SYMPTOM-ORIENTED
NEUROLOGY

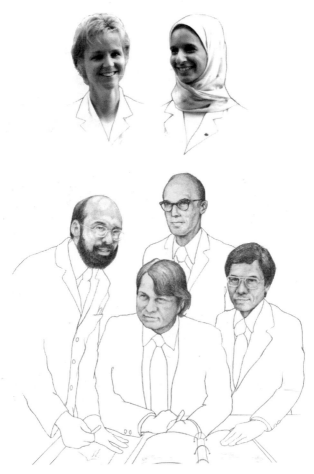

The first edition of this book (published by Charles C. Thomas) was conceived in the late 1970s by four faculty members of the University of North Dakota. A portrait of the original four authors—Dr. Roger Brumback, Dr. William Olson, the late Dr. Lee A. Christoferson, and Dr. Generoso Gascon—appeared on the inside cover of the original edition. The three remaining authors are approaching retirement age. Over the years, the book has proved invaluable to numerous primary care physicians. We now pass the torch to Dr. Kerri Remmel and Dr. Reem Bunyan, who are shown at the top of this page. We are confident that they will continue to emphasize the common and the practical in future editions.

HANDBOOK OF SYMPTOM-ORIENTED NEUROLOGY

KERRI S. REMMEL, M.D., Ph.D.
Assistant Professor
University of Louisville School of Medicine
Louisville, Kentucky

REEM BUNYAN, M.D.
Assistant Professor
University of Louisville School of Medicine
Louisville, Kentucky

ROGER A. BRUMBACK, M.D.
Professor and Chairman of Pathology
Creighton University School of Medicine
St. Joseph Hospital
Omaha, Nebraska

GENEROSO G. GASCON, M.D.
Professor of Clinical Neurosciences and Pediatrics
Brown University School of Medicine
Chief, Division of Pediatric Neurology;
Medical Director, Pediatric Epilepsy
Rhode Island/Hasbro Children's Hospital
Providence, Rhode Island

WILLIAM H. OLSON, M.D.
Professor of Neurology
University of Louisville School of Medicine
Louisville, Kentucky

THIRD EDITION

Illustrated by Gary Baune
with **286** illustrations

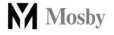

Mosby

An Imprint of Elsevier Science

St. Louis London Philadelphia Sydney Toronto

a mosby handbook

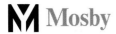

An Imprint of Elsevier Science

Acquisition Editor: Liz Fathman
Editorial Assistant: Paige Mosher Wilke
Publishing Services Manager: Pat Joiner
Associate Project Manager: Keri O'Brien
Designer: Mark A. Oberkrom
Cover Art: Gary Baune

THIRD EDITION
Copyright © 2002 by Mosby, Inc.
Previous editions copyrighted 1984, 1989

NOTICE
Pharmacology is an ever-changing field. Standard safety precautions must be followed, but as new research and clinical experience broaden our knowledge, changes in treatment and drug therapy may become necessary or appropriate. Readers are advised to check the most current product information provided by the manufacturer of each drug to be administered to verify the recommended dose, the method and duration of administration, and contraindications. It is the responsibility of the licensed prescriber, relying on experience and knowledge of the patient, to determine dosages and the best treatment for each individual patient. Neither the publisher nor the editor assumes any liability for any injury and/or damage to persons or property arising from this publication.

Mosby, Inc.
An Imprint of Elsevier Science
11830 Westline Industrial Drive
St. Louis, Missouri 63146

Printed in the United States of America

International Standard Book Number 0-323-01712-6

02   03   04   05   06   CL/FF   9   8   7   6   5   4   3   2   1

Foreword

I was first introduced to the *Handbook of Symptom-Oriented Neurology* when I was a medical student in 1985 during a clerkship in neurology at the University of Louisville (Kentucky). Since then, I have established a large private practice in central Kentucky and am a board-certified internist. This book has been of enormous help to me in treating my patients with neurologic complaints, and in the intervening years I have referred back to it on numerous occasions. Because the book is symptom oriented, I can go directly to the problem in a very brief period of time. Because of the press of time, I certainly can't do a complete neurologic examination on every patient, but the book alerts me to the most important 2 to 3 things that I need to ask in my history and my physical examination. This is especially helpful in a small community where neurologic consultation is not always available. When I do need a neurologic consultation, the book has enabled me to provide the specialist with the appropriate studies and, in most cases, therapeutic trial of medication so that the patient is treated in an expeditious manner.

I also appreciate the small size of the book so that it can fit easily into my pocket or examining bag, and because it is paperback and does not contain color illustrations, it is much less expensive than other neurologic textbooks.

I believe that ownership of this book would greatly enhance the quality of practice of any primary care provider.

Sincerely,

Stephen Hinton, M.D.

Preface

This is the fourth version of a book first published in 1980. The purpose now is the same as it was then: to assist the primary care physician in managing common, treatable, and emergency neurologic problems. No attempt has been made in this text to write an exhaustive treatise of neurologic disease, to present neurologic pathophysiology, or to detail the diagnosis of rare, untreatable neurologic conditions. We believe that this book will enable primary care physicians to take a neurologic symptom and, in most cases, arrive at a neurologic diagnosis and institute an appropriate therapeutic regimen. Where appropriate, we have attempted to provide the readers with the cost of medications and outcomes of treatment.

The content and philosophy of this manual was based on a paper by Dr. T. J. Murray (Concepts in undergraduate teaching, *Clin Neurol Neurosurg* 79[4]237-284, 1976), which addressed the issue of common neurologic complaints presenting to family physicians in Canada. Although at least 10% of all patients presenting to primary care physicians seen in family practice have neurologic problems, many physicians feel uneasy with neurologic problems because medical school curricula devote far less than 10% to these types of problems.

Plasmapheresis or IVIg is routinely used to treat myasthenia gravis and other autoimmune diseases, and various anticonvulsants are available on the market for the treatment of seizures. The treatment of Parkinson's disease has been improved with the introduction of a variety of dopamine agonists and decarboxylase inhibitors. Likewise, in the treatment of stroke, many centers are now using clot-busting techniques or directly attacking the problem vis-à-vis interventional neuroradiology.

Since 1980, there have been major advances in the clinical neurosciences. Superb images of the brain generated by either computed tomographic (CT) scans or magnetic resonance imaging (MRI) are available in most communities throughout the United States. Lumbar punctures are no longer necessary to determine if a stroke is hemorrhagic, and in most cases the diagnosis of multiple sclerosis is simple with MRI. Plasmapheresis is routinely used to treat myasthenia gravis and other autoimmune diseases, and in the near future at least a half dozen more anticonvulsants will be available for the treatment of seizures. The treatment of

Parkinson's disease has been improved with the introduction of dopamine agonists.

Since the first edition, two diseases—Alzheimer's disease and acquired immunodeficiency syndrome (AIDS)—have moved to the forefront of the health concerns of the general public. With our increasingly aged population, more and more cases of the progressive dementing disorder, Alzheimer's disease, are being recognized. With greater public awareness of this devastating and currently untreatable condition, it is imperative that physicians not only recognize the clinical symptoms and provide patient counseling, but also identify treatable conditions with similar symptoms. On the other hand, AIDS currently provides a much more difficult problem, since the causative viral agent is highly neurotropic and can produce a wide variety of symptoms related to the infection. In many respects this infection deserves the appellation once applied to syphilis—the "great imitator."

Special recognition needs to be given to Mr. Gary Baune, who continues to be our superb medical illustrator. We also wish to thank Asad Ismail, M.D., for his input into the chapters with psychiatric content.

Kerri S. Remmel
Reem Bunyan
Roger A. Brumback
Generoso G. Gascon
William H. Olson

Contents

Scattered throughout the text are triangular markers, ▶, which highlight the key diagnostic features for each specific disease.

HANDBOOK OF
SYMPTOM-ORIENTED
NEUROLOGY

1

Neurologic
Examination

Contrary to popular opinion, there is no "standard" neurologic examination. When we are requested to teach the neurologic examination, our response is, The neurologic examination of what? The ambulatory adult? The infant? The comatose patient? A neurologic examination should be *problem-oriented*, and in reality there are different examinations for different clinical situations. Therefore we have included many of our suggestions for the neurologic examination under specific chapter headings. In most circumstances common sense should prevail. For example, testing smell is of little help in the diagnosis of a primary muscle disease, and testing the anal wink is of little value in diagnosing the average patient with a headache. In essence, the neurologic examination is a process of gathering objective data relating to the hypotheses formed during the process of history taking. (For neurologic examination of the infant, see Chapter 16.)

This chapter is intended to provide hints on the more commonly used (and abused) portions of the neurologic examination. It is not a complete guide to the entire procedure. A more complete guide to the standard problem-oriented neurologic examination is found in the appendix.

SCREENING OF NEUROLOGIC ABNORMALITIES

Station and Gait

Table 1-1 outlines and Fig. 1-1 illustrates the procedure for station and gait testing, which usually can be performed in less than 1 minute. Box 1-1 emphasizes that virtually every aspect of the central and peripheral nervous system is tested. A patient with a normal station and gait is unlikely to have any serious structural neurologic abnormality. Twenty feet of straight walking space is desirable, and the patient should be barefooted and clothed only in underwear or a gown.

By observing the station and gait, a skillful examiner can obtain in 1 minute a glimpse of mental status (how well the patient comprehends and follows instructions), upper motor neuron function (posturing of

TABLE 1-1
Procedure for Station and Gait Testing

Instructions	Things to note
Walk the distance normally.	Asymmetric arm swing, abnormal arm and hand postures, and instability of the trunk should be noted.
Rapidly turn around and walk on tiptoe.	Extra steps while turning around and inability to rise completely on the tips of the toes should be noted.
Rapidly turn and walk on heels.	Foot drop should be noted.
Turn and walk with heels touching toes (tandem walk).	Instability characteristic of midline cerebellar lesions should be noted.
Turn and "walk on outsides of feet like a bowlegged cowboy does" (walking on lateral aspects of feet).	This maneuver specifically brings out hemiplegic posturing of an arm from subtle or old upper motor neuron damage.
Do a deep knee bend (preferably with hands on hips; if there is an obvious balance problem, patient may hold onto an object, such as a chair).	Loss of balance indicates cerebellar difficulties; inability to rise indicates proximal weakness.
Stand with feet together, eyes closed, and arms outstretched with palms facing ceiling and fingers spread apart.	Increased swaying with eyes closed indicates either posterior column disease or a peripheral neuropathy; with subtle hemiparesis the affected arm will pronate, whereas in more obvious hemiparesis the arm will pronate and then drift downward and outward.

BOX 1-1
Possible Abnormalities of Station and Gait

Abnormal mentation: Poor or slow ability to follow directions; need for examiner to demonstrate instructions; tendency for patient to continue doing same task (perseveration)

Hemiplegia: Decreased arm swing on affected side, circumduction of leg, pronation of arms when held outstretched with palms up, flexion of arm when walking on sides of feet

Cerebellar ataxia: Unsteadiness when turning around, in tandem walking, and in deep knee bending

Sensory ataxia: Increased swaying when eyes are closed (positive Romberg test)

Muscle disease: Difficulty with deep knee bend, waddling gait

Basal ganglia disorders: Abnormal postures and movement (e.g., Parkinson's syndrome, Huntington's disease)

Lumbar disc disease: Inability to walk on heels or toes on one side; spinal list

Peripheral neuropathy: Bilateral foot drop; inability to walk on heels

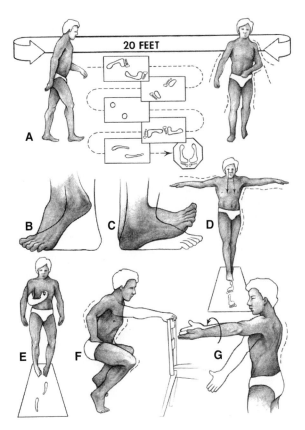

FIG. 1-1 Testing of station and gait. Pay particular attention to arm swing, arm posture, body posture, instability while turning around, and tendency to look at floor. See text for additional information.

arms and gait), lower motor neuron function (muscle atrophy and weakness), muscle disease (proximal weakness), basal ganglia function (abnormal posture and movement), cerebellar function (balance and tandem walk), and the sensory system (poor balance with eyes closed–the Romberg test). A patient who can perform all the maneuvers normally will rarely have a significant neurologic abnormality. Abnormalities noted can be more specifically tested in the remainder of the neurologic examination. For example, if station and gait testing suggests a cerebellar abnormality, more specific cerebellar tests should be performed.

Deep Tendon Reflexes (Muscle Stretch Reflexes)

The most difficult part of the neurologic examination to perform correctly (and the one that medical students think is easiest) is the evaluation of deep tendon reflexes (Figs. 1-2 to 1-5). If at all possible, have the patient undress and sit with legs dangling freely over the edge of the table. The reflex elicited will depend on the following:

1. Whether or not the tendon is struck
2. How hard the tendon is struck
3. How quickly the tendon is struck

To avoid striking an improper area, the examiner should first palpate the tendon. The lightest tap that will still elicit the response should be given. A hammer with a relatively soft rubber end and a flexible handle will best allow the rapid, light tap. The examiner will most often find asymmetry of reflexes rather than gross hyperactivity or absence of reflexes. Reflexes may be normal, hyperactive or hypoactive, clonic or absent, or symmetric or asymmetric and should be recorded as such.

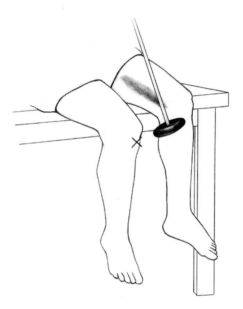

FIG. 1-2 The patellar reflex. Note that the legs do not touch the floor. The type of hammer illustrated was developed in England and is especially effective. Look not only for reflex contraction of the quadriceps but also contralateral contraction of the adductor muscle and the number of swings the leg makes. REMEMBER: Dysfunction of either the afferent or efferent nerves may diminish the reflex.

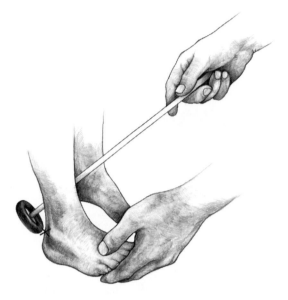

FIG. 1-3 Achilles reflex. While striking the tendon, have the patient apply *light* pressure with the sole of the foot to the palm of the examiner.

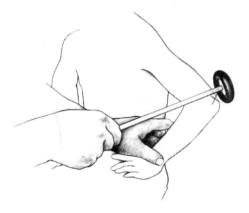

FIG. 1-4 Triceps reflex. This reflex is most easily elicited when the patient rests the arms on the hips.

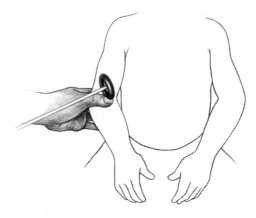

FIG. 1-5 Biceps reflex. It is very important to have the arms symmetrically flexed and relaxed as illustrated.

Recording pluses, minuses, or other symbols, unless carefully defined, does little to convey accurate information in the chart.

Babinski's Reflex

The Babinski's reflex (Fig. 1-6) is the eponym given to the plantar response, which may be present depending on the following:

1. The type of stimulation used
2. The rapidity with which the stimulus is delivered
3. The position of the patient

A sharp object (a safety pin or the sharpened end of some hammers) will produce little more than a withdrawal response, whereas too light a touch will produce no response. We find a key to be the most readily available, appropriate stimulus. The key is used to stimulate the *lateral* aspect of the plantar surface of the foot, beginning at the heel and moving up to the ball of the foot but staying lateral to the great toe. Examples of some responses to plantar stimulation are shown in Table 1-2.

Because the abnormal response is such an important sign of nervous system disease, the best approach to recording the results, if in doubt, is to record exactly the observed movements. It is inadequate to say simply, "Babinski absent." Of course he is; he died more than a half century ago.

Optic Fundus

Ophthalmoscopic examination of the optic fundus is the only opportunity the physician has to look directly at the brain, and it is imperative to do so on *every* patient with neurologic symptoms. This should be done even in difficult cases, such as a crying, hyperactive 4-year-old child. Men-

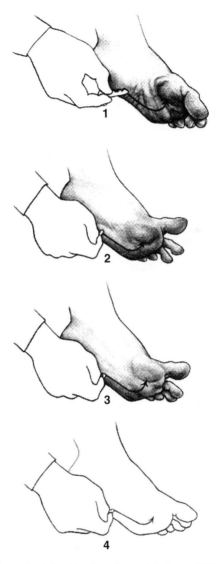

FIG. 1-6 Plantar stimulation. Note that only two of the five possibilities constitute a positive Babinski's response. See text for additional information.

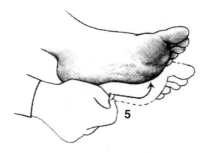

FIG. 1-6, cont'd

TABLE 1-2
Responses to Plantar Stimulation

Name	Observation	Interpretation
Normal response (flexor plantar response)	First movement of great toe is flexion.	Normal
Classic Babinski's reflex (classic extensor plantar response)	Extension of great toe with extension and fanning of other toes occur.	Most often seen in upper motor neuron lesions (below the foramen magnum)
Babinski's reflex (extensor plantar response)	First movement of great toe is extension (there may be subsequent flexion of great toes); other toes either show no movement or flexion.	Seen in all types of upper motor neuron lesions (especially above the foramen magnum)
Mute plantar response	Nothing happens.	Seen in severe sensory loss or paralysis of foot
Withdrawal	Patient pulls foot away.	Often seen in toxic-metabolic peripheral neuropathies
Asymmetric response	Mute plantar response on one side and flexor plantar response on other side occur.	Is indication of need to look for other signs of neurologic disease

tally make a list of those parts of the fundus that must be seen to confirm the hypotheses formed during the history. For example, in the patient with suspected multiple sclerosis, look particularly for temporal pallor of the optic disc. Adjust the size of the beam to match the size of the pupil (too large a beam causes light to reflect from the iris). Using too bright a beam may cause excessive pupillary constriction. In general, use the brightest light possible that still allows visualization of the retina. Darkening the room is usually not helpful, since it prevents the patient from fixating on a target. Pupillary dilating agents are generally not necessary.

Pharyngeal Reflex

The pharyngeal reflex (Fig. 1-7) should be tested on each side by stimulating the pharyngeal pillars with a cotton swab. After observing the motor response (elevation of the palate), ask the patient if the sensation was the same on both sides of the pharynx. (Simply jamming a tongue depressor down the patient's throat not only gives very little neurologic information but is downright rude.) The response is significant only if it is asymmetric; the normal gamut of responses runs from hyperactive to hypoactive.

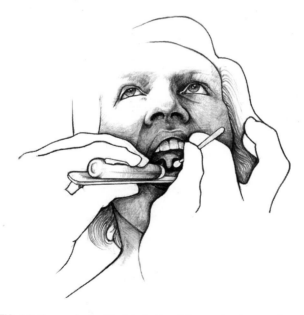

FIG. 1-7 Pharyngeal reflex. Touch both sides of the posterior pharynx and watch for elevation of the palate. Ask the patient if the sensation on both sides is the same. In some patients, it may be necessary, as illustrated, to press down on the tongue by holding the tongue blade and flashlight in one hand.

Sensory Examination

The sensory examination under most clinical conditions does not produce objective, "hard" data because it involves subjective judgments by both the patient and the examiner. Beginning medical students are often fascinated by the sensory examination and spend an inordinate amount of time performing it. If pinprick, vibration, light touch, and position sensation are present in the feet and if the patient can recognize numbers written on the palms of the hands with eyes closed, a major sensory

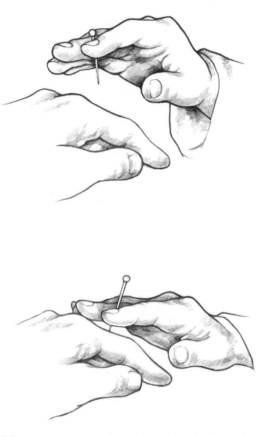

FIG. 1-8 Testing sensation of pain. Grasp the pin shaft and allow the pin to slide through the fingers until the pin makes contact with the skin. *Compare* a normal area (e.g., chest) with a suspected area of involvement (e.g., foot).

deficit is unlikely. On the other hand, if given a pin and a marking pencil, an intelligent, cooperative patient can often accurately define a circumscribed sensory deficit. Likewise, when looking for a sensory level, have the patient run his or her own finger up the body until sensation changes. When a peripheral neuropathy is suspected, ask the patient to compare a single pinprick proximally (such as on the chest) with a single pinprick distally (such as on the foot). Use a disposable pin and allow the shaft to slide through the finger to deliver a relatively quantitative response (Fig. 1-8). Simply comparing sharp and dull sensations on the foot is inadequate. The examiner should attempt to quantitate any difference between the proximal and distal stimulation sites. For example, ask, "If this [chest] pinprick is worth $100, how much is this [foot] pinprick worth?" and consider a response less than $75 as significant. A useful, objective sign of sensory loss is *summation;* that is, repeated quick pinpricks of the same intensity will suddenly become very painful and will result in the patient withdrawing the extremity and grimacing (normally, repeated pricking will not become more painful). This phenomenon is most frequently present in toxic-metabolic peripheral neuropathies such as those associated with diabetes mellitus.

Only when the examination basics—mental status, cranial nerves, reflexes, motor system, sensory system—have been thoroughly mastered are the "curiosities"(e.g., Hoffman reflex) and "toys" (e.g., optokinetic drums) used. In specialized situations these may be useful but need not be routinely used by the student or the time-pressed physician.

BIBLIOGRAPHY

Barrows H: *Neurologic examination,* Chicago, 1981, Division of Marketing Services, American Medical Association, (videotape).

Caselli RJ: Rediscovering tactile agnosia, *Mayo Clin Proc* 66:129-213, 1991.

DeMyer W: *Technique of the neurologic examination: a programmed text,* ed 4, New York, 1993, McGraw-Hill.

Goldberg S: Principles of neurologic localization, *Am Fam Physician* 23:131-141 1981.

Haerer AF: *DeJong's the neurologic examination,* ed 5, Philadelphia, 1992, JB Lippincott.

Mayo Clinic Foundation: *Clinical examinations in neurology,* ed 6, Philadelphia, 1991, WB Saunders.

Perkin D: *Atlas of clinical neurology,* Philadelphia, 1986, JB Lippincott.

Rodnitzky RL: *Van Allen's pictorial manual of neurologic tests,* St. Louis, 1988, Mosby.

2

Neurodiagnostic Procedures

A well-elicited history and an adequate neurologic examination should enable the physician to form a provisional diagnosis. Such a diagnosis will include the probable site of the lesion and the probable type or cause of the neurologic disorder. There will be a number of differential diagnoses, particularly with regard to the type of lesion, which can often be settled only by suitable investigative procedures. It is essential for the physician to have a clear idea regarding the indications as well as the specificity and sensitivity of the various procedures. The physician's goal would be to put the patient through minimal discomfort (by choosing the least invasive investigations) and to obtain the most specific information that will point to the correct diagnosis. The neurodiagnostic procedures may not only be diagnostic but may also serve as prognostic indicators. This chapter gives brief descriptions of common neurologic procedures, along with their indications and potential side effects. Table 2-1 lists various neurodiagnostic procedures and their indications.

LUMBAR PUNCTURE
Lumbar puncture (LP) is perhaps the most common neurodiagnostic procedure that a physician must personally perform.

Indications
1. When a central nervous system (CNS) infection (meningitis or encephalitis) is suspected; a cerebrospinal fluid (CSF) study should be done *without delay*.

Caution: If there are focal findings, such as a hemiplegia, or if there is papilledema, a computed tomographic (CT) scan or magnetic resonance imaging (MRI) is strongly recommended before performing the LP to identify mass lesions.

2. When a subarachnoid hemorrhage is suspected: Most cases of subarachnoid hemorrhage can be diagnosed by a CT scan. An LP is indicated in

TABLE 2-1
Diagnostic Tests in Neurologic Disorders

Test	Anatomic/physiologic basis	Most useful in
Electroencephalogram (EEG)	Spontaneous electrical activity of cerebral cortical neurons	Seizure disorders Metabolic encephalopathy Tumors Infectious encephalopathy Dementia Brain death determination
Visual evoked potentials (VEPs)	Arrival of electrical signals at the visual cortex through the visual pathways, when the retina is stimulated	Multiple sclerosis Disorders of optic nerve Lesions of optic tract, radiations, or occipital cortex
Brainstem auditory evoked potentials (BAEPs)	Passage of electrical signals through auditory nerve, auditory nuclei, lateral lemniscus, and inferior colliculus to auditory cortex	Acoustic neurilemmoma (neuroma) Brainstem tumor Brainstem infarct Multiple sclerosis
Somatosensory evoked potentials (SSEPs)	Passage of electrical signals through peripheral nerves to central somatosensory pathways (including dorsal columns, medial lemnisci, thalamus, thalamocortical pathways) and arrival at sensory cortex	Multiple sclerosis Spinal cord tumors Myelopathy
Nerve conduction studies	Conduction of electrical signals through myelinated nerve fibers (motor or sensory)	Peripheral neuropathy Nerve trauma Nerve compression (e.g., carpal tunnel syndrome)
Needle electromyography (EMG)	Electrical activity of muscle during rest and voluntary contraction	Denervating disease (e.g., amyotrophic lateral sclerosis [ALS]) Muscular dystrophy Polymyositis
Repetitive nerve stimulation test (Jolly test)	Neuromuscular transmission	Myasthenia gravis Lambert-Eaton (myasthenic) syndrome

Continued

TABLE 2-1
Diagnostic Tests in Neurologic Disorders—cont'd

Test	Anatomic/physiologic basis	Most useful in
Muscle biopsy	Morphology and histo-chemistry of muscle fibers	Muscular dystrophy Polymyositis Metabolic disorders
Nerve biopsy	Morphology of axons and myelin	Peripheral neuropathy
Cerebrospinal fluid (CSF) study	CSF pressure, bio-chemistry, cell count, serology, micro-biology	Meningitis Encephalitis Subarachnoid hemorrhage Multiple sclerosis Central nervous system (CNS) syphilis
Myelogram	Outline of spinal canal and its contents via radiopaque contrast in subarachnoid CSF space may be com-bined with computed tomography (CT)	Cervical or lumbar disc herniations Spinal cord tumors
Magnetic resonance imaging (MRI)	Different responses of protons in various tissues and com-partments of nervous system to high-intensity magnetic fields	Multiple sclerosis Tumors (especially in posterior fossa) Spinal cord lesions Infarcts Malformations
Computed tomography (CT)	Different x-ray absorp-tion coefficients of various tissues and compartments within nervous system	Hemorrhage Infarct Tumor Hydrocephalus Dementia Head trauma

those patients in whom the CT scan is negative and a hemorrhage is still suspected on clinical grounds.
3. When an LP should be done in those patients in whom alterations in CSF biochemistry can be of diagnostic value: e.g., Guillain-Barré syndrome (albuminocytologic dissociation), multiple sclerosis (oligo-clonal bands and myelin basic protein, elevated immunoglobulin G [IgG]).
4. When CNS involvement must be determined in cases of leukemia and lymphoma (cytology).

5. When CNS syphilis is suspected.
6. When contrast media or drugs must be introduced into the CSF.
7. When CSF pressure must be measured for the diagnosis and management of pseudotumor cerebri.

Contraindications

1. When there is local infection at the proposed site of puncture (if CSF sample must be obtained in a patient, a cisternal puncture or lateral cervical puncture can be done).
2. When a cerebral mass lesion is suspected based on signs of increased intracranial pressure such as papilledema: A sudden decrease in intraspinal CSF pressure can potentially lead to herniation of either the tonsils of the cerebellum through the foramen magnum or portions of the temporal lobe through the tentorium cerebelli. Such a complication, if not promptly detected and treated, will be fatal. This underscores the importance of examining the ocular fundi and doing a CT scan before doing an LP. There are two situations in which an LP may still have to be done despite the presence of papilledema: (1) when there is a high index of suspicion of meningitis and (2) when pseudotumor cerebri is strongly suspected. In either case, a neurologic or neurosurgical consultation needs to be made before an LP is done.
3. Coagulopathy.

Note: When future diagnostic studies, such as myelography, are contemplated, postpone the LP, since a sample of CSF can be obtained when the radiologic procedure is performed.

Technique

1. Explain the procedure thoroughly to the patient and be sure to ask for a history of allergy to local anesthetics or iodine.
2. Site of puncture: The LP is usually carried out at the L3 to L4 or L4 to L5 interspinous space (the L4 to L5 interspinous space is at the same level as the highest point of the iliac crest).
3. Position of patient: Have the patient lie on a hard surface on the side with the knees pulled toward the chest and the head flexed (fetal position) (Figs. 2-1 to 2-5). Make sure that the spine is straight and not curved (bent) sideways. Alternatively, make the patient sit up to easier locate the correct space for puncture. For patients who are agitated or delirious, restraint or sedation may be necessary; if sufficient personnel are not available, the patient may be trussed (Fig. 2-4).
4. Prepare the skin surface for puncture by vigorously rubbing the area with povidone-iodine (Betadine) or another equally effective anti-infective topical solution. A sterile technique, including gloves and drapes, is very important. Commercially available sterile disposable LP trays and disposable (rather than reusable) spinal needles are preferred. Always use a spinal needle with a stylet.
5. Using local anesthetic, make a skin wheal and then infiltrate more deeply, particularly around the bone.

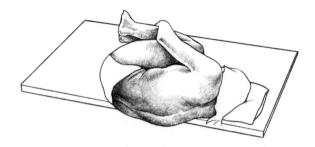

FIG. 2-1 Positioning for a lumbar puncture. Note that the patient is placed on a firm surface so that the spinal column is relatively straight. Once the subarachnoid space is entered, the legs should be greatly extended to relax the patient and relieve pressure on the abdomen.

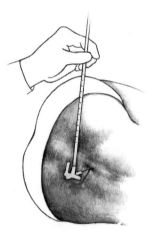

FIG. 2-2 Once the subarachnoid space is entered, place the stopcock in upright position and record the pressure. If a moderately high pressure is recorded (e.g., 250 mm of water), it is most often secondary to patient anxiety. Wait a few minutes and the pressure will frequently return to normal (<200 mm of water).

Insert the needle with the bevel parallel to the long axis of the body so that it separates rather than cuts through the fibers of the ligamentum flavum (Fig. 2-5). When the needle enters the subarachnoid space (you will feel a pop as it passes through the posterior spinal ligament and dura), withdraw the stylet, allowing only 1 drop of CSF to escape, verifying that the needle is indeed in the subarachnoid space.

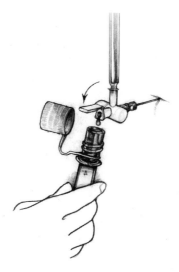

FIG. 2-3 After the pressure measurement is taken, turn the stopcock as illustrated and obtain an appropriate amount of fluid.

Reinsert the stylet immediately and tell the patient to relax; have an assistant extend the patient's head and legs. Attach the manometer and record the opening pressure. Normal CSF opening pressure is less than 200 mm of water. Opening pressure should not be measured when the patient is in a seated position. Closing pressure is of no clinical importance.

6. Keep the needle strictly parallel to the spine and the tip pointed toward the patient's umbilicus. If you encounter bone, withdraw the needle up to the subcutaneous tissue and then reintroduce it at a different angle. If the needle does not enter the subarachnoid space on the second attempt, try the procedure in the sitting position, which enables you to better gauge the midline. Do not make repeated, unsuccessful attempts to perform an LP; call for more experienced help or perform the procedure under fluoroscopy.

7. After measuring the opening pressure, remove the CSF for laboratory study. Know how much CSF is required before attempting the LP, so that enough fluid can be obtained for all studies. About 5 ml of CSF is required for biochemical studies for determination of glucose (0.5 ml), protein (1 ml), and protein electrophoresis (4 ml). Microbiologic studies require about 8 ml of CSF for a routine culture (1 ml), acid-fast and fungal cultures (2 to 3 ml), syphilis serology (1 ml), cryptococcal antigen and antibody (1 ml), and Gram's stain (1 ml). Cell count requires 0.5 ml. It is always a good idea to have an extra 2 ml of CSF labeled

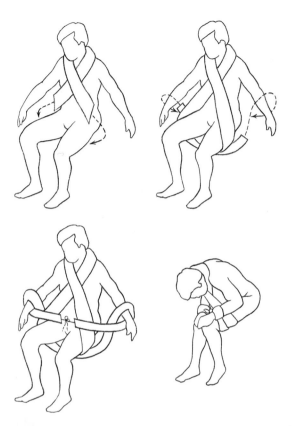

FIG. 2-4 Trussing with a sheet. An uncooperative patient may be restrained with a sheet as illustrated.

and frozen in case the quantity originally sent to the laboratory turns out to be insufficient for the tests ordered or if confirmation is desired. In general, the first collected tube should go for routine culture and the second tube for protein and other biochemical studies.

Caveat: At completion of the fluid collection and needle removal there is a hole through the dura into the subcutaneous paravertebral tissue. The continuously produced CSF (at the rate of about 20 ml/hr) can leak through this hole until normal repair processes obliterate the hole. With normal technique the leakage occurs for only a short period, but may amount to 30 ml or more. Continuing leakage can result in greater fluid

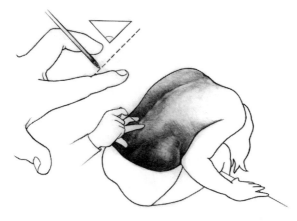

FIG. 2-5 When a difficult lumbar puncture is being performed, it may be necessary for the patient to be in a sitting position, which often makes the landmarks clearer. Increased hydrostatic pressure in the lumbar area tenses the dura, making needle penetration easier. Note that the needle must be inserted with the bevel parallel to the long axis of the spine. Once the needle has entered the subarachnoid space (and with the stylet in place), assist the patient into a lying position; appropriate pressure measurements may then be taken.

loss and cause post-LP headache. The fluid removed for the study constitutes only a small proportion of the extra fluid that can be lost with leakage. Therefore one should always be certain to collect adequate amounts for laboratory study and not be concerned about taking too much. The leakage can be minimized by keeping the bevel of the needle parallel to the long axis of the spine to avoid a dural and posterior ligament tear.

8. If the CSF appears bloody, spin the CSF sample down *immediately* and compare that tube in the sunlight with an identical tube containing water, looking down from the tops of the tubes (Fig. 2-6). If the LP was traumatic, the CSF should appear clear; if the patient has had a subarachnoid hemorrhage, the CSF should appear xanthochromic (yellow). Elevated levels of CSF protein (more than 100 mg/dl) or peripheral bilirubin can also result in xanthochromic fluid.
9. Cell count.
   a. A cell count should be done *immediately* (preferably by the physician), since white blood cells (WBCs) lyse quickly at room temperature (at room temperature, there is a 50% loss of cells in the first half-hour after collection).
   b. Red blood cells (RBCs) in the fluid can be lysed (leaving only the WBCs to be visualized in counting) by drawing acetic acid into a capillary hematocrit tube (or white cell pipette) and then blowing

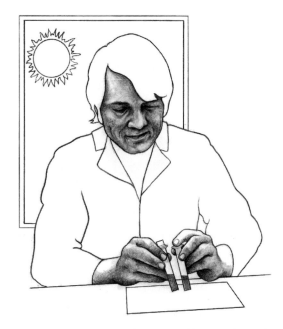

FIG. 2-6 Xanthochromia may best be appreciated by comparing cerebrospinal fluid with water in sunlight against a white sheet of paper.

it out; the capillary tube is then introduced into the CSF solution and the CSF drawn up into the capillary tube.

   c. It will be easier to see the cells if they are stained; crystal violet may be used (mix 0.1 g of crystal violet, 1 ml of glacial acetic acid, 50 ml of distilled water, and 2 drops of phenol). The solution is drawn up the into capillary hematocrit tube (or white cell pipette) and then blown out. The capillary tube is then introduced into the CSF solution. The CSF is drawn up into the capillary tube. After it mixes well, place the CSF into the counting chamber. Under these conditions RBCs appear green and WBCs appear purple.

   d. Normal CSF contains fewer than five lymphocytes and no polymorphonuclear leukocytes per microliter (mm^3). In addition to looking for WBCs and doing a differential count, you may want to use cytologic techniques to look for the presence of malignant cells. When meningitis or encephalitis is suspected, a Gram's stain and an acid-fast stain (on centrifuged sediment) need to be done.

10. Chemistries.

   a. The protein level is less than 40 mg/dl in the lumbar subarachnoid fluid and much lower (10 to 20 mg/dl) in fluid from the ventricles. Markedly increased protein levels (750 to 1000 mg/dl) can be seen in spinal block (Froin's syndrome), whereas mild to moderate elevation can be seen in Guillain-Barré syndrome, meningitis, diabetes, polyneuropathy, and certain types of brain tumors. In multiple sclerosis (MS) the elevation is seldom more than 80 to 100 mg/dl. An elevated CSF IgG percentage (normal is less than 13%) by CSF protein electrophoresis indicates the possibility of MS, tuberculosis, myeloma, or other inflammatory or immunologic disorders. An IgG index is a sensitive test of excessive IgG synthesis in the CNS; it is calculated by the following formula:

$$\frac{\text{CSF IgG/serum IgG}}{\text{CSF albumin/serum albumin}} \qquad [\text{normal} < 0.7]$$

Demonstration of oligoclonal (IgG) bands and myelin basic protein (>1.0 ng/ml) in the CSF is highly useful in the diagnosis of MS.

   b. If meningitis is suspected in a diabetic patient or a patient receiving intravenous (IV) glucose, it may be advantageous to compare the blood glucose and the CSF glucose levels. The blood should be drawn at least 1 hour before the LP for such comparison. The CSF glucose level is normally about two thirds of that in blood.

11. Microbiology. When CNS infection is suspected, prompt identification of the etiologic agent is crucial for initiation of appropriate therapy. The following CSF studies should be done:

   a. Gram's stain is positive in 90% of patients with bacterial meningitis, although *Haemophilus influenzae* or *Listeria monocytogenes* are difficult to identify.

   b. Culture is positive in 70% to 90% of untreated bacterial meningitis, but the percentage drops if oral antibiotics have been given before LP.

   c. Rapid detection of bacterial antigens by latex particle agglutination or countercurrent immunoelectrophoresis is useful in this context. The limulus lysate assay is useful when meningitis resulting from gram-negative bacteria is suspected.

   d. When tuberculous meningitis is suspected, special stains (such as the Ziehl-Neelsen method) should be ordered. Repeated culture or animal inoculation studies may also be necessary.

   e. When viral meningitis is suspected, a culture as well as detection of antibodies in CSF is useful.

   f. In suspected fungal meningitis, detection of antigen (e.g., cryptococcal antigen) and culture (with large volumes of CSF) are necessary.

   g. The CSF Venereal Disease Research Laboratory (VDRL) should be done when neurosyphilis is a possibility.

Complications of Lumbar Puncture

1. Post-LP headache occurs in about 10% to 20% of patients. The diagnostic feature is marked exacerbation of pain upon sitting up and dramatic relief on lying down. The onset is within 1 to 3 days after LP, and the headache lasts for days to weeks. Bed rest and liberal fluid intake are useful, but in persistent post-LP headache, an autologous epidural blood patch may be necessary.

2. Iatrogenic meningitis: this complication should not occur if adequate sterile precautions are taken.
3. Herniation: a CT scan easily identifies mass lesions that increase the probability of herniation.

Caveat: Millions of LPs were done safely before the invention of the CT scanner; the lack of a CT scan should never delay an LP when acute bacterial meningitis is suspected.

NEURORADIOLOGIC PROCEDURES
Computed Tomography Scan
Since its inception, the CT scan has revolutionized the practice of neurology. CT scans show important anatomic structures, even though they do not demonstrate most blood vessels adequately enough to exclude vascular pathologic conditions. They are most often used in acute stroke to demonstrate extravascular blood; an MRI shows a much wider range of pathologic conditions.

This radiologic examination uses narrow beams of x-rays to penetrate the head in multiple directions with quantification of the absorption of the x-rays by various structures and tissues. With computer analysis, an entire cross section of the brain can be depicted with clear differentiation of the densities of all areas. Such tomographic "slices" can be visualized as a picture on a cathode ray tube (television screen) where a gray scale shading of each picture point is proportional to its density. IV injection of iodinated contrast material ("IVP dye") may be used to enhance the density of vascular or pathologic structures. A pathologic structure such as an infarct will cause a breakdown of the blood-brain barrier, allow the contrast material to seep into normal brain tissue, and draw attention to abnormalities that might otherwise be inapparent on the CT scan.

Injection of a water-soluble iodinated contrast material into the subarachnoid space permits improved visualization of the spinal cord and subarachnoid space on a CT scan.

A CT scan is indicated in patients with focal neurologic deficits, altered mental status, head trauma, new-onset seizures, increased intracranial pressure, and suspected mass lesions or subarachnoid hemorrhage. A CT scan done after the injection of contrast material will improve diagnostic yield in the case of intracranial tumor, abscess, chronic subdural hematoma, infarct, and vascular malformation.

Although a CT scan is highly sensitive and somewhat specific in documenting many types of intracranial pathologic problems, its limitations include an inability to show small lesions or lesions that are isodense with brain tissue and the presence of bony artifacts that make evaluation of the posterior fossa difficult. For example, small plaques of MS may not be visible on CT scans, whereas they are easily visualized by MRI. Infarct in the first 24 to 48 hours may not be seen on a CT scan, and subdural collections that are bilateral and isodense can be missed by a CT scan.

Caveat: A normal CT scan does not rule out intracranial pathologic conditions. Also, a CT scan can show lesions that are not relevant to the patient's current illness (e.g., agenesis of corpus callosum, old infarcts in a patient with unrelated new symptoms). Remember that symptoms and signs must be correlated with lesions found on the CT scan.

Magnetic Resonance Imaging

MRI affords visualization of the anatomic structures of the brain and spinal cord with clarity and detail that is unmatched by any other test. Sagittal, coronal, and horizontal (axial) views can be obtained. The patient is placed in a powerful magnetic field that tends to make the protons of the tissues align themselves in the orientation of the magnetic field. A specific radiofrequency signal (RF pulse) is introduced into the magnetic field, which makes the protons resonate; subsequently, the protons return to their original positions when the RF pulse is stopped. By computer analysis of the RF energy emitted by the protons, an image of the tissue is created. Tissue-specific differences in the energy emission allow delineation of the different components such as white matter, gray matter, and CSF.

MRI is superior to a CT scan except for when imaging acute hemorrhage or bony detail. MRI is especially valuable in diagnosing MS, posterior fossa lesions, temporal lobe lesions, and spinal cord lesions. As with CT scans, IV contrast materials (paramagnetic agents such as gadolinium) add valuable information to the detection of disease processes. Further developments such as MR angiography (MRA) and tissue spectroscopy make the procedure even more valuable.

MRA is a technique that uses MRI and contrast material to specifically look at cerebrovasculature. It is particularly useful in identifying aneurysms and occlusions of larger cerebral blood vessels. It is also very useful in identifying carotid artery disease. If vasculitis is suspected as the cause of the neurologic deficit, a cerebral angiogram should be ordered.

MRI diffuse weighted imaging is particularly useful in identifying areas of ischemia in the first few hours after a stroke. It will identify approximately 90% of the lesions. It is also useful for differentiating tumor from radiation necrosis and will also accurately diagnose acute attacks of MS. The technology requires only an MRI and often can be included in an MR study at no additional cost.

Carotid Doppler Studies

A carotid Doppler study is routinely ordered in stroke victims to identify a carotid pathologic condition. It is 85% to 90% accurate in diagnosing stenosis. *Duplex* indicates that both wave forms and color forms are identified. It is less accurate than the MRA in identifying carotid ulcerations.

Single Photon Emission Computed Tomography

Single photon emission computed tomography (SPECT) is a poor man's positron emission spectroscopy (PET) scan and is rarely ordered. It is not useful in identifying subtle brain disease not seen on MRI, and its cost is only slightly less than that of a PET scan.

Computed Tomography Myelography

When an MRI is contraindicated, a CT scan with contrast material is indicated when external pressure on the spinal dura and its contents or when a mass within the subarachnoid space is suspected.

Myelograms using contrast media heavier than spinal fluid or with conventional radiography are rarely performed at the present time.

Cerebral Angiography

The most important indication for cerebral angiography (arteriography) is suspicion of an abnormality of the blood vessels of the brain that cannot be seen on a CT scan or MRI. The most common indications are suspected aneurysm or arteriovenous malformation (AVM), evaluation of extracranial and intracranial portions of cerebral blood vessels in patients with a transient ischemic attack (TIA) before surgical treatment, arteritis involving intracranial vessels, and assessment of vascularity and vessel configuration in tumors such as meningioma.

During angiography the catheter is inserted into the femoral artery and threaded up the aorta. At the aortic arch the carotid and vertebral arteries and their branches are selectively catheterized. A series of radiographs is taken during injection of a radiopaque contrast material. Fine detail of cerebral vessels as well as the configuration of the larger arteries in the chest and neck can be seen. Arteriography is the "gold standard" for demonstrating aneurysms, AVMs, tumor vascularity, occlusive vascular diseases, and abnormal vascular shunts (such as the subclavian steal phenomenon). In addition to anatomic detail, much physiologic detail, including collateral circulation and the primary feeding vessels to AVMs and tumors, can be assessed. Interventional angiography can obliterate AVMs and aneurysms when particles are injected or coils are inserted into the lesions through special catheters, at times making surgery unnecessary.

Spinal Radiographs

Spinal radiographs (x-ray films) are often taken for any complaint referable to the spine or the spinal cord.

Radiographs of the spine are only as useful as the technical competence of the x-ray technician in obtaining correctly positioned views and as the ability of the radiologist to interpret the films. Especially important in cervical spine radiographs are views of all seven vertebrae. In cervical and lumbar spine radiographs, good oblique views are important. Remember when ordering the radiographs that the segmental spinal cord levels are higher than the vertebral spine levels (in adults, the spinal cord ends at approximately vertebral level L2). Pathologic conditions producing changes seen on spinal radiographs include congenital lesions (e.g., fusion, anomalies, syringomyelia), tuberculosis, fractures, spondylolisthesis, tumors, metabolic bone disease, and degenerative disc disease. Osteosclerotic myeloma lesions may not be seen on any other forms of imaging.

Skull Radiographs

Skull radiographs (x-ray films) are most useful in assessing abnormalities in cranial bones, pituitary fossa, abnormal calcifications, and shifts of normal calcified structures. They are occasionally useful in picking up abnormalities in facial bones, vertebrae, and pericranial structures. They usually are not necessary when a patient has had a CT scan or MRI of the head.

Pathologic conditions producing abnormalities that can be seen on skull radiographs include changes in bone structure (single or multiple areas of destruction as in metastases and multiple myeloma), fractures, intracranial calcifications (normal: e.g., pineal, choroid plexus; or abnormal: e.g., tuberous sclerosis, Sturge-Weber syndrome, certain tumors), increased intracranial pressure, craniostenosis, cerebellopontine angle tumor, enlarged sella from pituitary masses, sinus changes, and congenital or acquired disorders of the skull base. If the odontoid process is not seen on spine radiographs, it should be included in the skull series. There is controversy about the need for routine skull radiographs for minor head injuries, since the yield of therapeutically useful information is very low.

Isotope Cisternography

Isotope cisternography, formerly called *radioiodinated serum albumin (RISA) scan,* consists of the injection of a radioactive nuclide into the lumbar subarachnoid space. The substance used most often is technetium 99m, which can be useful in the investigation of normal pressure hydrocephalus (NPH), CSF leakage, and the patency of ventricular shunts.

Positron Emission Spectroscopy

The PET scan is currently available in many major medical centers and is particularly useful in oncology. It involves injecting a proton emitter, fluorodeoxyglucose (FDG), then computer-mapping the relative metabolism of various areas of the brain. In neurology, the scan is useful for identifying seizure foci and differentiating radiation necrosis from tumor recurrence. It is also thought to be fairly specific in diagnosing the early onset of Alzheimer's disease, which will become more important as specific therapies are developed. Positron emitters are relatively short-lived, and the major technologic hurdle for this technology is an on-site cyclotron.

Magnetic Resonance Spectroscopy

MR spectroscopy has not yet received widespread community applicability; in some centers it is used to differentiate radiation necrosis from tumors. It is also useful in differentiating epileptic foci and recurrent brain tumors.

NEUROPHYSIOLOGIC TESTS

Electroencephalography

Electroencephalography (EEG) records the spontaneous electrical activity of the brain. Electrodes are placed on the scalp in a specific pattern, and the electrical voltage fluctuations between any pair of these electrodes are amplified and recorded permanently on moving paper. Indications include (1) finding the origin and type of electrical discharge associated with clinical seizures and more often in detecting epileptiform abnormalities between seizures (interictal tracing); (2) localizing and assessing changes resulting from trauma, neoplasm, infection, or vascular disease; and (3) assisting in the diagnosis of coma and dementia. This technique is only as good as the skills of the technician recording the tracing and the physician (electroencephalographer) interpreting the tracing. In addition, during the short time of the recording, an intermittent abnormality (e.g., epileptiform abnormality) may not occur.

Caveat: A normal EEG does not rule out an epileptic seizure.

To increase the chances of recording epileptiform abnormalities in the interictal EEG, recommend that the patient be sleep-deprived on the previous night and that both awake and sleep tracings be obtained. Other measures include the use of special electrodes such as nasopharyngeal and sphenoidal electrodes, long-term ambulatory cassette EEG monitoring, or in-hospital video EEG with or without telemetry.

Electromyography

Electromyography (EMG) refers to the recording of the electrical activity of muscle fibers through a needle electrode inserted into the muscle belly. Abnormal spontaneous electrical activity in the form of fasciculations, fibrillations, or positive sharp waves may be recorded. Fasciculations are seen most often in chronic anterior horn cell disorders such as amyotrophic lateral sclerosis (ALS). Fibrillations and positive sharp waves are detected 3 to 6 weeks after the motor nerve is injured. Reinnervation of denervated muscle fibers may be documented by detecting polyphasic motor units during volitional contraction. Changes in the morphologic make up of motor units are helpful in the detection of myopathies and neurogenic disorders. Certain EMG abnormalities, such as myotonia (myotonia congenita, myotonic dystrophy), are diagnostic.

The site of the lesion (nerve, plexus, nerve root, anterior horn cell) can be accurately localized by delineating the distribution of denervation changes among different muscles. For instance, in doubtful cases, objective evidence for a nerve root compression can be obtained by documenting denervation changes limited to those muscles supplied by that particular nerve root. Recovery from a nerve injury can also be predicted or confirmed on the basis of serial EMG studies.

Nerve Conduction Study

A nerve conduction study consists of stimulating a nerve (motor or sensory) at different points and calculating the velocity of conduction of the propagated impulse. The measured velocity is that of the fastest conducting nerve fibers (large myelinated axons) and will be normal if the myelin sheath is intact. Demyelination leads to a decrease in conduction velocity. However, there may be no slowing if the conduction measurement is not through the area of myelin destruction. For example, a conduction study distal to the site of pressure injury to the nerve may initially be normal. In Guillain-Barré syndrome, in which the nerve roots are involved early in the course of the disease, distal conduction may be normal, whereas proximal conduction (measured as F-wave latency or H-reflex latency) tends to be abnormal.

Nerve conduction studies are useful in the following:

1. Diagnosing entrapment neuropathies: i.e., median nerve at the wrist (carpal tunnel syndrome), tibial nerve at the ankle (tarsal tunnel syndrome), ulnar nerve at the elbow
2. Confirming the presence of peripheral neuropathies and distinguishing predominantly demyelinating from predominantly axonal polyneuropathies (see Chapter 15)
3. Localizing the site of injury and following up on recovery in nerve trauma

Remember: Normal nerve velocity does not rule out the existence of polyneuropathy; it only excludes a demyelinating neuropathy involving the larger, thickly myelinated nerve fibers. Small fiber neuropathies (involving only thinly myelinated or unmyelinated nerve fibers) or axonal neuropathies may not significantly slow nerve conduction.

Evoked Potentials

Evoked potentials are a recording of the electrical activity in the CNS produced by stimulation of peripheral sensory receptors. Signals are recorded by placing electrodes over the scalp (as in an EEG) or over the spine; the signals are analyzed by a computer that averages and amplifies them. Auditory stimuli are delivered by clicks through earphones and visual stimuli by stroboscopic flash or, more reliably, by a changing checkerboard pattern on a television screen (pattern-shift visual evoked potential). For somatosensory evoked potentials, electric stimuli are delivered to peripheral nerves, such as the median, peroneal, or tibial nerves.

Neurosonography

Diagnostic ultrasound was originally used to detect the shift of midline structures or hydrocephalus (A-mode echoencephalography). With the advent of the CT scan, this methodology was abandoned. High-resolution, portable, real-time ultrasound scanners have become available and have proved useful in detecting intracranial hemorrhage in premature infants (ultrasound is passed through the fontanels).

Duplex scan: B-mode ultrasound with pulsed Doppler ultrasound has been frequently used to investigate the extracranial carotid arteries. This noninvasive technique gives a graphic image of the arterial wall and analyzes the velocity pattern of the blood flow, providing information about stenosis and plaques.

Transcranial Doppler

Transcranial Doppler (TCD) ultrasonography uses high-energy, pulsed-wave Doppler to image blood flow through the middle cerebral artery, anterior cerebral artery, and the carotid arteries for the evaluation of stenosis, collateral blood flow, and emboli.

Muscle and Nerve Biopsy

Muscle and nerve biopsy specimens are very fragile, and special care must be taken in obtaining and processing the tissue. Muscle biopsies should be done only where the specimen can be quick-frozen and histochemistry performed. Nerve biopsy should be done only where facilities are available for electron microscopy and teased-fiber preparation of the specimen.

Note: Muscle and nerve biopsies should be done under local anesthetic, since general anesthesia in susceptible patients may precipitate malignant hyperthermia (see Chapter 15).

Muscle biopsy may be of value in the following:
1. Evaluating congenital weakness, proximal or distal weakness, or muscle wasting without sensory loss
2. Diagnosing lipid and glycogen storage diseases, sarcoidosis, vasculitis, and inflammatory myopathies
3. Searching for microscopic changes seen in myotonic disorders, endocrine myopathies, and congenital myopathies

Nerve biopsy may be of value in the following:
1. Showing infiltration of peripheral nerves as in amyloidosis, vasculitis, myeloma, carcinoma, sarcoidosis, and leprosy
2. Characterizing congenital hypertrophic neuropathies

BIBLIOGRAPHY

Aminoff MJ: *Electrodiagnosis in clinical neurology,* ed 3, New York, 1992, Churchill Livingstone.

Bronen RA, Sze G: Magnetic resonance imaging contrast agents: theory and application to the central nervous system, *J Neurosurg* 73:820-839, 1990.

Davis KR, Kistler JP, Buonanno FS: Clinical neuroimaging approaches to cerebrovascular diseases, *Neurol Clin* 2:655-665, 1984.

Duffy FH, Iyer VG, Surwillo WW: *Clinical electroencephalography and topographic brain mapping: technology and practice,* New York, 1989, Springer-Verlag.

Fishman RA: *Cerebrospinal fluid in diseases of the nervous system,* ed 2, Philadelphia, 1992, WB Saunders.

Gilman S: Advances in neurology, *N Engl J Med* 326:671-675, 1608-1615, 1992.

Grant EG, White EM: Pediatric neurosonography, *J Child Neurol* 1:319-337, 1986.

Jablecki CK: Electromyography in infants and children, *J Child Neurol* 1:297-318, 1986.

Kirkwood RJ: *Essentials of neuroimaging,* New York, 1990, Churchill Livingstone.

Kovanen J, Sulkava R: Duration of postural headache after lumbar puncture, *Headache* 26:224-226, 1986.

Kughn MJ: *Atlas of neuroradiology,* New York, 1992, Gower Medical Publishers.

Longworth C, Honey G, Sharma T: Science, medicine, and the future: functional magnetic resonance imaging in neuropsychiatry, *Br Med J* 319(7224):1551-1554, 1999.

Mazziotta JC, Gilman S: *Clinical brain imaging,* Philadelphia, 1992, FA Davis.

Miller GM, Forbes GS, Onofrio BM: Magnetic resonance imaging of the spine, *Mayo Clin Proc* 64:986-1004, 1989.

Patten J: *Neurological differential diagnosis,* ed 2, New York, 1996, Springer.

Sato S, Rose DF: The electroencephalogram in the evaluation of the patient with epilepsy, *Neurol Clin* 4:509-529, 1986.

Sidhu PS, Allan PL: The extended role of carotid artery ultrasound, *Clin Radiol* 52(9):643-653, 1997.

Stokes HD, O'Hara CM, Buchanan RD, Olson WH: An improved method for examination of cerebrospinal fluid cells, *Neurology* 25:901-906, 1975.

Zisfein J, Tuchman AJ: Risks of lumbar puncture in the presence of intracranial mass lesions, *Mt Sinai J Med* 55:283-287, 1988.

3

Headache

Headache is one of the most common conditions for which patients seek medical treatment and is the fifth most common reason for outpatient visits. Remember that headache is *a symptom, not a disease,* and successful therapy depends on correct diagnosis. The physician who simply prescribes an analgesic or tranquilizer does the patient no service and runs the risk of causing an iatrogenic drug dependency problem. *Never* treat chronic or recurrent headaches with narcotics. A minimum of 30 minutes should be scheduled and spent with each patient complaining of headache. The primary aim is to differentiate serious or life-threatening conditions that present with headache (e.g., brain tumor, subarachnoid hemorrhage, meningitis) from relatively benign conditions (e.g., migraine, tension headache) and to develop appropriate strategies for treatment.

THE PATIENT WITH HEADACHE

The determination of the cause of headache is most often made from the patient's history. During the course of the interview (avoid leading questions), the following information should be obtained:
1. Location of pain
   a. Frontal, temporal, occipital, or vertex
   b. Unilateral, bilateral, or shifting
2. Type of pain
   a. Constant or throbbing
   b. Mixed (constant and throbbing, which is first?)
3. Duration and timing of pain
   a. Worse in morning or evening
   b. Worse with a Valsalva maneuver (bowel movement, coughing, sneezing); suggestive of increased intracranial pressure
   c. Consistent associations (premenstrual, weekends, emotional stress, alcohol intake, seasonal, specific foods)
4. Severity of pain: pain severe enough to wake the patient from sleep may be seen with increased intracranial pressure, cluster headache, and intracranial hemorrhage. On the other hand, the patient may find it difficult to go to sleep with any form of severe headache.

5. Associated symptoms preceding, accompanying, or following the headache (visual changes, dizziness, or other sensations may precede classic migraine)
6. Family history (migraine, epilepsy, psychiatric illness)
7. Past medical history (hypertension, infection, allergy, head trauma, recent lumbar puncture [LP])
8. Medication history (vasodilators, oral contraceptives, alcohol, or street drugs)

Caution: Sudden onset of a severe headache without past history of headaches should be considered ominous and warrants immediate exclusion of potentially life-threatening conditions such as subarachnoid hemorrhage or meningitis.

Caveat: Ask the patient to describe the last headache: time of day, preceding symptoms, etc., will often make diagnosis.

On examination, particular attention should be given to the following signs:
1. Blood pressure, pulse rate, temperature (headache or hypertension, infection)
2. Sharpness of optic discs, intact venous pulsations, presence of retinal hemorrhages (increased intracranial pressure)
3. Tenderness of temporal arteries (temporal arteritis)
4. Presence of spasm and tenderness in cervical muscles (greater occipital neuralgia)
5. Altered sensation in the scalp (greater occipital neuralgia)
6. Tenderness to percussion of spinous processes in the upper cervical area (greater occipital neuralgia)
7. Tenderness to percussion over sinuses (sinus headache)
8. Asymmetry of reflexes or other focal neurologic signs (intracranial mass)

HEADACHE OF INCREASED INTRACRANIAL PRESSURE

▶ 1. *The most important diagnostic clue* is a bilateral, nonthrobbing headache that is worse in the morning.
2. The headache is an initially mild and intermittent, increasing in severity to steady, nonthrobbing pain.
3. It may awaken the patient at night.
4. It is worse with the Valsalva maneuver.
5. When severe, it is associated with vomiting.
6. Papilledema is present early (see Chapter 13).
7. It is often associated with focal neurologic signs (asymmetric reflexes, palsy of extraocular muscles, pupillary asymmetry).

Treatment: Immediate hospitalization and additional diagnostic studies such as a computed tomographic (CT) scan or magnetic resonance imaging (MRI) are necessary. Treat the underlying cause.

The outcome depends on intracranial pathologic condition. If the patient is a young, obese girl and the CT scan is normal, the most probable diagnosis is pseudotumor.

MIGRAINE

Migraine is a periodic or cyclic disorder in which recurrent headaches occur usually associated with photophobia and autonomic disturbances such as nausea and vomiting. It is considered to be a disorder involving both intracranial vascular regulation and a neuronal electrical disturbance. If the diagnosis of migraine is made, always discontinue birth control pills.

1. Classic Migraine

▶   a. *The most important diagnostic clue* of a classic migraine is an aura followed by the sudden onset of a unilateral throbbing headache.

    b. The aura may consist of transient visual (scotoma, monocular blindness, or hemianopsia), sensory, or motor (paresthesia, weakness) phenomena or simply an indescribable feeling; prodromal symptoms (sometimes preceding the headache by several days) include changes in mood and appetite.

    c. Although unilateral, the headache often shifts sides with different attacks; it is commonly temporal, orbital, frontal, or rarely, occipital.

    d. It occurs at any time of the day.

    e. It is almost always associated with nausea and often with vomiting, photophobia, and phonophobia.

    f. It is relieved by sleep or vomiting.

    g. The onset is often in the teens; the frequency and severity may diminish after 50 years of age.

    h. It is commonly premenstrual in women and is usually less frequent during pregnancy.

    i. It may be precipitated by certain foods or chemicals (especially monosodium glutamate, chocolate, cheddar cheese, red wine, or sodium nitrite as in hot dogs) or with fasting.

    j. Onset or exacerbation often follows the administration of oral contraceptives or reserpine-containing drugs.

    k. A family history of headaches is common.

    l. There is a past history of motion sickness or cyclic vomiting as a child.

    m. The results of the neurologic examination are normal; if they are abnormal, the patient should have further studies such as an electroencephalogram (EEG) and a CT scan or MRI to exclude a structural lesion.

Caution: If the headache is always on the same side, if seizures and headache occur together, if the neurologic examination is abnormal, or if a cranial bruit is heard, consider the possibility of an arteriovenous malformation (AVM). Refer the patient for further study, including magnetic resonance angiography (MRA) and cerebral angiography.

Treatment:
1. General measures
    a. Migraine sufferers often are intelligent, obsessive-compulsive indi-

viduals; thus a thorough explanation of the pathophysiologic factors of the headache is an important part of therapy.

b. Always discontinue oral contraceptives and look for other triggering factors such as alcohol and specific foods, taking appropriate measures to reduce exposure.

2. Specific management

Patients with migraine fall into two categories: those who have frequent attacks (one or more per week) or attacks of such severity as to interfere with their lifestyle or work and those who have infrequent or sporadic attacks. Patients in the first category need regular prophylactic or interval therapy to prevent recurrence of the attacks, whereas patients in the second category need only abortive treatment at the onset of a headache.

a. Abortive treatment: To be effective, treatment should be given at the earliest warning of an impending attack. The following measures are usually recommended:

1) In children and in those in whom the attacks are seldom severe, prompt administration of analgesics such as acetaminophen should be tried as the initial measure. In some patients, sleep alone may abort the attack. If nausea or vomiting is a prominent feature, combine analgesics with metoclopramide (Reglan) hydrochloride 10 mg orally or intramuscularly (IM) or promethazine (Phenergan) hydrochloride suppositories.

2) The mainstay of abortive treatment is the 5-hydroxytryptamine (5-HT_1) receptor agonists. They are so effective that if the headache is not aborted, the diagnosis of migraine is doubtful. They should be prescribed *only* when the diagnosis of migraine is certain and only when attacks are occasional.

These are potentially dangerous, expensive drugs and should be used with caution. Contraindications include coronary artery risk factors, including hypertension, smoking, obesity, men over 40 years of age, peripheral vascular disease, ischemic bowel disease, selective serotonin reuptake inhibitors (SSRIs), and many others.

The following drugs are probably of equal efficacy:

Naratriptan (Amerge): 1- and 2.5-mg tablets. Maximum 5 mg in a 24-hour period. Cost: 9 1-mg tablets $139.64.

Rizatriptan (Maxalt): 5- and 10-mg tablets. Maximum 30 mg in a 24-hour period. Cost: 6 5-mg tablets $87.83.

Zolmitriptan (Zomig): 1-, 2-, and 5-mg tablets. Maximum 10 mg in a 24-hour period. Cost: 6 2.5-mg tablets $79.51.

Sumatriptan (Imitrex): 25- and 50-mg tablets. Maximum 200 mg in a 24-hour period. Cost: 9 25-mg tablets $124.32.

Sumatriptan (Imitrex) nasal spray: 5 and 20 mg. Maximum 40 mg in a 24-hour period.

Sumatriptan (Imitrex) injection: 6 mg/0.5 ml. Do not repeat dose in a 24-hour period. Administer at beginning of aura. Cost: 5 vials $211.83.

3) If the previously outlined measures fail to stop an attack and the pain persists continuously for a prolonged period, try the following:
   (a) Dihydroergotamine mesylate (DHE-45) 0.75 mg intravenously over 10 minutes. Repeat every half hour with 0.5 mg as necessary up to three times. This should be combined with metoclopramide 10 mg IM every 6 hours. Cost: 1 ampule $17.50. Oxygen administered by mask may also help abort the acute attack. See Table 3-1 for other ergot preparations used for abortive attacks; seldom used.
   (b) Narcotic treatment should only be a last and desperate measure because of its potential for addiction. If pain is severe enough to require narcotics, meperidine (Demerol) hydrochloride 50 to 100 mg IM may be given.
   (c) Occasionally, a patient who is resistant to these measures and goes into "status migrainosus" may respond to high-dose, short-term corticosteroid therapy.

Caution: Keep in mind that a patient known to have migraine can develop other conditions that cause severe headache; if there is any question about the diagnosis, a CT scan or MRI may be necessary.

b. Interval and prophylactic treatment: For patients with one or more attacks per week or those in whom the attacks are of such severity as to interfere with lifestyle and work, prophylactic treatment should be instituted. Historically numerous prophylactic medications are moderately effective (Table 3-2); however, in the year 2002, gabapentin (Neurontin) and topiramate (Topamax) are recommended because of their effectiveness and relatively benign side effect profile. Although widely used, they are not approved by the Food and Drug Administration (FDA) for migraine prophylaxis.
   1) Gabapentin: Usually effective at 400 mg in evening, lower doses are not effective. Gabapentin does not interact with other drugs but potentiates benzodiazepines and narcotics. It may be titrated up to 3600 mg (an epileptic dose), but this is rarely necessary.
   2) Topiramate: 25 mg in the evening. A relatively common side effect is mental confusion. The dosage for epilepsy control is 100 mg twice a day, but this is not necessary in migraine prophylaxis.
c. Patient and physician information about migraine can be obtained from the National Headache Foundation, 428 W. St. James Place, 2nd Floor, Chicago, IL 60614-2750; (888)NHF-5552; website: www.headaches.org.

2. Common Migraine

Common migraine (migraine without aura) is a diagnosis commonly used when the physician can think of no other. The criteria are inexact. A single dose of a 5-HT$_1$ agonist (see abortive treatment) may be used as a therapeutic trial. The headaches are usually accompanied by nausea and start at a young age.

TABLE 3-1
Commonly Used Ergot Preparations

Form	Brand name	Constituents	Dosage
Oral	Cafergot Wigraine	Ergotamine tartrate 1 mg and caffeine 100 mg	2 tablets at onset followed by 1 tablet every half hour to maximum of 6 tablets per attack
Suppository	Cafergot Wigraine	Ergotamine tartrate 2 mg and caffeine 100 mg	1 at onset followed by 1 every half hour up to a maximum of 3 suppositories per attack
Sublingual	Ergostat	Ergotamine tartrate 2 mg	1 tablet at first warning of impending attack followed by 1 tablet every half hour if needed to maximum of 3 tablets per attack or 5 tablets/wk
Parenteral	DHE-45	Dihydroergotamine mesylate 1 mg/ml	1.0 ml intramuscularly (IM) at first warning of attack followed by 1.0 ml every hour to maximum of 3.0 ml per attack or 6.0 ml/wk; for more rapid effect, initial dose may be given intravenously

TABLE 3-2
Common Drugs Used in Migraine Prophylaxis

Drug class	Dosage
β-BLOCKERS	
Atenolol	50-120 mg/day
Metoprolol	50-100 mg/day
Nadolol	40-240 mg/day
Propranolol	40-320 mg/day
Timolol	10-30 mg/day
ANTIDEPRESSANTS	
Tricyclics	
Amitriptyline	10-250 mg/day
Doxepin	10-150 mg/day
Nortriptyline HCl	50-150 mg at bed time
Protriptyline	5-10 mg twice a day
Selective Serotonin Reuptake Inhibitors (SSRIs)	
Fluoxetine	10-80 mg/day
Paroxetine	10-50 mg/day
Sertraline	50-200 mg/day
CALCIUM-CHANNEL BLOCKERS	
Diltiazem	120-360 mg/day
Nifedipine	30-180 mg/day
Verapamil	240-720 mg/day
SEROTONIN AGONISTS	
Methylergonovine maleate	0.2-0.4 mg 4 times a day
Methysergide	2-8 mg/day in divided doses up to 14 mg/day
Pizotifen	1-6 mg/day
ANTICONVULSANT	
Divalproex sodium	500-3000 mg/day

Treatment: A low dose of gabapentin or topiramate, prophylactically, is often effective (see section on abortive treatment).

3. Complicated Migraine

A complicated migraine is a headache associated with significant neurologic complications (such as hemiplegia), presumably secondary to ischemia from intracranial vascular constriction. The neurologic complications may outlast the headache phase, and the headache phase may be relatively minor. Very rarely there may be permanent neurologic sequelae. Before a diagnosis of complicated migraine is made, it may be necessary to rule out an underlying AVM (especially if the deficit always occurs in the same location). Prophylactic treatment, even when attacks are infrequent, is recommended in complicated migraines. The common types of complicated migraine are as follows:

a. **Hemiplegic migraine:** the hemiplegia often shifts from side to side during different attacks.

b. **Ophthalmoplegic migraine:** oculomotor paralysis occurs on the same side as the headache; recurrent painful oculomotor palsy in a child strongly suggests complicated migraine.

c. **Basilar artery migraine** occurs mostly in children and adolescents; vertigo, tinnitus, diplopia, and ataxia accompany occipital throbbing headache.

d. **Acute confusional migraine** occurs in adolescents and is manifested as recurrent episodes of confusion and disorientation along with headache.

e. **Retinal migraine** involves monocular visual disturbances lasting for days; it is not necessarily associated with a headache.

4. Cluster Headache

▶ a. *The most important diagnostic clue* of cluster headache (e.g., Horton's headache, histamine cephalgia, migrainous neuralgia) is the sudden onset of severe unilateral retroorbital lancinating pain that tends to occur repeatedly.

b. It is frequently associated with tearing or unilateral nasal discharge on the side of the headache; other features include partial ptosis and a smaller pupil (Horner's syndrome) on the side of the headache.

c. It may last from 30 minutes to several hours.

d. It often awakens the patient at night.

e. It tends to occur in a series, followed by remission for months or even years (hence the name *cluster headache*).

f. It is often precipitated by a small amount of alcohol.

g. It is usually familial and is more frequent in male patients.

Treatment: Patients with cluster headache need two forms of therapy: (1) abortive treatment for an attack and (2) prophylactic treatment to stop future attacks.

1) Abortive treatment: see section on migraine abortive treatment. Oxygen inhalation (100% oxygen through mask) for 10 to 15 minutes has been found to be effective in many patients.

2) Prophylactic treatment.

    (a) Gabapentin or topiramate should be tried (see section on migraine prophylaxis).

    (b) For patients who are resistant to these prophylactic agents, corticosteroid therapy may be useful; prednisone 60 mg daily for three days with the dose reduced progressively to the minimum is effective in stopping the attacks from recurring; continue for the duration of the attack.

(c) This type of headache may occur in chronic form on an almost daily basis; lithium carbonate treatment has been reported to be an effective therapy (300 mg 2 to 3 times a day to provide a blood level of 0.7 to 1.2 meq/l).

Note: Lithium carbonate has a number of side effects, so caution is necessary.

(d) In one variety of cluster headache, chronic paroxysmal hemicrania (CPH), in which the clusters are strictly unilateral (does not shift from side to side), indomethacin (Indocin) has been found to be highly effective (dosage may vary from 25 to 100 mg/day).

MUSCLE CONTRACTION HEADACHE

Muscle contraction headache (tension headache, greater occipital neuralgia) is the most common type of headache seen by the primary care physician.

▶ 1. *The most important diagnostic clue* is a bilateral, nonthrobbing, constant headache that begins in the occipital area and spreads to the frontal area. Scalp tenderness is common. The cause is compromise of the greater occipital nerve (C2) by bone or muscle.
2. Although the initial pain is viselike, it may eventually assume a vascular quality.
3. The pain is not affected by a Valsalva maneuver.
4. It is usually worse in the evening.
5. It may last for days.
6. It may occur in situations of tension, such as family problems and job stress. It is common in patients with a history of whiplash, cervical arthritis, and occupations in which the head is held for long periods in one position (as in secretaries using computers).
7. The patient may complain of scalp tenderness, especially when washing the hair.
8. The results of the neurologic examination are normal except for spasm and tenderness of cervical muscles, tenderness on percussion of the spinous processes in the high cervical area, and decreased sensation to pinprick over the scalp. Hyperalgesia of the scalp is occasionally found.

Note: Whatever the cause, pain is produced by irritation of C2, which becomes the greater occipital nerve innervating the scalp.

Treatment:
1. Explain to the patient that there is nothing wrong with the brain; it is simply a pinched nerve in the neck.
2. Have the patient alter precipitating situations (e.g., a computer screen adjusts up and down or right to left).
3. For most patients, gabapentin (because of its muscle relaxing activity) 400 mg in the evening combined with heat and massage to the back of the neck will provide adequate relief.

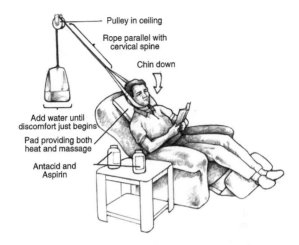

Pulley in ceiling

Rope parallel with
cervical spine

Chin down

Add water until
discomfort just begins

Pad providing both
heat and massage

Antacid and
Aspirin

FIG. 3-1 Modification of standard "over-the-door" traction for greater occipital nerve entrapment (tension headache) and cervical radiculopathy. Patients are compliant and comfortable.

4. Apply heat and massage to the cervical area.
5. Cervical traction (Fig. 3-1 of modified over-the-door traction apparatus) should be done in the evening. If used as directed, most patients will not stare at a blank door for a prolonged period of time.
6. Steroid injections in occipital area near exit of greater occipital nerve by a pain specialist is an effective last resort.

SINUS HEADACHE

▶ 1. *The most important diagnostic clue* of a sinus headache (nasal headache) is: a frontal, nonthrobbing headache with tenderness on percussion over the sinus.
2. Sinus headaches are rare without a predisposing nasal abnormality (structural defect, allergy, polyps).
3. They may be unilateral or bilateral; the location depends on the sinus involved.
4. Often, they are seasonal, particularly in allergic individuals.
5. They may be associated with nasal congestion and discharge, fever, malaise, and painful teeth.
6. Percussion over the sinuses exacerbates the pain.
7. Sinus radiographs show opacification. A CT scan or MRI shows the changes much better.

Treatment:
1. Systemic decongestant: pseudoephedrine (Sudafed) hydrochloride 60 mg 3 times a day or phenylpropanolamine hydrochloride (component of Entex LA).

2. Topical nasal decongestant: 0.25% phenylephrine (Neo-Synephrine) hydrochloride.

Caution: Decongestants should be used sparingly as tachyphylaxis, and rebound may develop.

3. Antihistamines: the allergic patient usually knows which works best. Fexofenadine (Allegra) 60 mg twice a day or astemizole (Hismanal) 10 mg every day is associated with less drowsiness than other agents.
4. Nonnarcotic analgesics such as aspirin, acetaminophen, or ibuprofen.
5. Systemic antibiotics cefaclor (Ceclor) 250 mg 3 times a day or amoxicillin 250 mg 4 times a day (or with clavulanate as [Augmentin] 250 mg 3 times a day) if patient has systemic manifestations such as fever.
6. Intranasal cromolyn sodium (Nasalcrom) 3 or 4 times a day and/or intranasal beclomethasone dipropionate (Vancenase) 3 or 4 times a day: for long-term prophylaxis.
7. Surgical drainage when headaches are chronic and severe.

POSTTRAUMATIC HEADACHE

1. Posttraumatic headaches occur after significant head trauma (loss of consciousness) and have both organic and psychologic components.
2. It may be indistinguishable from chronic, recurring tension headaches.
3. The duration is usually no longer than 6 months.
4. It may be associated with a sensation of "dizziness."
5. It may be part of postconcussion syndrome, which is characterized by anxiety, fatigue, irritability, and inability to concentrate.

Caution: Symptoms of a subdural hematoma can be insidious, and hence a CT scan or MRI should be done.

Treatment:
1. Nonnarcotic analgesics such as aspirin, acetaminophen, or ibuprofen.
2. Gabapentin 400 mg twice a day or topiramate 25 mg at bedtime may be helpful.

Caution: The physician should be alerted to emotional factors or to litigation problems in the patient with prolonged or treatment-unresponsive posttraumatic headache.

POST–LUMBAR PUNCTURE HEADACHE

▶ 1. *The most important diagnostic clue* of a post-LP headache is that it is precipitated by sitting or standing and relieved promptly by lying down.
2. It is often frontal or occipital, may be generalized, and may be associated with nuchal pain.
3. It occurs within 1 to 2 days of LP and is thought to be caused by leakage of cerebrospinal fluid (CSF) through the dural hole.

4. The duration varies from 1 to several days.
5. Predisposing factors may include poor LP technique, the larger size of the needle, and multiple punctures.

Treatment:
1. Strict bed rest with the feet elevated; let patient try to sit up every 12 hours to determine if headache reappears.
2. Adequate hydration (about 4 L/day).
3. Analgesics are usually ineffective.
4. With persistent headache, an epidural blood patch (usually done by the anesthesiologist) using the patient's venous blood may be highly effective.

SUBARACHNOID HEMORRHAGE HEADACHE

▶ 1. *The most important diagnostic clue* of a headache caused by sub-arachnoid hemorrhage is the abrupt onset of a severe occipital or generalized headache ("thunderclap headache") in a patient with no previous history of headaches.
2. It is usually not localized, but definite localization may suggest the site of an underlying leaking aneurysm.
3. It is associated with *stiff neck*, dizziness, nausea and vomiting, irritability, restlessness, convulsions, and drowsiness.
4. Altered consciousness is common.
5. Signs of localizing neurologic dysfunction may be *absent*.
6. Papilledema (see Chapter 13) may develop after hemorrhage depending on the location of hemorrhage and degree of impedance to venous return around the optic nerve. *Subhyaloid hemorrhages* are pathognomonic.

Treatment: A CT scan and angiography should be performed as soon as possible, since aneurysms tend to rebleed, leading to fatal outcome. Neurosurgical consultation should be obtained immediately.

TEMPORAL ARTERITIS

1. The onset of severe, continuous unilateral head pain in an elderly person is temporal arteritis until proved otherwise.
2. An elevated erythrocyte sedimentation rate (ESR) greater than 40 mm/h is present.
3. Tender swollen nonpulsatile temporal arteries are often, but not always, present.
4. The typical patient is 55 years of age and female.
5. Polymyalgia rheumatica (generalized muscle aches and pains) is frequently associated with temporal arteritis.

Treatment:
1. This is a neurologic emergency because arteritis may involve the ophthalmic or other intracranial arteries, leading to blindness and other focal deficits. Start steroid therapy with prednisone 60 to 80 mg *immediately.* Continue high-dose steroid therapy until the ESR returns to normal. Then gradually reduce the dose to 20 to 30 mg/day and

continue for 6 months to 1 year. Monitor the patient for complications of steroid therapy such as gastrointestinal bleeding, intercurrent infection, osteoporosis, and aseptic necrosis of the femoral head. Alternate-day therapy may reduce steroid-induced complications.
2. Diagnostic temporal artery biopsy should be scheduled within 2 to 3 days of presentation. A sufficient length of artery should be taken, since the arteritis tends to be focal and may be missed. Therapy should not be delayed, since instituting treatment with corticosteroids will not alter the histologic findings for a number of days.

CENTRAL NERVOUS SYSTEM INFECTION HEADACHE

1. Any headache associated with fever and altered mentation (abscess, encephalitis, meningitis) is a central nervous system (CNS) infection until proved otherwise.
2. There is a subacute or an acute onset of constant, increasingly severe pain.
3. The headache is usually generalized but may be worse in the occipital area.
4. It increases with physical activity.
5. It is associated with a stiff and painful neck, nausea and vomiting, irritability, and restlessness.
6. Altered consciousness may be present.
7. Photophobia, strabismus, ptosis, or pupillary inequality may be present.
8. LP is mandatory for the diagnosis and culture of the organism. A CT scan is recommended before the LP if the patient is not morbidly ill.

Treatment: Treatment depends on culturing the organism and determining its antibiotic sensitivity; broad-spectrum parenteral antibiotics should be used to treat the infection until the culture result returns. Consider isolation of the patient until the infectious agent is known (Chapter 14).

OCULAR HEADACHE

Ocular causes of headache include glaucoma, diplopia with accompanying orbicularis contraction, uncorrected refractive errors such as astigmatism, ocular or retroocular inflammations, and orbital tumors.

1. Ocular headache starts as a feeling of heaviness in the eyes, gradually becoming more severe.
2. It is absent on awakening, appears in afternoon and gradually worsens.
3. The pain may be dull, bursting, sharp, or throbbing, and it is often due to persistent muscle contraction.
4. The pain is bifrontal or periorbital in location.
5. It may be associated with prolonged reading or other use of the eyes.
6. It may be associated with altered visual acuity or reduced ocular motility.

Treatment: Measurement of intraocular pressure is necessary. Corrective lenses may be helpful. Obtain CT scans of the orbit if a retroocular lesion is suspected.

TRIGEMINAL NEURALGIA

1. Recurrent paroxysmal pain in the distribution of one or more branches of the trigeminal nerve is most probably trigeminal neuralgia (tic douloureux).
2. Pain may radiate to the jaw or teeth and present as a dental problem.
3. Trigeminal neuralgia is precipitated by minimal sensory stimuli to the affected side of the face (especially a localized area or trigger point, which may appear as a dirty or unshaven patch).
4. It occurs after 40 years of age; suspect multiple sclerosis (MS) when the onset is earlier.
5. There is no sensory loss in the trigeminal distribution; if there is sensory loss or decreased corneal reflex, look for tumors or vascular abnormalities involving the trigeminal nerve.

Treatment:

1. Carbamazepine (Tegretol-XR) 400 to 1200 mg daily is the drug of choice. Generic carbamazepine is not as effective as the long-acting preparation.
2. Phenytoin (Dilantin) 300 to 700 mg/day, adjusted to produce a blood level of 10 to 20 mg/ml may be effective in a few patients.
3. Gabapentin 400 mg twice a day may be titrated up to 3600 mg if necessary.
4. Surgical treatment may be considered in resistant cases. Trigeminal gangliolysis by percutaneous radiofrequency technique (80% chance of pain relief for 1 year), injection of glycerol around the gasserian ganglion, and suboccipital craniotomy with decompression of trigeminal nerve are some of the techniques used.

TEMPOROMANDIBULAR NEURALGIA

1. Temporomandibular neuralgia (TMJ syndrome) recurrent usually involves unilateral, severe, constant, aching facial pain around the temporomandibular joint sometimes radiating to the jaws associated with tenderness over the temporomandibular joint.
2. Pain is exacerbated by movement of the lower jaw (chewing, yawning).
3. The patient may report an associated clicking or grating sound.
4. This form of neuralgia may be associated with bruxism during sleep; depression or insomnia may also be present.
5. It occurs commonly in young women or in elderly patients with severe overbite resulting from the loss of back teeth, or it occurs after fracture.
6. Palpation of the temporalis muscle or direct pressure on the temporomandibular joint may result in pain.
7. Special x-ray techniques often reveal asymmetric temporomandibular joints with degenerative changes in the cartilage.

Treatment: Treatment is often unsatisfactory. Correction of dental malocclusion may or may not relieve the pain. Conservative therapy includes heat applied to the affected area, a diet of soft foods, limitation of mouth opening, dental protheses, mild analgesics, muscle relaxants, or antidepressants. Surgical replacement of the temporomandibular joint may be necessary.

TOXIC HEADACHE

1. Toxic headache has the characteristics of vascular headache.
2. Drugs causing headache include phenacetin, amyl nitrite, reserpine, lithium, dextroamphetamine, ephedrine, disulfiram, digitalis and imipramine.
3. Toxic headache may result after excessive intake of alcohol or coffee (caffeine).
4. It may appear on discontinuation of corticosteroids, barbiturates, ergot, or narcotics.
5. Occupational hazards include mechanics and farmers exposed to exhaust fumes (carbon monoxide), refrigerator repairmen exposed to refrigerants, coal miners exposed to mine gases, and individuals exposed to insecticides.

Treatment:
1. Headache will subside after removal of the patient from toxic exposure.
2. Caffeine-withdrawal headaches terminate with the administration of caffeine.

BIBLIOGRAPHY

Field AG, Wang E: Evaluation of the patient with nontraumatic headache: an evidence based approach, *Emerg Med Clin North Am* 17(1):127-152, 1999.

Jackson CM: Effective headache management: strategies to help patients gain control over pain, *Postgrad Med* 104(5):133-136, 139-140, 143-147, 1998.

Kulig J: Advances in medical management of asthma, headaches, and fatigue, *Med Clin North Am* 84(4):829-850, 2000.

Raskin N: Serotonin receptors and headache, *N Engl J Med* 325:353-354, 1991.

Saper JR: Headache disorders, *Med Clin North Am* 83(3):662-690, 1999.

Sjaastad O: *Cluster headache syndrome,* Philadelphia, 1992, WB Saunders.

Subcutaneous Sumatriptan International Study Group: Treatment of migraine attacks with sumatriptan, *N Engl J Med* 325:316-321, 1991.

Ward TN: Providing relief from headache pain: current options for acute and prophylactic therapy, *Postgrad Med* 108(3):121-128, 2000.

WEBSITES

American Headache Society: www.ahsnet.org

Migraine Awareness Group: a national understanding for migraineurs: www.migraines.org

National Headache Foundation: www.headaches.org

Pain: www.paincareplus.com, www.aapainmanage.org

Prophylactic treatment of migraine: www.neuroland.com/ha/migra_pro

Symptomatic treatment of migraine: www.neuroland.com/ha/migra_sym

4

Dizziness, Vertigo, and Lightheadedness: Problems of Spatial Disorientation

The dictionary definition of *dizziness* is: "a whirling sensation in the head, mental confusion, giddiness." Patients, likewise, use the word to describe the sensation they feel when they stand upright too quickly, when they look over the edge of a cliff, when they are unsteady on their feet, when they are seasick, or when they generally feel unwell. To some patients dizziness is the sensation one feels after rapidly spinning around or after receiving a severe blow to the head. The differences in these sensations are subtle, and most patients are not eloquent enough to differentiate between them. The term *vertigo* should be limited to the sensation of movement, either of oneself or of the environment; a clear-cut history of this type of sensation (vertigo) often indicates that the pathologic process is in the peripheral vestibular system.

THE DIZZY PATIENT

A major responsibility of the primary care physician is to identify the most common causes of dizziness, such as postural hypotension, hyperventilation, multiple sensory deficits, and postinfectious vertigo, and thus avoid costly and time-consuming evaluations by a specialist. The following historical information should be obtained from the patient:

1. Attempt to define the complaint of "dizziness"; a practical approach is to have the patient choose the sensation closest to the complaint from the examples previously listed.
2. The duration and description of the *first* attack is usually most helpful. The frequency of subsequent attacks should also be determined.
3. Associated symptoms include progressive hearing loss, diplopia, paresthesias of the hands and feet, and tinnitus.

4. Positional factors should be determined; dizziness on arising from a seated to a standing position, dizziness with sudden movement of the head, or dizziness associated with hyperextension or rotation of the neck.
5. Precipitating factors should be noted; dizziness associated with stressful situations, excessive or low salt intake, or direct relationships to meals may be diagnostic.
6. Past medical history should be ascertained; severe head trauma, antecedent viral infections, diabetes, atherosclerotic phenomena, and psychiatric difficulties are especially helpful diagnostic signs.
7. All present and past medications should be reported; particular attention should be paid to antibiotics (especially streptomycin), anticonvulsants, antihypertensives, and high-dose salicylates.

Classic Complaints That Are Nearly Diagnostic
Often the cause of dizziness is strongly suggested by the history, and under these circumstances a physical and neurologic examination should be targeted to a specific hypothesis. For example:
1. "I'm dizzy when I get up in the morning." (Patients tend to become dehydrated overnight, making postural hypotension most prominent in the morning.)
2. "I'm dizzy whenever I'm alone at night." (Hyperventilation is strongly associated with anxiety-producing situations.)
3. "Every time I'm dizzy I see double." (Intermittent diplopia is usually caused by ischemia of the midbrain, which suggests basilar artery insufficiency.)
4. "I can't use the phone in my right ear anymore, the right side of my face is numb, and I'm unsteady on my feet." (Unilateral hearing loss without a history of trauma or ear infection is an acoustic neuroma until proved otherwise.)
5. "I suddenly became dizzy, nauseous, and unsteady on my feet, and my left face and right arm felt funny." (Symptoms on one half of the face and opposite side of the body strongly suggest brainstem disease; in this case infarction in the distribution of the posterior inferior cerebellar artery.)
6. "I've had diabetes for many years, I can't read the newspaper because of my cataracts, and my grandchildren tease me about being drunk all the time." (Elderly patients with multiple sensory deficits commonly complain of dizziness.)
7. "I've had fullness in my ear for a week and then suddenly I became so dizzy I had to lie in bed and hold on for fear of falling out." (Ménière's disease presents with a prodrome and dramatic vertigo.)

On examination special attention should be given to the following:
1. A cardiovascular evaluation should be done (blood pressure in both arms, lying and standing, peripheral pulses, carotid bruits, heart murmurs, and arrhythmias).
2. Examine ears with otoscope looking for impacted cerumen, and evidence of infection.
3. Have the patient *hyperventilate* to see if the symptoms are reproduced. The sitting patient should take a deep breath every 2 seconds for 3 to

5 minutes. At the end of this time, ask the patient if this is the same sensation as the presenting complaint.

4. Cerebellar function can be tested by having the patient tandem-walk and perform rapid alternating movements and the finger-to-nose test.

5. Cranial nerves should be examined carefully. Pay particular attention to nystagmus when testing extraocular movements. Nystagmus is a rhythmic, involuntary eye movement, present at rest or induced by eye movement but persisting after eye movements cease. Usually there is a slow deviation of the eye in one direction with a quick jerk in the opposite direction. Nystagmus is named for the quick component. Table 4-1 may be helpful in differentiating peripheral (labyrinthine) from central nervous system (CNS) nystagmus. Specific types of nystagmus include the following:

   a. **End-point or physiologic nystagmus** will result if the normal patient gazes too far laterally. The examiner should have the patient gaze laterally only to the point in the adducting eye where the limbus meets the lacrimal punctum (Fig. 4-1).

   b. **Toxic-metabolic nystagmus** is symmetric in both eyes, equal in both directions of gaze, and primarily horizontal.

   c. **Asymmetric lateral nystagmus** (absent or reduced in one direction of gaze compared with the opposite direction of gaze) could indicate either CNS or peripheral dysfunction.

   d. **Dysconjugate nystagmus:** The abnormal movement is greater in one eye than the other. This always indicates CNS disease.

   e. **Upward-gaze, downward-gaze, or rotatory nystagmus** usually indicates CNS disease.

   f. **Positional nystagmus** induced by the Nylen-Bárány maneuver often indicates peripheral vestibular disease. The Nylen-Bárány maneuver is performed by seating the patient on the examining table and suddenly lowering the patient to a supine position with the head held 45 degrees backward over the end of the table and turned 45 degrees to one side (Fig. 4-2).

6. Evaluation of trigeminal nerve (cranial nerve V) function: *corneal reflex* is a sensitive index of fifth cranial nerve function; an abnormality may suggest a lesion such as acoustic neuroma.

TABLE 4-1
Differentiating Labyrinthine and CNS Nystagmus

Labyrinthine (peripheral) nystagmus	CNS nystagmus
Horizontal or horizontal-rotary	Often vertical or rotary
Fatigable	Persistent
Suppressed by visual fixation	May increase with visual fixation
Latency of onset after head motion	Occurs immediately after head motion
Associated with vertigo	Not directly associated with dizziness
Always conjugate	May be dysconjugate

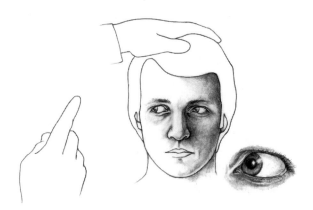

FIG. 4-1 When testing for lateral-gaze nystagmus, do not force the limbus of the iris beyond the lacrimal punctum to avoid end-point nystagmus. Nystagmus at this point is usually abnormal.

Caution: Be sure to touch only the cornea and not the sclera and also avoid producing a blink by threat reflex (Fig. 4-3).

7. Evaluation of the function of the auditory and vestibular portions of the eighth cranial nerve can be determined by the following tests:
   a. **Auditory acuity** is quickly tested by rubbing the fingers lightly several inches from the patient's ear. If an abnormality is present, perform the Weber's and Rinne tests.
   b. **Weber's test:** place the base of a vibrating tuning fork on the patient's forehead. Ideally, a 512-Hz tuning fork should be used, but often only a 256-Hz tuning fork is readily available. Normally the sound from the tuning fork is heard nearly equally in both ears. With eighth cranial nerve or cochlear destruction (sensorineural deafness), the sound is heard best on the side of normal acuity. With middle ear or outer ear disease (conduction deafness), sound lateralizes to the involved ear (Fig. 4-4).
   c. **Rinne Test** (Fig. 4-5). Lightly tap a 256-Hz tuning fork and place it firmly against the mastoid process. Ask the patient to indicate when it is no longer heard. Then place the fork in front of the external auditory meatus and note the period of time during which it is heard. A normal individual will have a positive Rinne test, in which the tuning fork is heard twice as long by air conduction as by bone conduction.
   d. **Caloric test:** Examine the auditory canal to check that the eardrum is intact and that there is no blood or impacted cerumen. With the patient sitting, tilt the head to one side and inject approximately 2 ml of cold water from a syringe equipped with a small-caliber soft

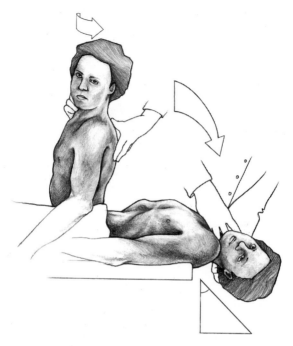

FIG. 4-2 Nylen-Bárány maneuver. Have the patient turn the head 45 degrees over the end of the table and observe the eyes for nystagmus. The patient is instructed to keep the eyes open. The onset and direction of nystagmus is noted. Note also whether the patient experiences vertigo. This maneuver is repeated with the head turned to the opposite side.

polyethylene catheter directed at the posterior wall of the external canal. Start a stopwatch at the beginning of the injection. After 20 seconds, evacuate the water from the ear, tilt the patient's head backward 60 degrees, and have the patient look at the examiner's finger from a distance of approximately 3 feet (Fig. 4-6). An ophthalmoscope can also be used to observe the nystagmus: in a darkened room visualizing a small-caliber retinal blood vessel permits detection of subtle nystagmus (with a slight rotatory component). In the alert patient, the eyes normally drift slowly toward the ear irrigated with cold water followed by the quick corrective component of the nystagmus back toward the primary position. Abnormal responses include the absence of nystagmus or a marked difference in nystagmus between the two ears. (NOTE: wait 15 minutes after irrigation of one ear before irrigating the other ear.)

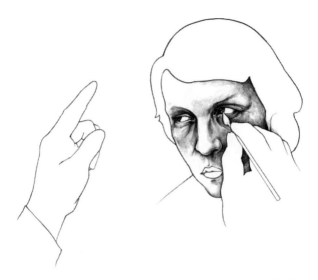

FIG. 4-3 Testing the corneal reflex. With the patient looking to one side, bring a wisp of cotton (a few strands pulled out from a cotton-tipped applicator) from the opposite side and touch the *cornea*. The patient should blink.

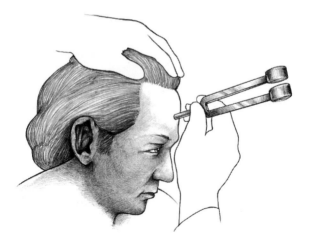

FIG 4-4 Weber's test. Place a tuning fork on the forehead and ask, "Is the sound the same in both ears?"

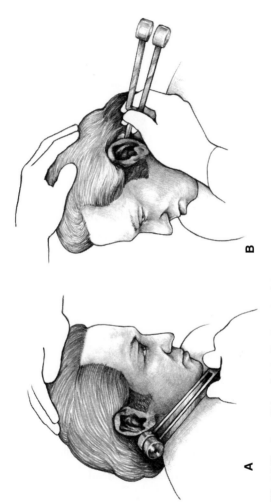

FIG. 4-5 Rinne's test. Using a lightly vibrating tuning fork, ask the patient if the sound is loudest in position **A** or position **B**.

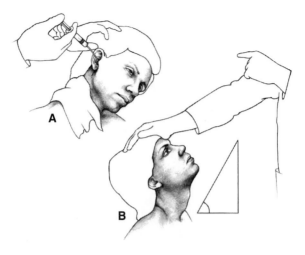

FIG. 4-6 Caloric test. **A,** have the patient sit in a chair with the head tilted to one side and inject 2 ml of water into the external canal. **B,** remove the water, tilt patient's head backward 60 degrees, and observe and time the nystagmus. Quick movements will be directed away from the cold ear.

Instillation of warm water into the ear produces the opposite findings but is ordinarily not necessary. (For caloric testing in the comatose patient, see Chapter 13.)

Laboratory Investigations

Because the causes of dizziness are so varied, we cannot suggest a standard laboratory investigation of all dizzy patients. The following choice of laboratory procedures should be tempered by the history and physical examination:

1. A complete blood count, erythrocyte sedimentation rate (ESR), and analysis of electrolytes and blood components are necessary because dizziness is so often equated with "unwellness."
2. Audiometry should be performed in all patients with significant hearing loss or tinnitus.
3. A glucose tolerance test is performed if hypoglycemia is considered in the differential diagnosis.
4. When the patient reports palpitations, consider performing carotid sinus massage during an electrocardiogram (ECG).
5. Electroencephalography (sleep-deprived, with nasopharyngeal electrodes) is performed when there is a suspicion of complex partial seizures.

6. Brainstem evoked responses are an inexpensive screening test in identifying acoustic neuromas and brainstem abnormalities.
7. Magnetic resonance imaging (MRI) identifies virtually all acoustic neuromas and cases of multiple sclerosis.

DIZZINESS OF PSYCHOLOGIC ORIGIN
Hyperventilation Syndrome
1. Hyperventilation is a common cause of dizziness (lightheadedness).
2. It may be associated with circumoral paresthesias, paresthesias of the fingers, and carpal-pedal spasm (muscle cramps in the hands and feet).
3. Patients with this syndrome frequently are anxious.
4. The diagnosis is usually confirmed when the symptoms are reproduced by having the patient hyperventilate.

Treatment:
1. Explain the cause of the dizziness and reassure the patient. Have the patient breathe into a paper bag (rebreathing) during attacks.
2. Psychologic or psychiatric evaluation is not necessary in most cases.

Psychogenic Dizziness
1. In psychogenic dizziness the patient is inconsistent in regard to history, description of the dizziness, and factors affecting the dizziness. If the dizziness is injury or event related, the circumstances of the injury or events are described in explicit detail.
2. The patient may note dizziness in all body positions.
3. The history may be misleading if the patient has had previous exposure to leading questions by other examiners; sometimes the patient may consciously mislead the examiner.
4. There may be associated symptoms of anxiety or depression; hyperventilation is common.
5. During the examination, there are inconsistencies in many of the tests, and often all of the test maneuvers reproduce the symptoms.
6. The sensation of acrophobia or claustrophobia is described by many patients as dizziness.

Treatment: A psychologic or psychiatric evaluation is indicated.

DIZZINESS AND VERTIGO OF VESTIBULAR ORIGIN
Symptomatic treatment of dizziness of vestibular origin involves the following drugs (remember that all of these drugs may cause excessive drowsiness):
1. Scopolamine (Transderm-Scōp) (a disc impregnated with scopolamine 1.5 mg and placed behind the ear, 4 patches, $21.51) is the drug of choice for motion sickness and other peripheral labyrinthine disorders. Each disc lasts 3 days.
2. Meclizine (Antivert) hydrochloride 25 to 100 mg daily in divided doses (30 25-mg tablets, $21.48) may be effective.

3. Dimenhydrinate (Dramamine) 50 mg every 4 hours may be effective for adults (over the counter).
4. Trimethobenzamide (Tigan) hydrochloride 100 to 250 mg 3 or 4 times a day is usually effective for controlling nausea (30 100-mg tablets, $19.56).

Benign Positional Vertigo

▶ 1. *The most important diagnostic clue is* recurrent transient vertigo precipitated by head motion whether the patient is standing or lying down.
2. Vertigo is often associated with nausea; auditory symptoms are absent.
3. Examination shows the following:
   a. Nystagmus in the Nylen-Bárány maneuver occurring after a latency period of a few seconds and disappearing after approximately 1 minute. The phenomenon is less apparent on repetition of the maneuver (fatigable). This finding is virtually diagnostic of benign positional vertigo.

Caveat: If there is no latency period before onset of nystagmus and if the phenomenon does not become less apparent on repetition, suspect posterior fossa tumor.

   b. Caloric tests are normal in 50% of patients.
4. This is a self-limited benign syndrome, initially severe, but gradually improving over days to weeks.
Treatment: Scopolamine (Transderm-Scōp)

Posttraumatic Vertigo

1. Skull fractures
   a. A lengthwise fracture through the petrous pyramid usually involves structures of the middle ear. The patient often has bleeding from the ear.
   b. Transverse fractures through the petrous pyramid involve the bony and membranous labyrinth. The patient has facial paralysis, vertigo, and spontaneous nystagmus.
2. Acceleration-deceleration injuries
   a. Severe positional vertigo, especially with the involved ear pointing downward, is caused by an inorganic deposit in the semicircular canal (cupulolithiasis).
   b. A persistent leak of perilymph from oval window to middle ear space occurs.
   c. Whiplash injuries may result in dizziness, with objective findings referable to the vestibular system.
Treatment: MRI of the posterior fossa and brainstem evoked responses may localize the lesion. A thorough otolaryngologic examination is indicated because of the possibility of surgical correction.

Ménière's Disease

▶ 1. *The most important diagnostic clue of Ménière's disease is* severe, dramatic (explosive onset), episodic vertigo lasting from hours to days associated with tinnitus (like a seashell held to the ear) and decreased hearing in the affected ear.

2. Ménière's disease is often preceded by an aura consisting of a fullness or pressure in the affected ear.
3. This is a disease primarily of middle age, affecting one side in 75% of cases.
4. Although hearing loss may fluctuate, it is progressive.
5. Some patients note that an attack may be precipitated by heavy salt intake.
6. The disease runs a prolonged course over many years, and the vertiginous attacks tend to decrease as the deafness increases. Ultimately the patient becomes deaf, and the vertiginous attacks cease.
7. Examination shows the following:
   a. A decreased caloric response occurs on the affected side.
   b. Loss of hearing, especially low tones, occurs.
   c. Spontaneous nystagmus toward the affected side may be present during the attack.
   d. Definitive diagnosis should be made with an audiologic examination requiring specialized equipment.

Treatment:
1. The armamentarium of vasodilators, diuretics, low-salt diets, vitamins, antihistamines, and tranquilizers suggests that no treatment is really effective.
2. A shunt procedure (between the membranous labyrinth and the subarachnoid space) is rarely used.

Note: There is a tendency to overdiagnose Ménière's disease. Other causes of severe acute vertigo include occlusion of the vestibular artery or the posterior inferior cerebellar artery, acute toxic labyrinthitis, and vestibular neuronitis. However, these causes of dramatic vertigo are usually not recurrent.

Acute Toxic Labyrinthitis

1. Acute toxic labyrinthitis is characterized by acute onset of vertigo that peaks in 24 hours and subsides in 7 to 10 days.
2. It is often associated with a nose or throat infection. Other associations include allergy or ototoxic medication.
3. Vertigo is exacerbated by head motion.
4. Examination shows the following:
   a. Caloric tests are abnormal in 50% of patients.
   b. Examination of the nose or throat may show evidence of infection.
   c. Spontaneous nystagmus may be present.

Treatment:
1. Throat culture if clinically indicated
2. Limitation of movement (bed rest)
3. Symptomatic drug treatment
4. Discontinuing drugs that may be vestibulotoxic

Postinfectious Vestibular Neuronitis

1. Postinfectious vestibular neuronitis is symptomatically very similar to acute labyrinthitis. The differentiating feature is that it is associated with the influenza syndrome and may occur epidemically.
2. This disease may have a longer recovery period (2 to 6 weeks) than acute labyrinthitis.

Motion Sickness

Some normal individuals have an increased sensitivity to the stimulus of motion.

Note: Adults with migraine frequently have a history of motion sickness in childhood.

Treatment: The application of Scopolamine (Transderm-Scōp) before the patient is in a situation in which motion sickness is likely to occur is especially effective.

DIZZINESS OR VERTIGO OF CENTRAL ORIGIN

Cerebrovascular Disorders

Dizziness or vertigo of central origin is a common complaint of patients with many types of cerebrovascular disorders (especially those involving the posterior fossa). The symptom of vertigo is related specifically to cerebrovascular diseases affecting the blood supply to the brainstem. The diagnosis is rarely easy, unless there are focal neurologic signs during or after the attacks. In many cases of vertebrobasilar transient ischemic attacks (TIAs) the patient is normal between attacks. A magnetic resonance angiogram (MRA) or a four-vessel cerebral angiogram performed by an experienced neuroradiologist can confirm the diagnosis.

1. **Vertebrobasilar insufficiency:** the onset is abrupt and often associated with loss of consciousness. Initial neurologic symptoms may include diplopia, slurred speech, numbness, dysphagia, visual field defects, or motor or sensory losses.
2. The **subclavian steal syndrome** may include attacks of vertigo, especially on exercising the arm on the affected side. A clue to the diagnosis is asymmetric blood pressure in the arms. This is a particular type of vertebrobasilar insufficiency in which there is an occlusion proximal to the origin of the vertebral artery.
   Treatment: If an occlusion is demonstrated, surgical correction can be considered, but in many cases the symptoms subside spontaneously.
3. **Ischemic damage** to vestibular nuclei or their connections often includes damage to other parts of the brainstem. Elderly hypertensive patients with diabetes, heart disease, or hyperlipidemia are likely candidates. Focal neurologic signs are present; caloric response is absent or asymmetric.
4. **Lateral medullary syndrome** is a specific type of ischemic damage to vestibular connections resulting from brainstem infarction in the distribution of the posterior inferior cerebellar artery. The patient

experiences vertigo, nausea, hiccups, and dysarthria. Abnormal neurologic signs include ipsilateral loss of pain and temperature sensation in the face, contralateral loss of pain and temperature sensation in the body, ipsilateral cerebellar ataxia, and ipsilateral Horner's syndrome. Note that there is no paralysis of arms or legs. The prognosis for complete recovery is especially good with this type of infarction. These patients usually have a history of hypertension.

Treatment: See Chapter 12.

Acoustic Neuroma (Cerebellopontine Angle Tumor)

▶ 1. *Suspect acoustic neuroma* (schwannoma, neurilemmoma) in any patient who develops insidious unilateral hearing loss unless it is clearly associated with trauma or infection. This tumor accounts for 10% of all primary intracranial tumors. High-pitched unilateral tinnitus can be an initial symptom.

2. The most common vestibular symptom is unsteadiness; true vertigo is rare. Occasionally, symptoms are episodic.

3. As the disease progresses patients develop other neurologic complaints such as facial numbness, facial weakness, clumsiness, and headache.

4. Examination shows one or more of the following:
   a. On the same side as the tumor:
      1) Sensorineural hearing loss (air conduction greater than bone conduction; tuning fork on forehead louder in normal ear)
      2) Decreased caloric response on affected side
      3) Loss of corneal reflex and sensory disturbance over the face
      4) Facial weakness involving the forehead
      5) Decreased sensation in the external auditory canal
      6) Ipsilateral cerebellar findings
   b. Café au lait spots with or without cutaneous neurofibromas suggest neurofibromatosis. This disease has an association with bilateral cerebellopontine angle tumors.
   c. Papilledema may be seen with large tumors.

5. Diagnostic studies: MRI with contrast should identify virtually all tumors.

Treatment: When diagnosis is confirmed, surgical exploration is necessary.

Other Posterior Fossa Tumors

Posterior fossa tumors are especially common in children, and although vertigo may be present, cerebellar and brainstem signs, cranial nerve abnormalities, and signs of increased intracranial pressure are usually more prominent. If these problems are suspected, referral to a neurologist or neurosurgeon is indicated.

Complex Partial Seizures

Vertigo, dizziness, or a feeling of unsteadiness may be an aura for complex partial seizures. For further diagnostic information and treatment, see Chapter 11.

Note: This type of seizure disorder is not necessarily associated with loss of consciousness or tonic-clonic movements.

Basilar Migraine

Basilar migraine usually occurs in children and young women and lasts for minutes. Symptoms may include attacks of vertigo, which can be associated with visual disturbance, ataxia, tinnitus, and sometimes sudden loss of consciousness. For further diagnostic information, see Chapter 3.

Multiple Sclerosis

Patients who later are diagnosed as having multiple sclerosis (MS) may have altered sensation of balance, but this is seldom true vertigo. Dizziness may also be the result of multiple sensory deficits. For further diagnostic information, see Chapter 10.

Multiple Sensory Deficits

1. Elderly patients often have altered sensory input: visual (cataracts) and proprioceptive, touch, pressure (from peripheral neuropathy, often diabetic, or cervical cord involvement in cervical spondylosis). Vestibular abnormalities may occur secondary to basilar artery insufficiency or premature aging of the vestibular nuclei.
2. The diminished sensory input causes dizziness (out of touch with the environment), especially when walking or turning.
3. Additional sensory cues, sometimes as simple as carrying a cane, during maneuvers that produce dizziness usually reduce the symptoms.

Treatment: Medications often make this condition worse. If possible, devise ways of increasing sensory input (e.g., cataract operation, moving slowly, walking stick).

DRUGS AS A CAUSE OF DIZZINESS

The vestibular nerve and the vestibular apparatus can be damaged by commonly used drugs. Some drugs produce reversible dysfunction, whereas others produce irreversible destruction. If the patient is taking one of the following drugs, it should be considered as a possible cause of the dizziness:

1. Antibiotics
   a. Aminoglycosides (such as streptomycin)
   b. Polypeptides (polymyxin B)
   c. Semisynthetic penicillin (ampicillin)
   d. Sulfonamides
   e. Synthetics (chloramphenicol)
2. Diuretics (furosemide)
3. Salicylates (aspirin)
4. Antiinflammatory drugs (phenylbutazone)
5. Antimalarials (quinine)
6. Anticonvulsants (phenytoin)
7. Antihistamines

SYSTEMIC DISORDERS
Cardiovascular Disturbances

1. **Orthostatic (postural) hypotension:** on standing, the patient experiences faintness from a fall in blood pressure. The magnitude of the drop in blood pressure is less important than the association of the faintness in moving from a lying to a standing position. The differential diagnosis of possible causes is lengthy but includes the following:
   a. Hypovolemic states
   b. Peripheral neuropathy (especially if the autonomic nervous system is affected as in diabetes)
   c. Lower-extremity venous pooling (as in severe varicose veins)
   d. Antihypertensive drugs
2. **Cardiac arrhythmias** may be recognized by auscultation or routine ECG, but 24-hour Holter monitoring may be required.
3. **Carotid sinus hypersensitivity**
   a. The patient may relate a history of faintness or syncope with neck motion or pressure on the neck; examples include faintness while backing a car out of a driveway or faintness associated with shaving the neck. This syndrome is most common in children and adolescents and in older patients with atherosclerotic disease involving the carotid bifurcation.
   b. The faintness or dizziness disappears rapidly (lasting about 15 seconds).
   c. The diagnosis is confirmed by reproducing symptoms by lightly massaging the carotid sinus (do not occlude the carotid artery) and monitoring both the blood pressure and the heart rate (ECG). A pause of more than 3 seconds in the heart rate or a decrease in systolic blood pressure greater than 50 mm Hg is considered abnormal. Valsalva maneuvers may also precipitate cardiac slowing and a fall in blood pressure (micturition syncope); this can be checked at the same time as the carotid massage.

Caution: Do not massage the carotid artery of patients with known carotid artery or intracranial cerebrovascular disease because of the risk of precipitating stroke. Cardiac arrest may also occur.

4. **Hypertension:** patients with severe hypertension in the early phases of hypertensive encephalopathy may experience faintness and dizziness.

Caution: The patient with symptoms of dizziness and rapidly elevating blood pressure may have an expanding mass lesion in the posterior fossa (see Chapter 13).

Vasovagal Phenomena

1. **Common vasovagal syncope:** this is the common fainting that occurs in normal persons and that is often precipitated by emotional stress or warm, crowded conditions. It is preceded by an aura of nausea and

sweating. The loss of consciousness may be prevented by assuming a supine position and elevating the legs.

2. **Reflex vasovagal syncope:** this is similar to the common vasovagal syncope, but the fainting spell is precipitated by a stimulus (e.g., venipuncture). There may be a family history of similar stimulus-precipitated syncope, breath-holding spells, or migraine. This syndrome must be differentiated from a seizure by lack of either postictal sleepiness or tonic-clonic movements.

3. **Breath-holding spells**
   a. A form of vasovagal syncope in children 6 months to 6 years of age, breath-holding spells may be of the following two types:
      1) They begin with crying; the child holds his or her breath and turns blue (cyanotic type).
      2) After a minor startle or sudden painful stimulus, the child turns white and loses consciousness (pallid type).
   b. The period from onset through loss of consciousness usually lasts less than 60 seconds. There may be a few seconds of tonic stiffening at the end of the period of unconsciousness, which may be mistaken for a seizure.
   c. At the termination of the breath-holding spell, the child immediately awakens, usually with no apparent postictal symptoms (no headache, confusion, or lethargy).
   d. If the physician thinks an electroencephalogram (EEG) is necessary, it should be done with monitoring of respiration and ECG to differentiate seizures from breath-holding spells.

Treatment: Breath-holding spells are benign, with the child outgrowing the disorder, such spells do not lead to epilepsy. Parents should be reassured of the benign prognosis.

OTHER MEDICAL CONDITIONS ASSOCIATED WITH FAINTNESS AND DIZZINESS

Almost any medical condition may be associated with dizziness; this chapter assumes that the general health of the patient is good.

1. Anemia causes dizziness as a result of hypovolemia or decreased oxygen-carrying capacity of the blood
2. Hypoglycemia, especially common in diabetics
3. Endocrine disorders, especially thyroid and adrenal insufficiency
4. Visual disorders, especially after a change in prescription for lenses, during diplopia, or after cataract surgery
5. Allergies: allergic reactions may cause a sensation of fullness in the head, lightheadedness, or faintness. This diagnosis should be pursued in patients with a strong allergy history. Remember that many of the drugs used to treat allergies also cause dizziness.

BIBLIOGRAPHY

Baloh RW: Vertigo, *Lancet* 352(9143):1841, 1998.

Drachman DA: A 69-year-old man with chronic dizziness, *JAMA* 280(24):2111, 1998.

Froehling DA, Silverstein MD, Mohr DN, Beatty CW: Does this dizzy patient have a serious form of vertigo? *JAMA* 271(5):385, 1994.

Furman JM, Cass SP: Benign paroxysmal positional vertigo, *N Engl J Med* 341(21):1590, 1999.

Hoffman RM, Einstadter D, Kroenke K: Evaluating dizziness, *Am J Med* 107(5):468, 1999.

Hotson JR, Baloh RW: Acute vestibular syndrome, *N Engl J Med* 339(10):680, 1998.

Jacob G, Atkinson D, Jordan J et al: Effects of standing on cerebrovascular resistance in patients with idiopathic orthostatic intolerance, *Am J Med* 106(1):59, 1999.

McGee S, Abernethy WB III, Simel DL: Is this patient hypovolemic? *JAMA* 281(11):1022, 1999.

5

Sleep Disorders

It has been estimated that each year, almost 10 million Americans consult their physicians for sleep problems. To diagnose and treat sleep disorders successfully, the physician needs to have an understanding of the normal sleep cycle, the pharmacology of hypnotics and related medications, and the various disorders of sleep and arousal.

NORMAL SLEEP PATTERN

Sleep Stages

1. On the basis of electroencephalogram (EEG) and other physiologic parameters, two categories of sleep can be recognized: nonrapid eye movement (NREM, e.g., slow wave, or spindle sleep) and rapid eye movement (REM, e.g., active, paradoxical) sleep. NREM sleep can be further divided into four stages on the basis of the EEG pattern (Table 5-1).
2. Certain sleep stages may affect underlying medical disorders adversely. For example, during REM sleep, angina of coronary heart disease and the pain of duodenal ulcer may be exacerbated; stage I sleep (the transition between wakefulness and sleep) is most prone to enhance abnormal EEG activity or clinical seizures in patients with seizure disorders.

Sleep Cycle

1. In the young adult the normal sleep cycle is made up of 20% to 25% REM, 5% to 10% stage I, 50% stage II, and 20% stages III and IV. Typically sleep begins with stage I and progresses through Stages II, III, and IV and back through stages II and III. Then, about 70 to 100 minutes after the onset of sleep, the first REM period occurs.
2. This cycle is repeated approximately every 90 minutes with a total of four to six cycles every night. Toward morning the REM periods lengthen, and NREM sleep progresses only to stages II and III.

Normal Variations

1. There are specific variations in the sleep cycle with age. A newborn may spend as much as 50% of sleep in REM, with the amount of time the child spends in REM reaching adult proportions by the third year. Children have a high percentage of stages III and IV sleep, whereas the

TABLE 5-1
Sleep Cycle

Category	Stage	Patient appearance	Physiologic characteristics	Pathologic disturbances
REM	REM	Very still, deep sleep; body apparently paralyzed; REM	Bursts of REM; irregular respiration; high BMR; inhibited peripheral muscle activity (except diaphragm); dreaming; penile tumescence; bursts of sympathetic nervous system activity	Narcolepsy; nightmares; REM behavior disorder
NREM	I	Drowsiness	Sleep myoclonus	Excessive sleep myoclonus; seizure activity
	II	Light sleep	Sleep spindles	
	III	Deep sleep	EEG slow waves	
	IV	Deep sleep	EEG slow waves	Sleepwalking; night terrors; enuresis

For NREM stages II, III: Decreased body temperature, pulse, and respirations; peripheral muscle activity present; Increased vagal tone

REM, Rapid eye movement; *BMR,* basal metabolic rate; *NREM,* nonrapid eye movement.

elderly have virtually no stage IV sleep. The elderly also often have frequent and lengthy awakenings.
2. There is also considerable amount of individual variation in the sleep cycle and total duration of sleep. Most adults require 7½ hours sleep during the same period of a 24-hour cycle.

APPROACH TO SLEEP DISORDERS

A large number of clinical conditions affect sleep. The major categories include patients with disorders of initiation and maintenance of sleep and those with excessive daytime sleepiness. Clinical evaluation of the patient with sleep disorders should include the following steps:
1. Interview: the first and most important step in evaluating a patient with a sleep disorder is the interview.
   a. It is important to determine whether the sleep-related complaints are real or subjective. Patients tend to overestimate sleep complaints. A bed partner can give valuable information during the interview. A sleep log (written record kept by the patient and the patient's bed partner that charts bedtime, time of onset of sleep, awakenings during sleep, time of awakening, and other sleep habits such as snoring, apnea, bruxism, and myoclonus) could offer further insight into the sleep pattern of the individual.
   b. Obtain the following information without asking leading questions:
      1) Sleep habits: when, where, how long, naps
      2) Sleep problems: difficulty in falling asleep, use of sleep aids; awakening during night, frequency and length; cause of awakenings (e.g., dreams, movement, pain, anxiety)
      3) Daytime somnolence: how often, duration, history suggestive of cataplexy (sudden loss of power in limbs while laughing or when emotionally upset)
      4) Medications and drug history: sedatives, stimulants, street drugs, alcohol
      5) History suggestive of seizure disorders, anxiety neurosis, depression, or affective disorders
      6) Medical history: any medical condition that may lead to disturbances in sleep (e.g., cluster headache, asthma, cardiac failure, hyperthyroidism)
2. Physical examination: obesity, hypertension, cardiac abnormalities, neurologic deficits, evidence of endocrine dysfunction, such as thyrotoxicosis or hypothyroidism.
3. Investigations
   a. A decision regarding investigations should be made only after detailed consideration of the history and physical findings. Patients with transient sleep problems or poor sleep hygiene do not need costly investigations such as polysomnography.
   b. If an underlying medical disorder such as intracranial disease or endocrinopathy is suspected, perform the relevant investigations (such as a computed tomographic [CT] scan, magnetic resonance imaging (MRI), EEG, or biochemical tests for endocrine disorders).

TABLE 5-2
Laboratory Investigations in Sleep Disorders

Test	Procedure	Indications
Multiple sleep latency test (MSLT)	During an 8- to 9-hour period, the patient is allowed to sleep for five 20-min periods; the average sleep latency and any REM-onset sleep are documented	Excessive daytime sleepiness, particularly narcolepsy
Polysomnography	Simultaneous recording of electroencephalography (EEG), electrooculography (EOG), electromyography (EMG), respirations electrocardiography (ECG), and oxygen tension during all-night sleep readings; may also be combined with video recording	Sleep apnea syndrome, sleep myoclonus, and other sleep-related disorders; differentiation of nocturnal seizures from night terrors, nightmares, sleepwalking, and apneic spells

c. Patients with persistent sleep disorders often need polysomnography (recording of EEG along with other physiologic parameters such as respiration, electromyography [EMG], electrocardiography [ECG], and electrooculography [EOG]). This will require referral to a sleep disorders laboratory (Table 5-2).

DISORDERS OF INITIATING AND MAINTAINING SLEEP

In evaluating a patient with a disorder of initiating and maintaining sleep (DIMS; insomnia), one should take into account the normal variations as well as the effects of age on the architecture of sleep stages and cycle. Remember that there is significant variation from person to person regarding the optimal duration of sleep. It is important to ascertain whether the patient feels alert and is performing well despite a shorter duration of sleep, since this may simply be the normal pattern for that person.

Transient Insomnias

The characteristic features of transient insomnias are: insomnia lasting less than 3 weeks and the presence of a clear precipitating cause such as emotional shock (e.g., the death of a loved one, divorce) or depression or anxiety provoked by circumstances such as change of job, tests, interviews, or sleeping in unfamiliar surroundings (e.g., the hospital).

Treatment:
1. Reassurance and, if necessary, crisis intervention and counseling
2. Temporary use of hypnotics, mainly to ensure rest and to prevent chronic insomnia

Persistent or Chronic Insomnia
1. When insomnia persists for more than 3 weeks it is considered as chronic insomnia
2. It may evolve from situational insomnia, or there may be no obvious factors
3. It is characterized by difficulty in falling asleep, frequent awakenings, or early morning awakenings
4. Somatization of anxiety and negative conditioning to sleep have been considered possible underlying factors, but it is necessary to exclude insomnia caused by underlying neurologic disorder, major psychiatric illness, chronic sedative or alcohol use, or periodic leg movements

Treatment:
1. General measures for sleep hygiene include establishing regular schedules for bedtime and waking, improving sleep environment, late afternoon or early evening exercises, avoidance of alcohol and caffeine-containing drinks in the evening, and stress management.
2. Continual use of hypnotics should be avoided because they can be addictive, usually lose their effect within a few days (leading to escalation of dosage), tend to produce rebound insomnia when withdrawn, and may be dangerous if taken in larger-than-prescribed doses. Occasional use of hypnotics is permissible in insomniacs experiencing a run of sleepless nights to avoid panic and other psychologic problems. Of the hypnotics, benzodiazepine derivatives are considered to be the drugs of choice. Table 5-3 lists the benzodiazepines currently approved as hypnotics.

Psychiatric Disorder Insomnia
Psychiatric disturbances constitute major causes of insomnia. The underlying condition may be excessive tension with somatization of symptoms, anxiety neurosis, depression, or major psychiatric disorders such as schizophrenia.

Treatment: Treatment should be directed toward the underlying cause (see Chapter 9).

Caution: Do not simply prescribe sedatives or hypnotics without adequate treatment of the underlying psychiatric disorder.

Medical Insomnia
Underlying medical problems that disturb sleep may account for insomnia in about 20% of patients. Such conditions include chronic pain from

TABLE 5-3
Benzodiazepine Hypnotic Agents

Drug	Usual dose (mg)	Duration of sedative effect (hours)	Remarks
Estazolam (ProSom)	1-2	6-8	Useful for sleep-onset and sleep-maintenance insomnia
Flurazepam (Dalmane)	15-30	12 or more	Useful for insomnia and daytime anxiety; metabolite has long elimination half-life, resulting in tendency to accumulate with prolonged administration; daytime sedation is major problem
Temazepam (Restoril)	15-30	6-8	Useful for frequent nocturnal awakenings; slow onset of action
Triazolam (Halcion)	0.125-0.25	6-7	Useful for sleep-onset insomnia as a result of rapid onset and short duration of action; can cause early morning rebound insomnia; with higher doses anterograde amnesia may occur

cancer, arthritis, peripheral neuropathy, metabolic disorders such as uremia, and endocrine disorders such as hyperthyroidism.

Treatment: The underlying medical problem should be identified and appropriately treated. Sedatives can be used as an adjunctive treatment if necessary.

Insomnia Associated with Drug and Alcohol Use

1. When sedatives or hypnotics such as barbiturates, glutethimide, chloral hydrate, or methaqualone are taken regularly, they lose their effectiveness in about 2 weeks, leading to a need for increased dosage. Then tolerance develops and sleep becomes disturbed with frequent awakenings. Abrupt withdrawal leads to more marked insomnia.

2. The use of central nervous system (CNS) stimulants can cause problems. Excessive intake of caffeine-containing beverages, excessive use of weight-reducing agents, drug abuse (amphetamines, cocaine), or ingestion of other stimulants (e.g., pemoline and ephedrine) can lead to insomnia.

3. Chronic alcohol abuse leads to insomnia, especially during withdrawal.

Other Insomnias

Insomnias associated with nocturnal myoclonus, restless leg syndrome, and sleep apnea syndrome are discussed in the section on disorders of excessive somnolence.

DAYTIME SOMNOLENCE

Daytime somnolence disorders manifest as inappropriate sleepiness while awake, frequent naps, incomplete arousal in the morning, and sometimes, cognitive dysfunction. Any condition that impairs nocturnal sleep may lead to daytime sleepiness. In addition, there are a number of disorders that lead to periodic or persistent daytime somnolence. The two most important causes of persistent daytime somnolence are narcolepsy and sleep apnea syndrome.

Narcolepsy

1. Narcolepsy is the manifestation of an imbalance between wakefulness and sleep in which the REM stage appears to be dominating over wakefulness.
2. Irresistible "sleep attacks" occur at any time and usually last less than 15 minutes.
3. As part of the narcolepsy syndrome, the patient may also experience one or more of the following (11% to 14% of patients may show all the features):
   a. Cataplexy is a sudden loss of muscle tone (patient may fall down without warning) that is often precipitated by laughter or any strong emotion. If cataplexy persists for more than 60 seconds, the patient may go into REM sleep.
   b. Sleep paralysis occurs during the transition between sleep and waking and is characterized by an inability to move even though awake.
   c. Hypnagogic hallucinations (vivid visual or auditory perceptions) occur at the time of falling asleep.
4. The onset is usually in adolescence or young adulthood.
5. There may be a family history of similar problems.
6. The diagnosis is confirmed by special studies such as the multiple sleep latency test (MSLT), which shows a reduced sleep latency and REM-onset sleep.
7. There is a close relationship between narcolepsy and human leukocyte antigen (HLA)-type DQW1 and DR2.

Treatment:

1. Explain the nature of the symptoms to the patient. This is crucial in long-term management.
2. Impress on the patient the need to exercise extreme caution while driving an automobile or operating heavy machinery.
3. Scheduled naps of 15 minutes in the morning and afternoon may reduce the number of sleep attacks.
4. Modafinil (Provigil) 200 mg by mouth in the morning may be helpful.

5. Pemoline (Cylert) 18.75 to 75 mg/day or methylphenidate (Ritalin) hydrochloride 5 to 60 mg/day divided into morning and early afternoon dosages may control the irresistible sleepiness. Start with a small dosage (e.g., methylphenidate 10 mg once or twice a day), and find the smallest effective dose for that particular patient.

6. Imipramine (Tofranil) hydrochloride 50 to 200 mg/day may benefit cataplexy, sleep paralysis, and hypnagogic hallucinations, but it has minimal effect on irresistible sleep attacks. Protriptyline (Vivactil) hydrochloride 15 to 30 mg/day is an alternative.

7. Patient information materials may be obtained from the National Sleep Foundation, 1522 K St. NW, Suite 500, Washington, DC 20005; e-mail: nsf@sleepfoundation.org; website: www.sleepfoundation.org.

Sleep Apnea Syndrome

1. Sleep apnea may result from problems with neural control of respiration (central apnea), from obstruction of the upper airway (obstructive apnea), or from a combination of the two (mixed apnea). *Apnea* is defined as cessation of airflow at the nose and mouth lasting 10 seconds or more. A considerable number of such episodes occurs in patients with sleep apnea syndrome.

2. Obstructive apnea is due to sleep-related upper airway obstruction (relaxation of muscles around the upper airway during sleep leads to the obstruction). It occurs predominantly in older men. It is characterized by extreme restlessness during the night with severe snoring, snorting, and frequent respiratory pauses and excessive daytime sleepiness. Once asleep, arousal may be difficult and accompanied by confusion, disorientation, and ataxia. Predisposing factors for sleep-related upper airway obstruction include enlarged tonsils and adenoids, micrognathia, retrognathia, macroglossia, and endocrinopathies (such as hypothyroidism and acromegaly).

Note: Sleep apnea syndrome may cause both insomnia and excessive daytime sleepiness.

3. A number of associated symptoms and complications are reported with sleep apnea syndrome: cardiac arrhythmias, right-sided heart failure, hypertension, obesity, night sweats, and morning headache. A drop in oxygen tension may lead to cardiac arrhythmia and arousals. In children, nocturnal enuresis, learning difficulties, and hyperactivity interrupted by hypersomnolence may be seen.

4. CNS dysfunction that occurs only during sleep leads to lack of respiratory drive in patients with central apnea. Such patients experience frequent nocturnal awakenings. The syndrome may have some overlap with sudden infant death syndrome (SIDS).

5. Consider in the differential diagnosis: intracranial lesions (e.g., diencephalic tumor), nocturnal seizures, hypothyroidism, acromegaly, and drug dependence.

6. The diagnosis should be confirmed by nightlong polysomnographic recording (Table 5-2).

Treatment:

1. Factors such as the degree of daytime sleepiness, level of oxygen desaturation during the apneic spells, cardiac status, and type of apnea (central or obstructive) should be taken into consideration in charting the treatment plan.
2. Weight reduction, alcohol withdrawal, and sleeping in a position other than supine is helpful in many cases.
3. Respiratory stimulants such as theophylline, protriptyline, and progesterone have been tried with varying results.
4. Nasal continuous positive airway pressure (CPAP) is being used more frequently in obstructive and mixed apnea. The positive pressure tends to splint the upper airway, keeping it open during sleep. Dramatic improvement in the daytime functioning of the patient is often seen after using CPAP.
5. Some patients with airway obstruction are helped by surgery (i.e., tonsillectomy, adenoidectomy, uvulopalatopharyngoplasty, or removal of an intrathoracic goiter).
6. Permanent tracheostomy, which can be kept closed during the day and opened at night, gives relief in severe cases with marked upper airway obstruction and cardiac decompensation.
7. No effective treatment has been found for central sleep apnea. In severe cases the feasibility of pacing the diaphragm by electrophrenic stimulation is being evaluated.

Caution: Do not prescribe hypnotics in sleep apnea because they will aggravate the apnea and the daytime sleepiness.

Sleep-Related Abnormal Movements

1. Sleep-related (nocturnal) myoclonus is characterized by abrupt jerking of the feet and legs, which may be frequent enough to cause symptoms.
   a. The myoclonic jerks may be violent enough to awaken the individual. Occasionally the patient may not be aware of the movements, and the complaint may come from the bed partner.
   b. Both insomnia and excessive daytime sleepiness can result from this disorder.

Treatment: Gabapentin (Neurontin) 400 mg by mouth at bed time often gives dramatic results. Clonazepam (Klonopin) 0.5 to 2.0 mg at bedtime has been found to be helpful, particularly when troublesome insomnia accompanies abnormal movements. Cost: 0.5-mg tablets, 30 tablets $24.06.

2. "Restless legs syndrome" is characterized by an indescribable, unpleasant sensation in the legs with an irresistible urge to move them.
   a. Movement seems to relieve the discomfort.
   b. Sleep-related myoclonus may also be present; insomnia may be a prominent complaint.
   c. There may be a family history of similar complaints.

   d. It is sometimes associated with peripheral neuropathy (e.g., uremic neuropathy, diabetes).

Treatment:

1. Gabapentin 400 mg orally at bedtime may help.
2. Phenytoin (Dilantin) 300 to 700 mg/day or carbamazepine (Tegretol-XR 400 to 1200 mg/day) may be useful in some patients. Cost: Phenytoin 90 caps $122.70.
3. Clonazepam 0.5 to 2.0 mg at bedtime has been tried with varying success.
4. Treatment of neuropathy should be directed at the underlying condition (e.g., diabetes or uremia).

Periodic Disorders with Daytime Somnolence

Kleine-Levin syndrome

The Kleine-Levin syndrome of periodic hypersomnia is very rare and is characterized by recurrent episodes of markedly prolonged sleep (several weeks) with intervening periods of normal sleep and wakefulness. It may also be associated with a periodic increase in appetite for food and sex. It occurs in adolescence and young adulthood, more commonly in men. Consider lesions (inflammatory and neoplastic) involving the diencephalon or limbic system in the differential diagnosis.

DISORDERS OF SLEEP-WAKE SCHEDULE

The following are disorders of the circadian or 24-hour biologic clock:

Jet Lag

With the rapid time zone change (jet lag) syndrome, the patient's sleep-wake schedule does not adjust immediately to the new time zone; hence, sleepiness and fatigue occur during wakefulness, whereas insomnia occurs during the new sleep period. Symptoms last an average of 2 days.

Treatment: Morning wake time is a strong cue to reset the biologic clock. The wake-up time should be adjusted to suit the new environment. The use of a hypnotic for the first 2 nights may also be helpful.

Shift Work Change

When the work period is shifted to normal sleeping hours, the person is sleepy, performance is suboptimal, and the new sleep period disrupted. At least several days are required to adjust.

Delayed/Advanced Sleep-Phase Syndrome

Delayed/advanced sleep-phase syndrome includes conditions in which the patient's biologic clock is set differently from the norm, such that the circadian rhythm is out of phase with socially prescribed bedtime.

Treatment: Chronotherapy, which involves "resetting the biologic clock," consists of going to bed 3 hours later each day (e.g., functioning on a 27-hour day until the individual has advanced to the normal 10 or 11 PM bedtime).

PARASOMNIAS

The parasomnias include the following conditions that occur either exclusively during sleep or are exacerbated by sleep:

Bed-Wetting (Enuresis)

1. Primary enuresis (child never toilet-trained)
   a. Primary enuresis is often due to maturational lag.
   b. A total of 10% to 15% of children 4 to 5 years of age continue to wet the bed; this rarely continues into adulthood.
   c. There is often a family history of this disorder. Enuresis occurs in all sleep stages.

Treatment:
1. Advise parents against overreacting to the situation, and reassure them that children usually outgrow it. Patience and understanding are important.
2. Rewarding the child for a dry bed is helpful.
3. Various behavior-modification methods can be applied in difficult cases with the aid of experienced child psychologists.
4. Imipramine (Tofranil), 10 to 75 mg at bedtime, is often effective in preventing bed-wetting but is not recommended for prolonged usage. The antidiuretic hormone (ADH) analogue desmopressin administered intranasally in doses of 10 to 40 mg at bedtime has been found to be useful.

2. Secondary enuresis (relapse to bed-wetting after a dry period of several months to years):
   a. Secondary enuresis is often due to psychologic factors such as childhood depression.
   b. Organic disease must be ruled out, even if a psychologic cause is obvious.

Treatment:
1. Psychologic evaluation and family counseling are often necessary.
2. Imipramine, a tricyclic antidepressant, in doses of 0.5 to 2.0 mg/kg/day at bedtime is effective in reducing the frequency of bed-wetting. It is most effective when childhood depression is associated with the enuresis; with other causes the response is not as good. There is a tendency to relapse when the drug is withdrawn, and it is not recommended for prolonged use.
3. Behavioral techniques, such as bladder-control exercises, rewards for dry beds, and wetting alarms, frequently improve the enuresis.

Remember: An important organic cause of enuresis is urinary tract infection, and all children with enuresis should have urinalysis and a culture tests. Other rare possibilities to consider include seizures in sleep, diabetes, congenital anomalies of the bladder, urethral obstruction, and ectopic ureter.

Sleepwalking (Somnambulism)

1. The prevalence of sleepwalking is estimated at 1% to 6%.
2. It occurs mostly in children and usually disappears by 14 to 15 years of age.
3. There is often a family history of sleepwalking.

4. Episodes last several minutes with total amnesia for the incident.
5. Episodes occur during stages III and IV sleep.
6. Sleepwalkers have a high incidence of enuresis.
7. The onset of sleepwalking in older age groups should arouse suspicion of a psychiatric disorder or medication effect. Nocturnal delirium ("sundown syndrome") may manifest as sleepwalking in the demented elderly.

Treatment:
1. Protect the patient from injury by locking the doors and windows and avoiding other dangerous situations. Advise parents that children usually outgrow sleepwalking.
2. Benzodiazepines, such as diazepam (Valium) 2 to 5 mg at bedtime, which suppress sleep stages III and IV, may be helpful for chronic and frequent sleepwalking.
3. In adult sleepwalkers, psychologic disturbances are frequent, unless there is a strong family history. Thorough psychologic evaluation and treatment are recommended.

Night Terrors

1. Night terrors occur early in the night during slow-wave sleep, most frequently at ages 4 to 6 years.
2. Sudden apparent awakening is accompanied by extreme physiologic arousal (increased heart rate, respiratory rate, and sweating), and the child will scream and cry but cannot be awakened.
3. The incident is usually not remembered, although the child may recall a single frightening image or a sense of doom.

Treatment:
1. Advise the parents that children usually outgrow night terrors, and medication is generally not necessary.
2. Night terrors may be abolished by diazepam 2 to 5 mg for children or 5 to 20 mg for adults. Long-term use is not recommended.
3. Other medical conditions causing distress and disturbing stage IV sleep may result in night terrors. Correction of this condition may decrease the frequency of night terrors.
4. Psychiatric referral is indicated for night terrors past 14 years of age.

Nightmares

1. Nightmares (dream anxiety attacks) are frightening dreams occurring in REM sleep, more frequently toward morning.
2. The degree of physiologic arousal is much lower than in night terrors.
3. Patients often have detailed recall of dream content.

Treatment:
1. Usually reassurance is all that is necessary.
2. In cases in which nightmares are frequent and disabling to the patient, psychotherapy and behavioral treatment may be effective.

Sleep-Related Epileptic Seizures

1. While seizures may occur predominantly or exclusively during sleep in epileptic patients, conditions such as enuresis, night terrors, and

sleepwalking may be triggered by seizures originating in the temporal lobe.

2. Seizure monitoring (EEG recording with split-screen video monitoring) will confirm the diagnosis.

Treatment: Anticonvulsant therapy (see Chapter 11).

REM Behavior Disorder

REM behavior disorder is a rare condition in which the normal loss of muscle tone fails to occur during REM sleep, such that the patient may actually "act out" dreams resulting in injury to the self or to the bed partner.

Treatment: Responds readily to clonazepam 0.5 to 1.5 mg at bedtime.

OTHER CONDITIONS AFFECTING SLEEP

Gastric Acid Secretion

Patients secrete 3 to 20 times more gastric acid during REM sleep.

Treatment:

1. Decrease acid production. Cost: famotidine (Pepcid) 30 20-mg tablets $51.71; cimetidine (Tagamet) 500-mg tablets, 60 tablets $53.66; omeprazole (Prilosec) 40-mg capsules, 30 capsules $156.72.

2. Try to minimize sleep disruptions.

3. Antidepressants (e.g., amitriptyline and doxepin, in low dosage) may prove helpful for both the sleep disturbance and the hyperacidity.

Angina

Angina is more likely to occur during REM sleep.

Asthma

Bronchial asthma attacks often occur during REM sleep.

Caution: Do not prescribe hypnotics to patients with bronchial asthma.

Thyroid Dysfunction

Hyperthyroidism and hypothyroidism may cause excessive sleepiness or insomnia, both of which are treated by correcting the thyroid dysfunction.

Pregnancy

Sleep time is increased in early pregnancy and decreased in later pregnancy, but normal sleep patterns should be recovered a few weeks after delivery. Drugs should be avoided during pregnancy.

Alcohol

Alcohol depresses REM sleep and results in REM rebound during withdrawal. Chronic alcoholics show fragmented, shallow sleep. Insomnia is also associated with alcohol withdrawal.

BIBLIOGRAPHY

Chiappa KH, Hill RA: Evaluation and prognostication in coma, *Electroencephalogr Clin Neurophysiol* 106(2):149-155, 1998.

Coleman RM, Roffwarg HP, Kennedy SJ et al: Sleep-wake disorders based on a polysomnographic diagnosis, *JAMA* 247:997-1003, 1982.

Feske SK: Coma and confusional states: emergency diagnosis and management, *Neurol Clin* 16(2):237-256, 1998.

Gillin JC, Byerley WF: The diagnosis and management of insomnia, *N Engl J Med* 322:239-247, 1990.

Hauri P, Esther MS: Insomnia, *Mayo Clin Proc,* 65:869-882, 1990.

Kryger MH: Management of obstructive apnea, *Clin Chest Med* 133:481-492, 1992.

Liu GT: Coma, *Neurosurg Clin N Am* 10(4):579-586, 1999.

Miller K, Atkin B, Moody ML: Drug therapy for nocturnal enuresis, *Drugs* 44: 47-56, 1992.

Reite ML, Nagel KE, Ruddy JR: *The evaluation and management of sleep disorders,* Washington, 1990, American Psychiatric Press.

Scharf MB, Flexcher KA, Jennings SW: Current pharmacologic treatments of narcolepsy, *Am Fam Physician* 38:1-6, 1988.

Treatment of sleep disorders in older people: NIH consensus development conference statement, 1990.

6

Diminished Mental Capacity and Dementia

Dementia is a general term for the progressive impairment of mental functioning. It is a syndrome characterized by a decline in two or more of the following: language, memory, visuospatial skills, executive abilities, and emotions. Dementia is acquired, not developmental, and is distinguished from mental retardation or low intelligence by a *decline* from a prior higher level of mental functioning. The task of a physician caring for a demented patient is twofold: (1) identify dementias that are treatable and (2) educate and support the family of the patient with incurable dementia.

DIAGNOSIS OF DIMINISHED MENTAL CAPACITY

Suspect dementia when the patient exhibits any of the following signs:
1. Confusion as a result of slight provocation such as a change in schedule or surroundings
2. A tendency toward repetition during the process of history-taking
3. Slowness in following commands during the physical examination (e.g., the examiner may have to demonstrate the tasks of station and gait)
4. Emotional lability or irritability

If dementia is suspected or if the patient or the patient's family complains of mental deterioration, a mental status evaluation *must* be performed. Conduct it so that the patient does not become defensive. Usually, it can be worked in during the history and presented in an easy conversational style, such as, "I'm going to ask you some questions that may sound silly, but it's part of my examination."

The Folstein Mini-Mental Status Examination (MMSE) is the standard screening mental status evaluation (Box 6-1).

In addition to the MMSE, make specific notation of the following signs:
1. Appearance and behavior
   a. Dress and grooming: Clean? Neat? Appropriate?
   b. Attention: Alert? Dull? Apathetic? Distracted?

BOX 6-1
Mini-Mental Status Examination

The Mini-Mental Status Examination (MMSE) is a brief, 30-point scale that screens cognition in the following areas:

- Orientation (time: date, year, month, season; and place: location, floor, city, county, state)
- Registration (repeating three words)
- Attention and calculations (spelling *world* backward or subtracting serial sevens)
- Recall (recalling the three words from the registration section)
- Language (naming two common objects, repeating a simple phrase such as, "No ifs, ands, or buts," following a three-stage command, following a written command, and writing a sentence)
- Construction (copying intersecting pentagons)

---

   c. Movements: Slow? Hyperactive? Restless? Tremor?
   d. Discretion: Inhibited? Discusses intimate topics without restraint?
   e. Affect: "I don't know" responses are seen in dementia associated with depression. The degree is important, because many patients with neurologic abnormalities also have depression; see Chapter 9.
   f. Insight: Demented patients have limited insight about their problems.
2. Language abnormalities
   a. Quantity: Talkative? Noncommunicative?
   b. Content: Simple or complex sentence structure? Has trouble finding words?
   c. Perseveration: Has trouble changing topics? Uses words from earlier sentence inappropriately in a new sentence?
   d. Appropriateness: Irrelevant? Illogical?
   e. Comprehension: Follows verbal commands without cues? Answers questions directly?

Caveat: Aphasic or schizophrenic patients may appear to be demented. Patients with a motor aphasia have a paucity of speech and difficulty finding words and are aware of their problem. Patients with a sensory aphasia or schizophrenia may produce many words that make no sense (see Chapter 12).

ABNORMALITIES SOMETIMES SEEN IN DEMENTED PATIENTS
Diagnostic Considerations

Caveat: The following abnormalities do *not* diagnose dementia, but one or more of them are often seen in demented patients. The diagnosis is made on the basis of a decline in multiple areas of mental functioning.

1. Expressionless or masklike facies; facial grimacing
2. Bruns' frontal ataxia: a broad-based gait with short steps and feet placed flat on the ground as if on ice; a tendency toward retropulsion increases the risk of falling; occurs in patients with frontal lobe deficits
3. Abnormal posturing and movement
4. Primitive reflexes:
   a. Grasp reflex: lightly stroking the palm of the patient's hand elicits a grasp response and reluctance to let go (Fig. 6-1)
   b. Rooting reflex (sometimes incorrectly called *suck reflex*): the patient turns the lips toward a stroking stimulus at the corner of the mouth (Fig. 6-2)
   c. Snout reflex: the patient puckers the lips in response to gentle percussion of the lips (Fig. 6-3)
   d. Active jaw reflex (Fig. 6-4)
5. Paratonic rigidity (gegenhalten): advise the patient to relax his or her limbs. Passive manipulation of the patient's arm in unpredictable di-

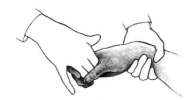

FIG. 6-1 Grasp reflex. The patient will squeeze the examiner's fingers as the examiner rubs his or her fingers along the patient's palm from the hypothenar eminence toward the thenar eminence (normal response in infants).

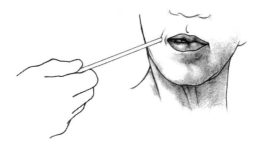

FIG. 6-2 Rooting (suck) reflex. Stroking away from the corner of the patient's mouth elicits lip movements and movement of the mouth toward the stimulus (normal response in infants).

rections feels as if he or she is consciously resisting every movement of the examiner (Fig. 6-5)

6. Motor perseveration: when asked to perform a task such as rapid alternating movements, the patient continues for an inappropriate length of time
7. Motor impersistence (inability to persist in a motor task):
   a. Keeping eyes closed
   b. Keeping tongue out
   c. Fixating gaze

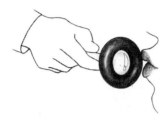

FIG. 6-3 Snout response. Lightly tapping the patient's closed lips causes the lips to pucker.

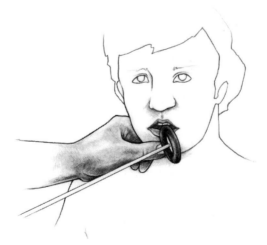

FIG. 6-4 Jaw reflex. With the patient's mouth slightly open, the examiner places a finger on the patient's chin and strikes the finger, causing the jaw to close momentarily.

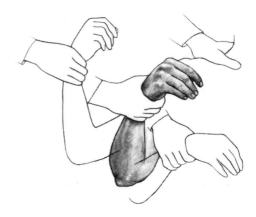

FIG. 6-5 Gegenhalten. After instructing the patient to relax the arm "like a rag doll," the examiner moves the patient's arm in unpredictable directions. With gegenhalten, the examiner notes resistence as though the patient is actively attempting to prevent movement.

    d. Sustaining "ah" or "ee" sound
    e. Maintaining hand grip

Note: In position sense testing, demented patients tend to peek. (They are unable to sustain eye closure.)

EVALUATION OF DEMENTIA

Box 6-2 lists some of the disease processes of diminished mental capacity that may either be cured or have the progression stopped. The box suggests that the following studies should be considered in every patient with dementia:

1. Laboratory studies:
    a. Complete blood count and erythrocyte sedimentation rate (ESR): abnormalities may suggest infection, vitamin deficiency, or autoimmune disease.
    b. Blood chemistry testing: blood chemistry testing is essential in diagnosing secondary metabolic encephalopathies.
    c. Serum studies: serum vitamin B_{12}, serum folate, and red blood cell (RBC) folate levels are especially important in patients with chronic ulcer disease or postgastrectomy. Serum methylmalonic acid levels are more accurate than serum vitamin B_{12} levels.
    d. Endocrine studies: hypothyroidism is the most common endocrine cause of dementia. A determination of thyroid stimulating hormone (TSH) levels is recommended. Other studies should be ordered as suggested by the history and physical examination.

BOX 6-2
Selected Treatable Causes of Dementia

Toxins and drugs
Nutritional deficiency states
Metabolic or endocrine disorders
Hypoxia
Normal-pressure hydrocephalus
Intracranial mass lesions
Central nervous system infections
Atherosclerotic cerebrovascular disease

---

    e. Human immunodeficiency virus (HIV) titer if indicated from history: HIV/AIDS (acquired immunodeficiency syndrome) encephalopathy is a common clinical syndrome associated with HIV infection.

2. Lumbar puncture (LP): An LP is necessary for the diagnosis of indolent infections and neurosyphilis if suggested by the history or meningeal enhancement on magnetic resonance imaging (MRI). When normal-pressure hydrocephalus is suspected from a computed tomographic (CT) scan or an MRI, remove 40 or 50 ml of cerebrospinal fluid (CSF) to evaluate the patient for immediate improvement of gait.

3. Neuroimaging: MRI with and without contrast (the CT scan is less sensitive) shows mass lesions, multiple infarcts, normal-pressure hydrocephalus, cerebral atrophy, and white matter disease.

4. Electroencephalography (EEG): The EEG is often normal in dementia; however, characteristic findings can be seen in certain conditions. A periodic spike-and-wave pattern is seen in Creutzfeldt-Jakob disease (CJD), triphasic waves are seen in metabolic encephalopathy associated with hepatic or renal failure, periodic lateralizing epileptiform discharges are seen in herpes encephalitis, focal slowing and focal epileptiform discharges are seen with structural lesions, and generalized slowing is seen with many other causes of dementia.

TREATABLE DEMENTIAS

Vascular Dementia

1. Vascular dementia is also known as *multiinfarct dementia* or *Binswanger's disease.*

2. Patients frequently have a history of chronic hypertension.

3. Patients have a history of a "stepwise" progression (i.e., periods of stability with sudden decompensation).

4. MRI shows multiple small subcortical infarcts.

5. Patients have pseudobulbar palsy and emotional lability. They may burst into tears at a trivial incident, but when asked, they deny they are

sad. Neurologic examination shows generalized hyperreflexia, including a hyperactive jaw reflex. MRI shows multiple small infarcts.

Treatment: Progression may be controlled by blood pressure control. Patients with pseudobulbar palsy may benefit from fluoxetine 20 mg by mouth daily in the morning.

Mass Lesions

1. Patients with large brain tumors sometimes may have no symptoms or signs other than dementia, especially if the tumor is slow-growing (e.g., meningioma).
2. MRI of the brain with and without contrast easily diagnoses these conditions.

Alcoholism

1. Patients suffering from alcoholism usually have a history of daily alcohol intake.
2. Lability of mood is common.
3. Recovery of mental faculties is surprisingly good if alcohol consumption can be stopped.

Caveat: This dementia should be differentiated from Korsakoff's psychosis, which is a specific defect in acquiring new information, not a global defect (see Chapter 8).

Drugs

1. Many drugs, even when prescribed in conservative therapeutic doses, may cause diminished mental capacity. Examples include phenobarbital, phenytoin, and anticholinergic drugs.
2. Elderly patients are especially sensitive to medications; sedatives and antihistamines should be prescribed with great caution.

Subacute Combined Degeneration

1. Patients suffering from subacute combined degeneration (combined system disease, vitamin B_{12} deficiency) commonly have a history of ulcer disease or gastrectomy; older patients may develop gastric achlorhydria and fail to produce intrinsic factor.
2. Although patients may have four neurologic abnormalities (dementia, corticospinal tract signs, posterior column abnormalities, and peripheral neuropathy), dementia may be the most prominent finding (see Chapter 15).
3. Other vitamin deficiencies may produce dementia but rarely do so in the presence of an adequate diet.
4. Treatment is initiated with vitamin B_{12} 1000 μg intramuscularly (IM) daily for 5 days followed by 1000 μg IM every other day for 2 weeks. A regimen of 1000 μg monthly should then be maintained indefinitely.
5. With proper treatment, at least partial improvement can be expected in most instances. Most of the symptomatic improvement occurs in the first 6 months of treatment, although it may not be complete for a year or more.

Endocrine Abnormalities

1. Hypothyroidism: neurologic abnormalities include dementia and a slowed relaxation phase of the Achilles tendon reflex.
2. Hypoglycemia: the usual clinical setting is in a diabetic patient with repeated episodes of hypoglycemia precipitated by inappropriate doses of insulin or oral hypoglycemic agents. Acute attacks should be treated with intravenous (IV) glucose. Hypoglycemia can cause permanent brain damage. The dementia can be made worse if care is not taken to prevent further hypoglycemic attacks.
3. Both hyperparathyroidism and hypoparathyroidism may be misread as dementia. Hypoparathyroidism may be associated with basal ganglia calcification.
4. Any endocrine abnormality, if severe enough, may cause mental slowness; this includes Cushing's syndrome and panhypopituitarism.

Toxic-Metabolic Encephalopathy

1. Toxic-metabolic encephalopathy is usually subacute at onset. A general physical examination, blood chemistry tests, and blood gas determinations usually reveal the cause. Common causes include chronic obstructive pulmonary disease, an acute infectious process, a drug overdose, and hepatic and renal failure. The EEG often shows generalized slowing.

Chronic Infection

1. AIDS: HIV infection causes dementia from the virus itself or from opportunistic infections of the brain.
2. Tuberculosis and fungal meningitis: tuberculous and fungal meningitis may produce dementia both by destroying the brain parenchyma and by thickening the posterior fossa meninges and causing obstructive hydrocephalus. The patient may have no other signs of infection, such as fever, and the diagnosis can be excluded only by examining the CSF. Neuroimaging may show meningeal enhancement (see Chapter 14).
3. Tertiary central nervous system (CNS) syphilis: the presence of typical pupillary abnormalities (Argyll Robertson pupil) may suggest the diagnosis. The blood Venereal Disease Research Laboratory (VDRL) test may be nonreactive; the diagnosis is made with certainty only with a CSF VDRL test.

Normal-Pressure Hydrocephalus

1. Diagnosis
   a. The diagnosis of normal-pressure hydrocephalus should be considered with a subacute onset (months) of dementia associated with ataxia and urinary incontinence.
   b. Many patients have a history of a previous subarachnoid hemorrhage or meningitis.
   c. The neurologic examination shows hyperactive stretch reflexes in the lower extremities (sometimes with Babinski's reflex) and normal reflexes in the upper extremities.

d. A CT scan and MRI show large ventricles with no significant atrophy of the brain. The sulci are not prominent.

e. An LP to document normality of the opening pressure is a prerequisite for this diagnosis.

Treatment: If the patient shows improvement after removing 50 ml of CSF by LP, consider a permanent shunt; however, shunting does not guarantee improved cognitive function.

Dementia Associated with Depression

1. Diagnostic considerations

    a. The term *dementia associated with depression* was previously referred to as *pseudodementia* and refers to a major depressive disorder in the elderly (see Chapter 9).

    b. It is often mistaken for Alzheimer's disease. (Table 9-2 may help in distinguishing between the two.)

    c. Vegetative signs such as sleep disturbance (early morning awakening), motor slowness, and lack of energy are often present.

Treatment:

1. Fluoxetine 20 mg by mouth daily for depression with an associated reduced energy level

2. Paroxetine (Paxil) 20 mg by mouth daily for depression with associated anxiety

3. Sertraline (Zoloft) 50 mg by mouth daily for depression with associated insomnia

PROGRESSIVE DEMENTIAS

Alzheimer's Disease

1. Alzheimer's disease accounts for up to 70% of all cases of dementia, affecting 15 million people over 40 years of age and progressing from onset of symptoms to death in a mean of $8\frac{1}{2}$ years. The prevalence doubles every 5 years between 65 and 85 years of age. Alzheimer's disease costs society $100 billion each year.

2. Clinical diagnosis can be made with 85% accuracy using criteria from the *Diagnostic and statistical manual of mental disorders*, ed. 4. Alzheimer's disease is characterized by multiple deficits manifested by memory impairment and other cognitive deficits. Its course is gradual and progressive.

Caveat: Currently, a definitive diagnosis of Alzheimer's disease is made on the pathologic basis of significant β-amyloid–containing neuritic plaques and neurofibrillary tangles. An incorrect diagnosis deprives a patient of treatment of a curable dementia.

3. Associated symptoms include depression, sleep disturbance, psychosis, agitation, and aggression. Genetic risk factors for Alzheimer's disease exist in some families.

Note: Patients over 40 years of age with Down syndrome have neuropathologic changes of Alzheimer's disease and a progressive dementia.

4. Except for the finding of dementia, the findings from a neurologic examination of the cranial nerves, reflexes, sensation, and station and gait can be normal early in Alzheimer's disease.
5. MRI shows nonspecific cerebral atrophy.
6. The EEG is normal until late in the disease.
7. Management
   a. Family support, environmental manipulation, prevention of other medical illnesses, and proper nutrition and exercise can improve functioning of patients with Alzheimer's disease. Families should be counseled to obtain power of attorney and a living will early in the disease. Information may be obtained from the Alzheimer's Association.
   b. Pharmacologic treatment with acetylcholinesterase inhibitors is based on increasing the acetylcholine concentration in the brain. Studies have shown a reduction in the rate of cognitive decline and an improvement of global function in a majority of patients. Treatment can delay loss of activities of daily living (ADLs) by as much as 1 year.
   c. A second-generation cholinesterase inhibitor, donepezil (Aricept) was approved for treatment of mild to moderate Alzheimer's disease. Donepezil is started at 5 mg orally at bedtime, then increased to 10 mg after 6 weeks. The drug costs $126.45 for 30 5-mg tablets. If the drug delays nursing home placement and reduces family burden, the medication would be cost effective. No formal cost-effectiveness analyses have been conducted to date. Other second-generation cholinesterase inhibitors, rivastigmine, metrifonate, and galanthamine, are expected to be as effective as donepezil.
   d. Antioxidants: Vitamin E at 1000 IU orally twice daily can be used to possibly delay progression of the disease. No cost-effectiveness analyses have been conducted to date.
   e. Depression should be treated with antidepressants. Selective serotonin reuptake inhibitors (SSRIs) are first line drugs for depression. Avoid drugs with high anticholinergic activity, which can worsen the cognitive deficits.
   f. Psychosis is treated with neuroleptics. New atypical antipsychotics, such as olanzapine (Zyprexa) 2.5 to 5 mg daily or quetiapine (Seroquel) 12.5 to 25 mg once or twice daily, can be effective with treatment of aggression and agitation.

Frontotemporal Dementias

1. Clinical distinctions of frontotemporal dementias (FTDs) are personality changes, disinhibition, reduced speech output, and relatively spared memory functions. The onset is between 50 and 70 years of age. Progression of the disease is more rapid than that of Alzheimer's disease.
2. Three types include the following: Pick's disease characterized by neuronal Pick body inclusions, frontal lobe degeneration without Pick bodies, and dementia associated with motor neuron disease (frontal lobe degeneration–amyotrophic lateral sclerosis [ALS] complex).

3. A CT scan or MRI may show frontal and temporal lobe atrophy, which is out of proportion to the atrophy in the rest of the brain.
4. Some 20% of cases have a pattern of autosomal dominant inheritance.
5. Management is the same as for Alzheimer's disease.

Lewy Body Disease

1. Clinical distinctions of Lewy body disease (LBD) are parkinsonian features, early hallucinations, fluctuating mental status, and relatively preserved memory. Disease progression is more rapid than that of Alzheimer's disease.
2. The findings of a CT scan or MRI may be normal.
3. Management is symptom oriented. Patients with LBD are highly sensitive to neuroleptic medications.

Huntington's Disease

1. Dementia may precede the choreoathetosis and psychosis by many years. The correct diagnosis is most strongly suggested by a family history of dominantly inherited psychosis or dementia (see Chapter 7). Treatment is symptomatic.

Creutzfeldt-Jakob Disease

1. Clinical distinctions of CJD are dementia with generalized myoclonus.
2. The course is rapid, with death in 6 to 12 months.
3. The infectious agent is a prion (proteinaceous material).
4. The EEG shows characteristic periodic epileptic discharges, which may not be evident until late in the disease.

BIBLIOGRAPHY

Cummings JL, Trimble MR: *Neuropsychiatry and behavioral neurology,* Washington, 1995, American Psychiatric Press.

Drachman DA: Geriatric/behavioral neurology, *Curr Opin Neurol* Jan 2000.

Francis PT, Palmer AM, Snape M, Wilcock GK: The cholinergic hypothesis of Alzheimer's disease: a review in progress, *J Neurol Neurosurg Psychiatry* 66:137-147, 1999.

Mayeux R, Sano M: Treatment of Alzheimer's disease, *N Engl J Med* 341:1670-1679, 1999.

Molloy W, Caldwell P: Alzheimer's disease, New York, 1998, Firefly Books.

WEBSITES

Alzheimer's Association: www.alz.org

Alzheimer's Disease Clinical Trials Database: www.alzheimers.org/trials

Clinical pharmacology online: www.gsm.com

MEDLINEplus: health information: dementia: www.nlm.nih.gov/medlineplus/dementia.html

Patient Education Forum: dementia: www.americangeriatrics.org/education/forum/dementia.shtml

7

Movement Disorders

Accurate observation and description are essential for classifying movement disorders. The patient's abnormal movements and postures can often be observed during the interview; one look is worth a thousand words.

ABNORMAL MOVEMENTS

Tremor

A tremor is an involuntary, rhythmic movement across a joint. The tremor can be present at rest (static tremor), only apparent with motion (kinetic tremor), or at a specific posture (postural tremor).

Chorea and Athetosis

Chorea is an irregular, arrhythmic, unpredictable, brief movement involving the extremities in continuous, random sequence; *athetosis* is a slow, sinuous more proximal movement. In some cases the distinction between these two types of movement is unclear, and the term *choreoathetosis* is used. When chorea is seen in slow motion on a videotape, it often closely resembles athetosis.

Myoclonus

Myoclonus is a series of spontaneous, brief, shocklike contractions of one or more muscles, causing movement across a joint (think of the jerklike movements often seen in dogs, cats or people as they fall asleep).

Tics

Tics are repetitive, rapid, usually brief, seemingly purposeful, stereotyped movements. The movements are commonly complex and involve the face, axial muscles, and proximal limbs; they seldom involve fingers or toes.

Focal Motor Seizures

Focal motor seizures are relatively rhythmic movements, usually involving multiple joints and often persisting in sleep. (Tremors, choreoathetosis, and tics commonly disappear during sleep.)

Clonus

Clonus is a rhythmic movement precipitated by the sudden stretching of a tendon. Clonus is most commonly seen at the ankle, and is associated with upper motor neuron lesions.

Fasciculations

Fasciculations are very brief twitches of a group of muscle fibers, all innervated by the same anterior horn cell. They are best seen where subcutaneous fat is thinnest (e.g., the back or the tongue). Generally, fasciculations do *not* cause movement across a joint, but they can occasionally cause slight movement of the fingers.

Dystonia

Dystonia is sustained muscle contractions that frequently cause twisting and repetitive movement or abnormal postures.

THE PATIENT WITH A MOVEMENT DISORDER

History

1. Many movement disorders are *familial*.
2. It is important to elicit a drug and alcohol history. Alcoholism can cause cerebellar degeneration and alleviate familial tremor. Phenothiazines and other neuroleptics can cause Parkinson's syndrome or tardive dyskinesias. Excess thyroid hormone (endogenous or exogenously administered) can result in a metabolic tremor.
3. The medical history is important. Liver disease can cause asterixis, and Sydenham's chorea is associated with streptococcal infections.
4. A description of the movement disorder should include age at onset, rate of progression, symmetry, and exacerbating or alleviating factors (e.g., stress, drugs, sleep).

Neurologic Examination

1. Have the patient draw a spiral or connect dots as a permanent record of the motor dysfunction; this record can be used later to monitor the efficacy of treatment.
2. Muscle tone is the resistance of the muscle to passive movement. *Hypotonia* can be seen as floppiness of joints or an excessive number of swings after the patellar reflex is elicited when the patient is sitting on the examining table (Fig. 7-1). Increased tone, as in Parkinson's disease, can be seen in passive movement of the arm. When the patient draws an imaginary figure 8 in the air with the contralateral arm, abnormal tone is more evident.
3. Instruct the patient to point his or her index fingers (Fig. 7-2) to bring out some tremors and to differentiate proximal and distal tremors.
4. Abnormal postures are most often apparent during station and gait testing.

Caution: Never make the diagnosis of a movement disorder on the basis of a single finding. Table 7-1 illustrates this point by showing the overlapping features of Parkinson's syndrome, cerebellar tremor, and essential

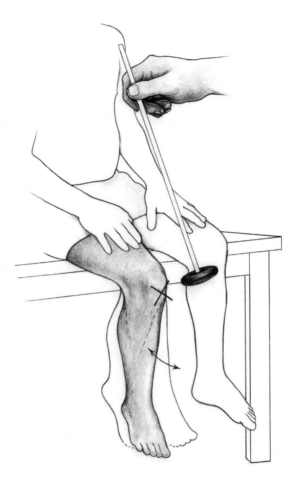

FIG. 7-1 The patient with cerebellar disease can have an abnormal number of swings of the leg when the patellar reflex is tested.

tremor. Also, note that on the finger-to-nose test (Fig. 7-3), both cerebellar tremor and essential tremor have an intentional component.

PARKINSONISM

Parkinson's *disease* is an idiopathic disorder associated with a progressive loss of neurons in the midbrain substantia nigra; Parkinson's *syndrome*

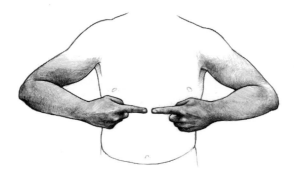

FIG. 7-2 Having the patient point (but not touch) his index fingers can differentiate between a proximal and distal tremor. With a proximal tremor there is flapping of the arms; with a distal tremor the fingers are constantly in misalignment.

TABLE 7-1
Overlapping Features of Various Types of Tremor

Feature	Parkinson's syndrome	Cerebellar tremor	Essential tremor
Present at rest	Yes	No	Yes
Increased tone	Yes	No	No
Decreased tone	No	Yes	No
Postural abnormality	Yes	Yes	No
Head involvement	Yes	Yes	Yes
Intentional component	No	Yes	Yes
Incoordination	No	Yes	No

involves entirely different pathophysiologic processes and is associated with dozens of other neurologic diseases, including repeated head trauma, multiinfarct state, Alzheimer's disease, and acute effect of neuroleptics such as chlorpromazine (Thorazine), haloperidol (Haldol), promethazine (Phenergan), prochlorperazine (Compazine), and metoclopramide (Reglan). Suspect Parkinson's *syndrome* (and refer to a neurologist) if the following are true:

1. Reflexes are abnormal (hyperactive in amyotrophic lateral sclerosis [ALS]–dementia–parkinsonism complex or olivopontocerebellar degeneration).
2. Significant dementia is present (Alzheimer's disease or Lewy body disease).
3. Downward or lateral gaze is impaired (progressive supranuclear palsy).

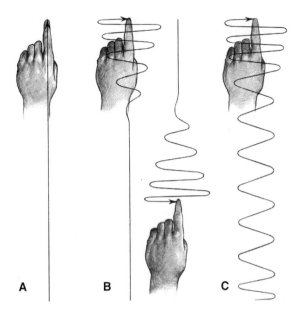

FIG. 7-3 Finger-to-nose test. **A,** The normal person is able to point to a target accurately and smoothly. **B,** The patient with cerebellar hemisphere disease shows a tremor that increases in amplitude as the target is approached. **C,** The patient with essential tremor shows a tremor throughout the range of motion. Note the increase in amplitude as the target is approached. **B** and **C** are easily confused.

4. Postural hypotension is present (Shy-Drager syndrome).
5. The patient does not respond significantly to combination carbidopa and levodopa early in the onset of the disease.

Early Symptoms

1. Voice changes (a decrease in volume and loss of melody): these are often not apparent to the examiner but are quite obvious to the family and close friends of the patient.
2. Sleep disturbances: frequent nocturnal awakenings, possibly secondary to loss of automatic motor movements during sleep, occur.
3. Wet pillow in the morning: saliva often is not swallowed during sleep even if there is no such problem during waking.
4. Rigidity: early in the disease, patients often complain of a tightness or pain in the neck and shoulders. Passively move the extremities; instruct the patient to relax the arm ("like a rag doll") and then passively move the arm. Increased tone (rigidity) is noted as increased resistance

throughout the range of movement (the so-called lead pipe rigidity); tremor can also be felt during this movement (the so-called cogwheel phenomenon). Ask the patient to draw a circle or a figure 8 in the air with the other arm to bring out the rigidity of the arm being moved passively. This is also manifest in facial muscles with reduction in frequency of blinking and masklike face.

Later Signs and Symptoms (Fig. 7-4)

1. *Tremor*

   a. Tremor is present at rest and is worse when the patient is experiencing emotional stress or when the examiner calls attention to it.

   b. The patient displays a "pill-rolling" motion, with the index finger flexing and extending in contact with the thumb, at approximately 4 to 10 Hz. This motion can involve the arm with rhythmic flexion-extension, abduction-adduction, pronation-supination, or a combination thereof.

   c. Tremor is present most commonly in the hands and fingers; it often begins unilaterally and distally and spreads proximally and to the other side over months or years.

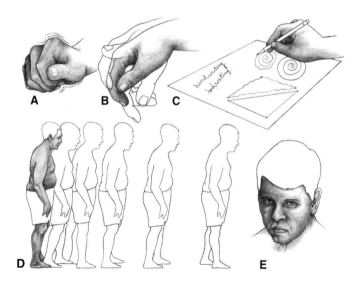

FIG. 7-4 The parkinsonian syndrome. **A,** The "pill-rolling" tremor. **B,** Tremor that can worsen with emotional stress. **C,** Handwriting abnormalities, which include micrographia. **D,** Typical posture and gait, which becomes faster (festination). **E,** Lack of facial expression as well as "stare" from decreased blinking.

2. *Postural changes* are observed during testing of station and gait. Changes include stooping of shoulders and slight flexion of the back, hips, and knees. Early loss of arm swing occurs. In starting to walk, the patient's steps are slow and small (the so-called marche à petit pas) and then rapidly increase. In turning, the patient's motion is not fluid but is done in a rigid whole-body fashion (en bloc) and is seemingly accomplished by "walking" rather than "pivoting." Later, postural reflexes and stability are lost, which puts patients at risk of falling and significant injuries.

3. *Bradykinesia* is a major problem manifested as difficulty in initiating movements (including bowel) and as slowed movements and thought processes (sometimes referred to as a *constipated mind*), or psychomotor slowing. Typically the family will notice the patient's lack of interest or involvement in many usual activities. (This can be confused with depression or dementia.)

4. Handwriting is slow and small with letters tightly bunched together (micrographia).

5. The basal ganglia are a center for automatic motor functions such as walking, maintenance of posture, maintenance of facial expression, clearing of saliva from the mouth, swallowing, rising from a chair, and regaining balance; many of the symptoms of Parkinson's syndrome can be explained in this context (i.e., a dysfunction of automatic motor behavior).

Treatment:

1. Treatment is directed toward relieving the symptoms of tremor and rigidity and slowing the progression of the disease. Especially in the elderly, initial doses of medication should be low and gradually increased to efficacy.

2. Patient education materials can be obtained from the United Parkinson Foundation, 833 W. Washington Blvd., Chicago, IL 60607; (312) 733-1893; or the National Parkinson Foundation, 1501 NW 9th Ave., Miami FL 33136; (305)547-6666 or (800)327-4545; website: www.parkinson.org.

3. Drug therapy (Table 7-1)
   a. General principles
      1) Begin selegiline (Eldepryl) as soon as the diagnosis is established. (A short course of carbidopa and levodopa can be necessary to establish diagnosis.)
      2) Avoid dopamine-blocking agents in a patient with Parkinson's disease.
      3) Delay administration of carbidopa and levodopa until symptoms are truly bothersome.
      4) Start drugs at a low dose and titrate slowly.
   b. Selegiline: selegiline is a monoamine oxidase-B (MAO-B) enzyme inhibitor that seems to retard Parkinson's disease, possibly by decreasing free-radical formation in neurons. The recommended *Physician's Desk Reference* dosage is 5 mg twice a day (given on awakening and at midday), but a single morning dose can be just as ef-

fective. A single 5-mg dose of selegiline inhibits MAO-B in platelets and the brain for 2 months; thus a 5-mg dose daily or weekly can be effective in slowing disease progression. Cost: 65-mg capsules, 5-mg capsules, 60 capsules $141.50.

  c. Dopamine agonists: these should be used as the initial treatment at the first symptoms of Parkinson's disease and can be the only medication needed for years. Clinical trials indicate that all of the dopamine agonists are equally efficacious. They follow:

  1) Bromocriptine mesylate (Parlodel): Start at 1.25 mg 3 times a day, increase dosage weekly until Parkinson's symptoms are tolerable or until 10 mg 3 times a day is reached. Cost: 5-mg capsules, 30 capsules $100.02.

  2) Ropinirole (ReQuip): Start at 0.25 mg 3 times a day to a maximum of 24 mg/day. Cost: 4-mg tablets, 90 tablets $169.54.

  3) Pramipexole (Mirapex): Start at 6.375 mg 3 times a day and increase to a maximum of 45 mg/day. Cost: 1.5-mg tablets, 90 tablets $176.66.

  4) Pergolide (Permax): Start at 0.05 mg every day and gradually increase to a maximum of 5 mg/day. Cost: 1-mg tablets, 90 tablets $326.57.

  d. Pergolide: pergolide is a direct dopamine receptor agonist with similar action to bromocriptine. The beginning dose is 0.05 mg 3 times a day, which can also be slowly increased.

  e. Carbidopa and levodopa (Sinemet) therapy

  1) Sinemet comes as a single tablet containing 25 mg of carbidopa and 100 mg or 250 mg of levodopa; the initial dosage is 1 tablet 3 times a day, but it can be increased to 1 tablet 5 times per day. Cost: 25- and 100-mg tablets, 90 tablets $71.58.

  2) Sinemet CR is a long-acting form of Sinemet and is supplied in tablets containing 50 mg of carbidopa and 200 mg of levodopa. The usual dosage is 1 tablet 2 or 3 times a day. Cost: 60 tablets $106.46. It can be useful in patients with advanced disease.

  3) If cost is a major factor, generic carbidopa 25 mg 3 times a day and levodopa can be prescribed separately.

  f. Adjunct medications:

  1) Anticholinergics such as benztropine mesylate (Cogentin) can be helpful in controlling the tremor. Cost: 5-mg tablets, 300 tablets $7.94. Start at a dosage of 0.5 mg/day and increase until tremor is subdued or until intolerable side effects occur.

Caution: Anticholinergic drugs can exacerbate constipation and result in urinary retention.

  2) Amantadine (Symmetrel) hydrochloride is a mild dopamine agonist. Start with a dosage of 50 mg every day and gradually increase to 100 mg twice a day. (Although capsules are available only in 100-mg size, a syrup is available that contains 10 mg/ml.) Cost: 100-mg tablets, 60 tablets $62.93.

3) Entacapone (Comtan) is a peripheral catechol *O*-methyltransferase inhibitor that "stabilizes" blood levels of L-dopa and gives smoother symptom control, especially in advanced cases. The dosage is 200 mg *per dose* of carbidopa and levodopa. Cost: $1.20 per pill.

4. Complications of drug therapy

   a. Patients with advanced Parkinson's disease respond poorly to L-dopa, because there are no longer sufficient cells in the substantia nigra to convert it to dopamine. Patients with Parkinson's syndrome respond poorly or not at all to L-dopa, because the defect is at the postsynaptic receptor or in the continuity of nigrostriatal fibers.

   b. Excess amounts of dopamine cause abnormal, excessive movements, most frequently involving the tongue (buccal-lingual dyskinesia). In this circumstance the dosage of dopaminergic agents should be reduced.

   c. Some patients, especially those receiving L-dopa for a long period of time, can have symptoms which change dramatically from hour to hour, the "on-off" phenomenon. One moment they can be virtually immobile and unable to walk, whereas the next they can be mobile but suffer from abnormal movements. The measures to combat this disabling condition include using direct dopamine receptor agonists, increasing the time at night when no dopaminergic medicines are used, and using multiple different dopaminergic agents in combination. Entacapone can also be helpful in this condition.

5. Exercise is an important part of therapy; walking or water aerobics is critical to keeping patients mobile and preventing joint contractures as the disease progresses.

ESSENTIAL TREMOR

1. Benign, familial, hereditary or senile tremor

   a. The tremor is a coarse, rhythmic, usually symmetric, movement which may be present at rest; is most noticeable in the fingers, usually beginning in hands; and may also involve the head but seldom the legs.

   b. It persists throughout the range of voluntary activity and often (like a cerebellar tremor) increases in amplitude as the limb approaches an object (finger-to-nose test, Fig. 7-1).

   c. It characteristically increases when the patient attempts to write or to bring liquids to the mouth to drink.

   d. Tremor increases markedly under stress (like a parkinsonian tremor).

   e. It often attenuates or disappears with a small amount of alcohol. This feature, if present, is almost diagnostic.

2. Onset can be in adolescence or early adult years; it is often called *senile tremor* if it develops late in life.

3. Autosomal dominant inheritance can be identified in most families.
4. Tremor increases in amplitude with age and may eventually interfere with fine movements.
5. The findings of a neurologic examination are normal except for tremor. Tremor can involve the head and neck or the voice. It is distinguished from parkinsonism by lack of rigidity and bradykinesia; it is distinguished from cerebellar lesion by lack of hypotonia and ataxia and persistence at rest.
6. Cerebellar and parkinsonian tremors rarely involve the head. Tremor similar to essential tremor can be seen in individuals with thyrotoxicosis and patients receiving lithium, epinephrine, or terbutaline sulfate. Fatigue and anxiety can cause a similar fine rapid tremor.

Treatment:

1. Reassurance is often all that is necessary. If the tremor interferes with social adjustment or activities of daily living, drug treatment may be necessary.
2. Propranolol (Inderal) hydrochloride is often effective. The long-acting form at an initial dose of 80 mg is convenient and more effective than the generic drug. Cost: 8-mg capsules, 60 capsules $68.51.
3. Some patients respond to primidone (Mysoline). The initial dose should be 50 mg at bedtime, and this is increased by 50 mg weekly until the tremor is controlled.

Caution: Primidone can occasionally cause nausea, vomiting, drowsiness, and ataxia even in small doses.

4. Gabapentin (Neurontin) 400 mg per day, titrating up to as much as 3600 mg/day, can help. Cost: 90 capsules $113.18.
5. Topiramate (Topamax) 25 mg/day, titrated up to 100 mg twice a day as needed, can also help. Cost: 25-mg tablets, 60 tablets $71.01.
6. Alcohol is often the most effective agent, but it is not recommended for chronic use. In fact, chronic alcoholism can occur in patients with essential tremor who attempt this form of treatment. Wine with dinner or about 20 minutes before a stressful event occasionally can be used for elderly patients with symptomatic senile tremor.

CEREBELLAR TREMOR

1. Cerebellar tremor is noted only during movement. It can be unilateral or bilateral and indicates disease of the cerebellar hemisphere.
2. In the finger-to-nose test, tremor increases as the finger reaches the target and is less noticeable between targets (Fig. 7-3).
3. Other signs of cerebellar hemispheric disease include the following:
   a. Ipsilateral (same side) difficulty with rapid alternating movements occurs. (Have patient rapidly alternate pronation and supination of hand against thigh or other hand.)
   b. Hypotonia manifested as a limp "rag doll" arm with passive motion and as a pendular patellar reflex (Fig. 7-1) occurs. Hypotonia can also be manifested by hyperextension of the fingers (Fig. 7-5).

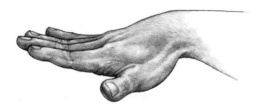

FIG. 7-5 "Spooning" of the hands is occasionally seen in cerebellar disease. Hyperextension of fingers in this manner can also exacerbate an essential tremor.

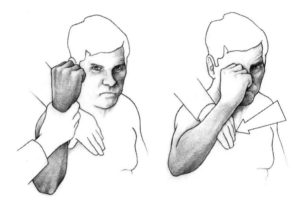

FIG. 7-6 Testing for rebound. Request that the patient pull against resistance, then suddenly release the arm without warning. **CAUTION:** If not protected by the examiner's arm, the patient with cerebellar disease will strike himself.

c. Rebound is commonly elicited by having the patient flex his or her arm against resistance from the examiner and then having the examiner suddenly let go of the arm; normally the arm remains relatively stationary, but with cerebellar disease, the arm will tend to rebound and strike the patient in the face.

Caution: The examiner must place his or her arm or hand so as to guard the patient's face (Fig. 7-6).

d. Occasionally, speech abnormalities occur, which consist of loss of normal speech melody. Speech tends to have an explosive quality (ataxic dysarthria or scanning speech). This can be demonstrated by having the patient vocalize a sustained "ah," which will have markedly variable volume and pitch.

Note: Disease of midline cerebellar structures can cause difficulty only in tandem walking (gait ataxia) with no abnormalities of finger-to-nose testing and no tremor or other signs of cerebellar hemisphere disease. This is commonly seen in chronic alcoholism, as a remote effect of carcinoma, or with phenytoin or carbamazepine intoxication. In children, medulloblastoma or a midline cerebellar tumor can cause similar abnormalities.

Treatment: Therapy must be directed at the underlying cerebellar disorder. Lesions of the cerebellum, including cerebellar atrophy, are best demonstrated by magnetic resonance imaging (MRI). Cerebellar tremor is commonly seen in patients with multiple sclerosis (MS) or brainstem strokes.

HUNTINGTON'S DISEASE (HUNTINGTON'S CHOREA)

▶ 1. Huntington's disease is a dominantly inherited disorder with abnormal involuntary movements, psychiatric disorders, and progressive dementia, with symptomatic onset usually after 30 years of age.
  2. The initial symptoms include clumsiness of movement, slowness of finger movements, and a tendency to drop objects. Abnormal movements, at first, can be converted to seemingly purposeful movements to conceal the abnormality.
  3. The abnormal movements are irregular rapid, jerky movements of the fingers and wrists associated with slower dystonic movements of the upper limbs.
  4. The gait is unsteady with a tendency to bob and weave.
  5. Facial grimacing with involuntary movements of the tongue are common; this produces a dysarthria.
  6. The abnormal movements can be exaggerated by sustained activity such as clenching a fist (milkmaid grip) or protruding the tongue (darting tongue).
  7. Patients can have subtle signs of intellectual deterioration, personality changes, or frank psychosis (depression and suicide attempts are frequent), with the movement disorder not being evident until many years later.
  8. The patient's family history is a very important diagnostic clue but can be exceptionally difficult to elicit; the family history can include mental deficiency, alcoholism, suicide, psychosis, and behavior disorders.

Treatment:
  1. There is no cure for Huntington's disease; genetic counseling is necessary. The genetic locus of this disease has been identified on the short arm of chromosome 4 as an expansion of CAG triplet repeat region as-

sociated with the huntingtin gene. Both in utero and presymptomatic diagnoses are available, but their use is controversial.

2. For improvement of the abnormal movements or treatment of the associated psychoses, the following can be used:

a. Haloperidol: 3 to 6 mg/day can initially be effective for the movement disorder and for behavior control. Cost: 0.5-mg tablets, 90 tablets $43.90.

b. Phenothiazines such as chlorpromazine (up to 150 mg/day), perphenazine (Trilafon) (10 to 16 mg 3 times a day), or trifluoperazine (Stelazine) hydrochloride (2 mg twice a day) are alternative treatments. Cost: thioridazine (Mellaril) 10-mg tablets, 90 tablets $37.78.

c. Olanzapine (Zyprexa) 5 mg every day and quetiapine (Seroquel) 100 mg twice a day have fewer extrapyramidal side effects but are expensive. Cost: 5-mg tablets, 30 tablets $162.63.

3. If serious depression is present, suicide precautions need to be taken.

4. Educational materials for patients and information about local support groups can be obtained from Huntington's Disease Society of America, 158 W. 29th St., 7th floor, New York, NY 10001; (212)242-1968 or (800)345-HDSA; website: www.hdsa.org.

SYDENHAM'S CHOREA

1. Sydenham's chorea (infectious or rheumatic) begins as an apparent restlessness, clumsiness, and behavior disorder characterized by involuntary movements, incoordination, and weakness in children and adolescents (more common in female patients) 5 to 15 years of age. It is often associated with rheumatic fever and a β-hemolytic streptococcal infection, which can precede the onset of chorea by days to months and is important to recognize because Sydenham's chorea has the same cardiac implications as rheumatic fever.

2. Choreic movements are nonrepetitive, abrupt, jerky, and purposeless; they are present at rest and accentuated by posturing; they are usually seen in the face and hands; and they can involve only one side of the body (hemichorea).

3. Facial grimacing, dysarthria, and explosive speech are common.

4. When asked to sustain a grip on the examiner's fingers, the patient will exhibit a "milking grip"; the patient cannot maintain a protruded tongue (darting tongue).

5. There may be decreased resistance to passive movements; reflexes can be hypoactive, delayed, or pendular.

6. The duration is usually 4 to 6 weeks; complete recovery is usual, but residua can be evident.

7. The patient may have an elevated erythrocyte sedimentation rate (ESR). Serum calcium and phosphorous levels should be obtained to rule out hypocalcemia. Electrocardiographic (ECG) changes or other features consistent with the Jones criteria for rheumatic fever should be sought, including throat culture for β-hemolytic streptococcal infection and serum antistreptolysin O (ASO) titers.

8. Some patients display mainly obsessive-compulsive symptoms and restlessness with little or no history of chorea. This variant form is termed *pediatric autoimmune neuropsychiatric disorders associated with streptococcal infections (PANDAS).*

Treatment:

1. Recommend bed rest in a tranquil environment.
2. Give haloperidol at an initial dose of 0.5 mg and gradually increase the dosage until movements are controlled. When movements are controlled for 3 to 4 weeks, slowly discontinue the medication.
3. Treat streptococcal infections with the appropriate antibiotics.
4. Prevent rheumatic complications (and recurrent choreic episodes) using *lifelong* prophylactic antibiotics. (Additional antibiotics can be necessary in situations in which there may be bacteremia [e.g., dental work].) Penicillin G benzathine is the recommended drug at the following dosages:

Age	Penicillin G dosage (units/month)
<6	600,000
6-12	900,000
>12	1,200,000

5. Frequent examinations are necessary to detect early signs of cardiac involvement.

CHOREA GRAVIDARUM

▶ 1. Chorea gravidarum occurs in approximately 1 in every 2000 to 3000 pregnancies. It occurs more commonly in first pregnancies and can recur in subsequent pregnancies. The cause is unknown, but it is often preceded by thyrotoxic chorea or Sydenham's chorea.
2. The average duration of chorea gravidarum is 1 to 2 months; it usually subsides spontaneously during pregnancy or shortly after delivery.

Treatment: Termination of pregnancy is rarely required. If the chorea is incapacitating, sedatives or neuroleptics can be used to control the movements, but use of such medications may pose a risk to the fetus.

SPASMUS NUTANS

1. Spasmus nutans is a rhythmic nodding or rotatory tremor of the head associated with pendular nystagmus.
2. It occurs in infants between 4 and 18 months of age.
3. It must be differentiated from the head tremor associated with congenital nystagmus (which is due to reduced visual acuity).
4. The tremor disappears when the infant is lying down.

Treatment: This disorder is rare but is important to recognize because it is self-limited and disappears by 2 years of age. Further workup is not necessary. The parents need reassurance.

KERNICTERUS

▶ 1. A jaundiced newborn at 2 or 3 days of age can show symptoms such as listlessness, poor sucking, fever, hypotonia, and weak cry and have Moro's and deep tendon reflexes that are difficult to elicit. Permanent symptoms appear after 18 months of age and can include choreoathetosis, dystonia, rigidity, tremor, upward gaze paralysis, mental retardation, spasticity, and hearing impairment.
2. Kernicterus is related to the combination of hyperbilirubinemia and cerebral ischemia/hypoxia in the newborn with resultant deposition of unconjugated bilirubin in the brain (primarily in the basal ganglia). This form of "cerebral palsy" is now rare because most infants are effectively treated early for hyperbilirubinemia, and good prenatal care prevents most causes of perinatal hypoxia.

Treatment: Attempt to prevent kernicterus by vigorously treating newborn hyperbilirubinemia using techniques such as phototherapy and exchange transfusion.

GILLES de la TOURETTE'S SYNDROME

▶ 1. Tourette's syndrome is characterized by motor and vocal tics with an onset usually between 6 and 15 years of age; it is more common in boys. Childhood hyperactivity can precede the onset of tics.
2. The initial symptoms include eye blinks, facial tics, and facial grimaces followed (in months and years) by sudden involuntary movements of the head, neck, shoulders, trunk, or legs. These movements can be repeated several times a minute and become worse with stress.
3. Frequently, movements are accompanied by phonic (vocal, respiratory) tics, which initially are grunts, snorts, or yells but eventually can develop into repeated obscenities yelled in a loud voice with no provocation (coprolalia). Phonic tics are a hallmark of the disease.
4. The character of the abnormal movements can change over the years.

Treatment:
1. Patients seem to be able to gain some voluntary control of the tics, but must, from time to time, "let it out." It should be emphasized that this is purely a social disability and has not prevented many patients with this disease from leading productive lives.
2. A dopamine receptor blocking drug, pimozide (Orap), has been found to be effective in suppressing the phonic and motor tics. The initial dosage is 1 to 2 mg/day, which can be gradually increased to achieve a maintenance dosage of less than 0.2 mg/kg/day.

Caution: An ECG study should be done periodically, since the drug prolongs the QT interval. Cost: 1-mg tablets, 60 tablets $39.87.

3. Haloperidol, at a recommended dosage of 0.25 to 10 mg daily, can result in improvement. Careful dose adjustment is important for long-term therapy. Cost: 0.5-mg tablets, 90 tablets $120.29.

Caution: Long-term use of a neuroleptic such as haloperidol can result in tardive dyskinesia.

4. Atypical neuroleptics such as risperidone and quetiapine can be effective for long-term therapy.
5. Educational material for patients and information about local support groups can be obtained from the Tourette Syndrome Association, Inc., 42-40 Bell Blvd., Bayside, NY 11361; (718)224-2999 or (800)237-0717; website: www.TSA-USA.org.

HEMIBALLISMUS

▶ 1. Hemiballismus is a rare disorder characterized by a sudden onset of violent involuntary movement (unilaterally and contralateral to the lesion), mainly of the arm; the appearance is similar to that of a baseball pitcher's windup.
2. Movement is worsened by stress.
3. It is caused by a lesion of the subthalamic nucleus, usually as a result of hemorrhage or infarction. The patient frequently suffers from chronic hypertension.

Treatment:
1. There is usually spontaneous recovery.
2. For long-term control of movement, oral diazepam alone or diazepam supplemented with reserpine or haloperidol has been used with variable success.

Caution: This disorder should not be confused with focal motor seizures (see Chapter 11).

MYOCLONUS

Myoclonus resembles the muscular twitching seen in dogs and cats as they drop off to sleep. Causes of myoclonus include central nervous system (CNS) degenerative disorders, benign hereditary myoclonus, cerebral anoxia, and metabolic disorders. The movement is indicative of a CNS disorder but has poor localizing value. For severe persistent myoclonus, pharmacotherapy (such as with clonazepam [Klonopin] or valproic acid) can be helpful. Cost: clonazepam 0.5-mg tablets, 30 tablets $24.06. Myoclonus should be differentiated from myoclonic seizures, which can also improve with these medications.

Caution: A demented patient with myoclonus can have Creutzfeldt-Jakob disease (see Chapter 6). The brains of such patients harbor an infectious prion.

ASTERIXIS

▶ 1. Asterixis is a movement disorder elicited primarily when the patient extends the arm forward with the wrist also extended. Irregular sudden flexion at the wrist (from gravitational pull) is followed by extension of the wrist back to the original position (Fig. 7-7). This movement has also been called *negative myoclonus*.
2. Although originally described in hepatic disease ("liver flap"), it occurs in patients with a wide variety of metabolic disorders (such as renal failure, pulmonary insufficiency, and malabsorption syndromes).

Treatment: Treatment of the underlying metabolic disorder is indicated.

DYSTONIA

Dystonia is a sustained abnormal posture. It can be generalized or focal. Focal dystonias are characteristically task specific and occur only when a particular task is performed (e.g., writing in writer's cramp). Co-contraction of agonist and antagonist muscles results in the abnormal movement. The most common form is spasmodic torticollis with persistent contraction of the neck muscles. Patients can also have sustained closure of the eyes (blepharospasm) or abnormal vocal cord movement during speech (spasmodic dysphonia). Medical treatment for dystonia is often ineffective, but chemodenervation using botulinum toxin A (Botox) or botulinum toxin B injected into an affected muscle can give relief that lasts several months. This should be done by an experienced practitioner. Electromyographic (EMG) guidance is often needed. Causes of dystonia include cerebral anoxia, birth injury, head trauma, or the rare syndromes of dystonia musculorum deformans and hepatolenticular degeneration (Wilson's disease).

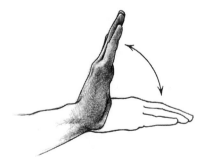

FIG. 7-7 Asterixis. The patient is unable to maintain wrist extension; intermittently there is a sudden loss of tone, causing the hand to flap in a "bye-bye" gesture.

MOVEMENT DISORDERS ASSOCIATED WITH NEUROLEPTICS

Acute Parkinsonism. The symptoms of acute parkinsonism often are dramatically relieved with diphenhydramine (Benadryl) hydrochloride 50 mg IV.

Tardive dyskinesias.

1. Tardive dyskinesias develop in a significant number of patients receiving long-term treatment with neuroleptic drugs (especially the more potent phenothiazines or haloperidol).
2. Symptoms include an oral-buccal-lingual stereotypy involving tongue protrusion, lip smacking, and facial grimacing. Abnormal movements of limbs and trunk can be seen.

Treatment:

1. In many patients, tardive dyskinesias remain refractory to all forms of treatment.
2. The new antipsychotic medications (e.g., olanzipine 5 to 20 mg/day) have fewer extrapyramidal side effects. Cost: 5-mg tablets, 30 tablets $162.63.
3. The best treatment is preventive (i.e., prescribing neuroleptics only for serious psychiatric disorders and monitoring patients carefully for the side effects). *Do not* prescribe for behavioral control in nursing homes or in patients with Parkinson's disease.

Akathisia. Akathisia is a *reversible* motor restlessness that is often confused with psychotic agitation. It is seen acutely with treatment with neuroleptics and with some antihistamines or as part of the tardive dyskinesia syndrome.

OTHER MEDICATIONS ASSOCIATED WITH MOVEMENT DISORDERS

1. CNS stimulants (amphetamine or methylphenidate) can produce tics.
2. Antihistamines, oral contraceptives (similar to chorea gravidarum of natural pregnancy), anticonvulsants, and chloroquine (Aralen) occasionally produce involuntary choreoathetosis, dystonia, or myoclonus.
3. The meperidine analogue (1-methyl-4-phenyl-1,2,3,6-tetrahydropyridine) MPTP, an illicit "designer" drug, damages the substantia nigra and produces parkinsonism.

BIBLIOGRAPHY

Bagheri MM, Kerbeshian J, Burd L: Recognition and management of Tourette's syndrome and tic disorders, *Am Fam Physician* 59(8):2263-2272, 2274, 1999.

Bain PG: Tremor assessment and quality of life measurements, *Neurology* 54(11 Suppl 4):S26-S29, 2000.

Conley SC, Kirchner JT: Medical and surgical treatment of Parkinson's disease: strategies to slow symptom progression and improve quality of life, *Postgrad Med* 106(2):41-44, 1999.

Findley LJ: Epidemiology and genetics of essential tremor, *Neurology* 54(11 Suppl 4):S8-S13, 2000.

Jankovic J, Brin MF: Therapeutic uses of botulinum toxin, *N Engl J Med* 324:1186-1194, 1991.

Louis ED, Ford B, Barnes LF: Clinical subtypes of essential tremor, *Arch Neurol* 57(8):1194-1198, 2000.

Mendis T, Suchowersky O, Lang A, Gauthier S: Management of Parkinson's disease: a review of current and new therapies, *Can J Neurol Sci* 26(2):89-103, 1999.

Pahwa R, Lyons K, Koller WC: Surgical treatment of essential tremor, *Neurology* 54(11 Suppl 4):S39-S44, 2000.

Quinn N, Schrag A: Huntington's disease and other choreas, *J Neurol* 245(11):709-716, 1998.

Robertson MM: Tourette syndrome, associated conditions and the complexities of treatment, *Brain* 123 (Pt 3):425-462, 2000.

Robertson MM, Stern JS: Tic disorders: new developments in Tourette syndrome and related disorders, *Curr Opin Neurol* 11(4):373-380, 1998.

Stocchi F, Brusa L: Cognition and emotion in different stages and subtypes of Parkinson's disease, *J Neurol* 247(Suppl 2:III):14-21, 2000.

8

Neurologic
Complications of
Alcoholism

In the United States, alcohol abuse accounts for a substantial percentage of hospital admissions, highway deaths, and psychiatric disturbances, yet alcoholic beverages are readily available and accepted by many Americans as a routine adjunct to social interaction. Identifying all pathologic users is one of the most common and difficult challenges facing the physician.

DIAGNOSING ALCOHOL ABUSE

1. Table 8-1 may be used as a basis for the patient interview. Positive responses in several categories make it likely that the patient is alcohol dependent.
2. The CAGE questionnaire has proved to be a specific and sensitive tool in the diagnosis of alcoholism. The acronym comes from *c*utting down, *a*nnoyance by criticism, *g*uilty feelings, and *e*ye openers. The questionnaire consists of the following four questions, put in conversational terms:
   a. Ever felt the need to cut down drinking?
   b. Ever felt annoyed by criticism of drinking?
   c. Ever had guilty feelings about drinking?
   d. Ever take morning eye openers?

Positive answers to two or more of these four questions correlates highly with alcoholism.

3. The diagnosis of alcoholism is associated with social stigmata. Patients from lower socioeconomic classes more often (unfairly) have the diagnosis on their medical charts than do more affluent patients from higher socioeconomic classes. A clear medical diagnosis of alcoholism may be a powerful incentive to reform.
4. Many alcoholics are extremely skillful (consciously or subconsciously) in camouflaging their addiction.

TABLE 8-1
Suggested Questions for Establishing the Diagnosis of Alcohol Dependence

Symptoms	Questions
Preoccupation	What are the occasions on which you have had a drink this past week (month)?
	When do you think about drinking?
	When during the day do you sometimes feel you need a drink?
	How often during the past week (month) did you crave a drink in the morning?
Increased tolerance	How often during the past week (month) have you been able to drink more than others and not show it?
	Has anyone ever commented on your ability to "hold your liquor?"
	Why do you think you are able to do this?
	How does this make you feel?
Gulping drinks	What strength drinks do you prefer?
	How long does it take you to finish your first drink?
	How many drinks do you usually have before going out to dinner or a party?
Drinking alone	When in the past week (month) did you have a drink alone?
	Where were you when you had a drink alone? (At home? In a bar?)
Use as a medicine	What are some of the reasons you drink? (Calm nerves? Reduce tension? As a nightcap to get to sleep? Relieve physical discomfort? Relieve feelings of inadequacy or depression?)
	Do you enjoy parties or events if there is nothing to drink?
Blackout	When during the past week (month) have you been unable to remember what happened the night before?
	When during the past week (month) have you been unable to remember how you got home after a night of drinking?
Physical	What reasons have doctors given for you to cut down or stop drinking?
	Where have you been hospitalized for drinking or a complication from drinking?
Social	How many of your friends drink?
	How has your group of friends changed since you began drinking?
	How have your hobbies and interests changed since you began drinking?

Continued

TABLE 8-1
**Suggested Questions for Establishing the Diagnosis
of Alcohol Dependence—cont'd**

Symptoms	Questions
	How often in the past week (month) have you been ashamed of what you did while you were drinking?
	What kind of things have you done that you were ashamed of while you were drinking?
	How do you act while you are drinking?
Family	Is there anyone in your family who is or was an alcoholic?

5. Any patient with a physical disability secondary to alcohol (peripheral neuropathy, cirrhosis, dementia, cerebellar degeneration) *is* an alcoholic.
6. Any patient with withdrawal symptoms from alcohol abstinence *is* an alcoholic.
7. The quantity of alcohol consumed does not necessarily define an alcoholic; body weight, nutrition, ethnic background, medical condition, and medical therapy all influence a patient's sensitivity to the acute and chronic effects of alcohol.
8. In making a diagnosis of alcoholism, the physician must make every effort to be *objective;* the alcoholic physician makes the diagnosis too seldom, and the teetotaler makes it too often.

Clinical Clues to Alcohol Abuse

1. **Physical Examination:** On the general physical examination the following signs may indicate a diagnosis of alcoholism:
   a. Excessive sweating, tachycardia, or flushed face (withdrawal syndrome)
   b. Bruises, cigarette burns, or other trauma often incurred with severe drunkenness
   c. Signs of liver disease such as palmar erythema, vascular spiders, or jaundice
   d. Neurologic abnormalities such as coarse hand tremor, peripheral neuropathy, forgetfulness or emotional lability
   e. Poor hygiene, dehydration, or poor nutrition
   f. Persistent or recurrent infections
   g. Odor of alcohol on breath at the time of examination
2. **Laboratory Findings:** On the laboratory profile the following abnormalities may indicate a diagnosis of alcoholism:
   a. A blood alcohol level of 150 mg/dl in a rational patient, which strongly suggests tolerance to alcohol, implying heavy and persistent alcohol ingestion
   b. Blood count showing a mean corpuscular volume (MCV) greater than 97 μL with round macrocytosis
   c. Elevated serum uric acid levels without history of gout

d. Elevation of serum alanine aminotransferase (glutamate pyruvate transaminase or GPT), serum aspartate aminotransferase (glutamic-oxaloacetic transaminase or GOT), and γ-glutamyltransferase (GGT or γ-glutamyl transpeptidase)

Stupor and Coma in Alcoholic Intoxication

A diagnosis of stupor or coma should be made *only* with a blood alcohol level greater than 300 mg/dl and *without* other causes for coma. *Most* comatose patients with an odor of alcohol on their breath will have some other cause for coma, such as diabetic ketoacidosis or another drug. Subdural hematoma, particularly bilateral subdural hematomas without localizing signs, must be suspected or ruled out in all cases of stupor or coma in an alcoholic.

Treatment:

1. Look for some other cause of coma and treat that cause appropriately.
2. Use the following immediate measures for the treatment of any coma: ensure clear airway; treat shock; check blood glucose levels; and administer thiamine 100 mg intravenously (IV), then glucose 1 amp IV, and then naloxone (Narcan) 0.4 mg IV every 2 to 3 minutes (see Chapter 13).
3. Gastric lavage is unnecessary; the bladder should be emptied and drainage instituted.
4. Check vital signs frequently; mechanical ventilation may be necessary.
5. In addition to blood levels for blood alcohol, obtain blood levels for other sedative drugs.

Alcoholic Blackouts

Alcoholic patients with blackouts may be suffering from seizures or may be having *simple alcoholic blackouts.*

1. Alcoholic blackouts are periods of amnesia during which the patient apparently functions normally but later has no recall for that period; they are related to the acute effect of alcohol.
2. Blackouts are not necessarily correlated with blood alcohol level.
3. They are usually of short duration.
4. Blackouts often are an early neurologic symptom of potential alcoholism.
5. They may rarely occur paradoxically in the nonalcoholic individual who consumes a large quantity of alcohol.
6. A related phenomenon is pathologic intoxication in which relatively small amounts of alcohol produce irrational and combative behavior for which the patient may later be amnesic.

Alcohol Withdrawal Syndrome

Chronic consumption of alcohol results in physical dependence. The following are at least four withdrawal syndromes:

1. Tremulousness
2. Alcoholic hallucinosis
3. Withdrawal seizures
4. Delirium tremens

Withdrawal symptoms (listed separately here but often occurring in various combinations) usually begin at any time, during which there is a falling blood alcohol level, and may occur as late as 7 days after cessation of alcohol intake. Prolonged or late withdrawal syndromes may occur in patients who abuse other drugs along with alcohol or in patients who are receiving tranquilizers or sedatives in a treatment program. The severity of the syndrome is affected by a variety of factors, including associated illness, other drug use or abuse, and environmental factors, as well as the amount of alcohol consumed and the duration of alcohol abuse.

In all of the withdrawal syndromes, treatment with atenolol is recommended in addition to the other therapy. The maximum dosage is atenolol 100 mg/day, with no drug given if the heart rate is less than 50 beats/min and 50 mg given when the heart rate is 50 to 70 beats/min. This regimen significantly reduces the duration of the withdrawal syndrome.

1. **Tremulousness**
   a. The "shakes" or "jitters" often occur the morning after a few days of excessive alcohol consumption and are frequently responsible for early morning alcohol consumption to relieve symptoms.
   b. Tremulousness is associated with general irritability and gastrointestinal (GI) problems (especially nausea and vomiting). There may also be overalertness, flushed facies, tachycardia, anorexia, or insomnia.
   c. A tendency to startle, uneasiness, jerkiness of movement, and insomnia may persist for as long as 2 weeks.

Treatment: In severe reactions benzodiazepines (such as lorazepam [Ativan] 1 to 2 mg by mouth every 2 hours as needed or diazepam [Valium] 5 to 10 mg by mouth every 2 hours as needed) may be instituted and can be withdrawn over several days.

2. **Alcoholic hallucinosis**
   a. The patient complains of terrifying hallucinations with no disorientation. Generally these are auditory hallucinations, lasting a brief time. Visual hallucinations are less common.
   b. Alcoholic hallucinosis may be related to rapid eye movement (REM) sleep rebound, since alcohol is known to suppress REM sleep.

Treatment:
1. Hospitalization is usually necessary; if the patient is not hospitalized, close supervision is necessary.
2. Lorazepam 1 to 2 mg by mouth every 2 hours as needed or diazepam 5 to 10 mg by mouth every 2 hours as needed may be used for sedation. An alternative drug is chlordiazepoxide (Librium) 50 to 100 mg by mouth every 4 hours as needed.
3. Institute a high-protein diet supplemented with multiple-vitamin therapy, including thiamine 50 mg by mouth twice a day. If the patient is hospitalized, use IV thiamine at 100 mg for 5 days.
4. Make every attempt to keep the patient oriented to reality by having a sympathetic individual present who can reassure the patient that the hallucinations are not real.
5. Occasionally, patients with alcoholic hallucinosis may enter a chronic stage of hallucinosis after the clearing of the alcohol-withdrawal process. Such a condition may require neuroleptic treatment.

6. During the phase of acute and remitting alcoholic hallucinosis, the patient may need treatment with a neuroleptic, which can be discontinued after remission of symptoms and a successful withdrawal regimen.

3. Withdrawal seizures

a. Withdrawal seizures ("rum fits") are characteristically brief, generalized convulsions with loss of consciousness.

b. They may be preceded by an aura of "fear" (anticipation of doom).

c. About one third of patients with alcohol-withdrawal seizures develop delirium tremens.

d. In patients with preexisting epilepsy, alcohol withdrawal may increase the frequency and intensity of seizures.

e. Alcoholics frequently have cortical scars from repeated head trauma, and these scars may trigger seizures during alcohol withdrawal.

Treatment:

1. Anticonvulsant medication is usually *not* necessary, since seizures cease before medication becomes effective; lorazepam 1 to 2 mg IV every 2 hours or diazepam 5 to 10 mg by mouth every 2 hours as needed for the treatment of other associated withdrawal symptoms may be preventive.

2. Rarely, a rum fit may result in status epilepticus, which should be handled as described in Chapter 11.

3. An alcoholic with epilepsy who continues to consume alcoholic beverages is a challenge to treat, since compliance is usually poor. If compelled to use long-term anticonvulsants because of frequent seizures, make phenytoin (Dilantin) your drug of choice. Phenobarbital should not be used, since abrupt withdrawal may cause seizures even in patients who are not epileptic.

4. Delirium tremens

a. Delirium tremens is characterized by profound confusion, delusions, extremely vivid visual hallucinations, tremor, agitation, and insomnia, as well as signs of increased autonomic nervous system activation (i.e., fever, tachycardia, and profuse sweating).

b. The patient is suspicious, restless, very disoriented, and difficult to distract; he or she carries on imaginary conversations or activities and may shout for hours or mutter inaudibly.

c. The peak incidence is between 72 and 96 hours after the cessation of alcohol consumption.

Treatment:

1. *This is a medical emergency, since the mortality rate may reach 15% in the untreated state.*

2. Maintenance of fluid and electrolyte balance is the most important consideration.

3. Treat with benzodiazepines, such as lorazepam 2 to 4 mg IV every 2 to 4 hours, chlordiazepoxide 50 to 100 mg IV every 6 hours as needed, or diazepam 5 to 20 mg by mouth every 2 hours as needed or diazepam 10 mg IV immediately and then 5 mg IV every 15 minutes until the patient is quiet but not asleep.

4. Carefully record all intake and output.

5. Administration of large quantities of IV fluids is necessary. Usually 6 L of IV fluids are required per day:
   a. IV thiamine 100 mg should be administered immediately.
   b. Glucose (at least 5%) must be included in each IV solution.
   c. Thiamine 100 mg must be included in each liter of IV solution.
   d. A therapeutic multivitamin preparation must be included in the first IV solution.
   e. Potassium, sodium, calcium, and magnesium must be added to the IV solutions based on the patient's laboratory determinations.
6. Restraints are almost always necessary, but a patient adequately sedated with benzodiazepines may need less restraint.
7. Search for associated injury or infection (especially cerebral laceration, subdural hematoma, pneumonia, and meningitis).
8. Seizures require treatment *if* they are repeated, prolonged, continuous, or life threatening. Anticonvulsants need not be continued past the withdrawal period, unless there is a preexisting seizure disorder.
9. Pancreatitis, cirrhosis, and renal disease frequently complicate the course of delirium tremens.

Caution: The symptoms of delirium tremens resemble those of carbon dioxide (CO_2) narcosis, which may occur in patients with delirium tremens who also have chronic obstructive pulmonary disease and have been given sedatives that can depress respirations.

NUTRITIONAL DISEASES SECONDARY TO ALCOHOLISM
Wernicke-Korsakoff Syndrome
This is an acute, subacute, or chronic disease of central nervous system (CNS) injury related to thiamine deficiency.
1. *Wernicke's syndrome* is the *acute* disorder, and is characterized by the following:
   a. An acute confusional state that may be associated with nystagmus associated with ataxia. The degree of mental status changes may vary from mild confusion to a comatose state.
   b. The confusional state is followed by paralysis of the extraocular muscles in any combination. *This is a neurologic emergency* and should be treated *immediately* with thiamine 100 mg IV followed by daily IV thiamine for 5 days. Prompt treatment will reverse the neurologic deficit. Oral administration of thiamine may be ineffective if the patient's GI absorption is compromised.
2. *Korsakoff's psychosis* results if Wernicke's syndrome is not treated.
   a. The outstanding feature of the mental disturbance is the inability to form new memories despite relatively intact immediate recall and relatively preserved remote memory. In effect, it is as though the patient's intellectual life was arrested at the moment of the onset of the pathologic condition.
   b. In conversation, the patient may discuss situations or give answers that sound very plausible but have little basis in reality (part

of the mental aberration known as *confabulation*). For example, when asked what was served for breakfast, the patient will describe a sumptuous feast when in reality there was no meal that day.

Treatment: Thiamine 50 mg twice a day should be administered to patients with Korsakoff's psychosis even though the disease is generally considered irreversible.

Peripheral Neuropathy Associated with Alcohol

1. Peripheral neuropathy is usually the earliest neurologic symptom of chronic alcoholism.
2. The disorder is secondary to nutritional deficiencies rather than the direct toxic effect of alcohol.
3. It is primarily a sensory neuropathy, with the patient complaining of burning or painful feet (see Chapter 15).
4. Very hypoactive or absent ankle reflexes are usually evident on examination before the patient notes any symptoms and should alert the physician to the diagnosis of alcoholism. Evidence of summation on sensory examination (see Chapter 1) as well as subjective symptoms of sensory loss is apparent later.
5. The patient's feet may have thin, atrophic skin devoid of hair.
6. Peripheral neuropathy is often seen in association with the Wernicke-Korsakoff syndrome.

Treatment: The disorder may respond to thiamine 50 mg twice a day, as well as abstinence from alcohol.

Alcoholic Dementia

1. Cerebral atrophy by a computed tomographic (CT) scan or magnetic resonance imaging (MRI) and deterioration of intellectual function are well documented in chronic alcoholics.
2. Alcohol abuse is one of the common causes of dementia. Fortunately *substantial recovery* of function may occur if the patient ceases alcohol consumption.

Alcoholic Cerebellar Degeneration

1. Alcoholic cerebellar degeneration is characterized primarily by truncal ataxia and difficulty in tandem walking, with lesser degrees of abnormality seen on finger-to-nose testing (see Chapter 7).
2. Subacute onset occurs over several weeks or months.
3. Its pathologic finding is degeneration of midline cerebellar structures.
4. It is not clearly related to thiamine deficiency.

Treatment: Abstinence from alcohol and oral thiamine 50 mg twice a day supplementation are recommended but are of no clear benefit.

Alcoholic Myopathy

1. The chronic form of alcoholic myopathy includes proximal muscle wasting and weakness. The creatine phosphokinase (CPK) level is mildly elevated, and muscle biopsy shows type II muscle fiber atrophy, necrosis, and other anatomic abnormalities.

2. The acute form has severe weakness, myoglobinuria, and rhabdomyolysis. This constitutes a medical emergency and should be treated with vigorous diuresis to prevent renal failure from the myoglobinuria; in addition, serum potassium levels must be closely monitored to prevent hyperkalemia.

Treatment: Alcoholic myopathy is potentially reversible if the patient abstains from alcohol.

Neurologic Disorders Caused by Liver Dysfunction

There are two syndromes of hepatic encephalopathy:

1. *Acute hepatic encephalopathy:* acute hepatic encephalopathy is a progressive state of altered consciousness, ataxia, dysarthria, asterixis, lethargy, and finally, coma. During this progression, characteristic electroencephalographic (EEG) abnormalities can be detected. This syndrome is reversible with appropriate treatment of the liver disease. The degree of coma does not necessarily correlate with the degree of hyperammonemia.
2. *Chronic hepatic encephalopathy:* after repeated episodes of hepatic coma with recovery, a chronic progressive dementia develops.

Treatment: Treatment should be directed at the underlying liver disease.

Chronic Alcoholism

The treatment of alcohol abuse (chronic alcoholism) has the goals of sobriety and amelioration of the psychologic problem underlying the abuse. The "cure" rate is dismal, and as a general rule, only those who want to stop will. A sign in the primary care waiting room stating, "If you think you consume too much alcoholic beverage, please discuss with me," will often open the door to those who are motivated. A discussion of the adverse effects of alcohol on health may then have a positive effect. At-risk drinking for men is greater than 14 drinks a week or 4 per occasion and for women, it is approximately half that. Sadly, many physicians treat only the complications of alcoholism, not the disease itself.

1. Alcoholics Anonymous (AA), a worldwide informal fellowship of recovering alcoholics, has been shown to be the most effective therapy for alcoholics. AA's philosophy is embodied in a series of steps to guide the alcoholic to recovery. There are also associated groups for the spouses of alcoholics (Al-Anon) and for teenage children (Al-Ateen). It is generally agreed that alcoholics should be encouraged to attend AA meetings on a regular basis. Each physician should identify a local resource person in AA to contact should the need arise. AA information may also be obtained from the general service office of Alcoholics Anonymous, Grand Central Station, PO Box 459, New York, NY 10163; (212)870-3400; website: www.aa.org.
2. Some alcoholics may need supportive individual therapy. For others, group and family therapy may be most effective. It is very important to encourage family support and employment when appropriate and realistic. When a mental disorder is associated with alcoholism, the

most likely condition is an affective disorder, either bipolar or unipolar depression: referral to a psychiatrist is necessary.

If there is lack of social support or if it is deemed necessary by a psychiatrist, live-in programs, such as halfway houses, may be appropriate. The physician must be aware of the current facilities available in the community, such as programs administered by local mental health centers and other local agencies.

3. A source of information on alcohol for both physicians and patients is the National Clearinghouse for Alcohol, PO Box 2345, Rockville, MD 20852; (301)468-2600.

BIBLIOGRAPHY

Burge SK, Schneider FD: Alcohol-related problems: recognition and intervention, *Am Fam Physician* 59(2):361-370, 1999.

Charness ME, Simon RP, Greenberg DA: Ethanol and the nervous system, *N Engl J Med* 321:442-453, 1989.

Ewing JA: Detecting alcoholism: the CAGE questionnaire, *JAMA* 252:1905-1907, 1984.

Fiellin DA, Reid MC, O'Connor PG: Outpatient management of patients with alcohol problems, *Ann Intern Med* 133:815-824, 2000.

Fiellin DA, Reid MC, O'Connor PG: Screening for alcohol problems in primary care: a systematic review, *Arch Intern Med* 160:1977-1988, 2000.

Ng SK, Hauser WA, Brust JC, Susser M: Alcohol consumption and withdrawal in new-onset seizures, *N Engl J Med* 319:666, 1988.

Saunders JB, Lee NK: Hazardous alcohol use: its delineation as a subthreshold disorder, and approaches to its diagnosis and management, *Compr Psychiatry* 41(2 Suppl 1):95-103, 2000.

9

Psychiatric Disorders in Neurologic Disease

Psychiatric and neurologic abnormalities often occur concomitantly in the same patient. Diseases once thought to be "emotional" now unquestionably have an organic basis. These diseases include schizophrenia and manic-depressive psychosis. The boundary between psychiatry and neurology is becoming less distinct. If a physician is able to recognize the common psychiatric disturbances, the diagnosis of many "neurologic" problems is facilitated, and unnecessary diagnostic tests and referrals will be avoided. Psychiatric conditions should never be diagnosed by exclusion. Positive evidence must be gathered from the history and physical examination; inconsistencies with known patterns of anatomy and physiology are major diagnostic clues. Unfortunately for the diagnostician, the presence of mental, emotional, or behavioral disturbances does not preclude the existence of another underlying organic abnormality. To convince a physician of the seriousness of the presenting complaint, patients sometimes embellish symptoms considerably. Psychiatric diagnosis should not be made lightly because such labels may preclude investigation of organic symptoms at a later date. The intent of this chapter is to illuminate the interrelationship between common neurologic and psychiatric disorders; it is not intended to be a definitive psychiatric text.

DEPRESSION

Depression is so pervasive in the population of ill adults that physicians may unwittingly accept it as the norm. This depression may be the basic underlying illness, the result of a chronic disease process or disability, or drug induced.

Grief Reaction

Grief reaction (bereavement, reactive depression) is the sadness that is a natural human emotion after personal loss. It is especially common in patients who have chronic diseases which in some way result in the loss of normal functional abilities and activities. Grief may also result from the death of, or separation from, a loved one. This type of depression does not usually respond to drug therapy.

Treatment:

1. Grief reaction is potentially a life-threatening situation; for example, the man who has just lost his wife and children in an automobile accident may commit suicide.
2. The patient needs the opportunity to discuss feelings and requires sympathetic support; this may be accomplished through a pastor, close friend, or professional counselor. If the family physician assumes this counseling responsibility, he or she must be available to the patient whenever things are not going well.
3. Drugs are usually not indicated; the disorder is self-limited and will gradually fade with time.

Major Depression

1. With major depression (endogenous depression) the patient has an "emptiness" that is not attributable to any life crises experienced. If questioned carefully, such patients reveal a mood alteration that is different in quality from the sadness experienced after personal misfortunes, bereavements, and tragedies.
2. Major depression may seem to be precipitated by some life event, but this is coincidence and not causation. In addition, positive changes in life circumstances do not improve depression.
3. Although patients with either major depression or grief reaction may have a variety of psychologic symptoms, it is the physiologic symptoms (Table 9-1) that often cause a patient to seek a physician's help. Common symptoms include headaches, chronic pain, sleep disturbances, fatigue, eating disturbances, confusion, and memory disturbances.
4. Major depression is the result of an alteration of central nervous system (CNS) biochemistry and thus responds to drug therapy. Usually the condition is idiopathic, but occasionally major depression can have a demonstrable cause.

Treatment: The patient with major depression can often be successfully treated by the primary care physician if depression is not severe and if the following guidelines are followed:

1. Take time to form a supportive relationship with the patient. Explain the nature of the illness and the fact that medications are not effective immediately and will probably not be magical. Schedule frequent return visits to discuss any problems, including troublesome side effects of the drugs and possible suicidal ideation.
2. Take suicidal thoughts and gestures seriously. Patients who talk about suicide will often attempt it. Clear suicidal ideation or attempts are stark testimony to the existence of a suicidal state and are considered an emergency. Such patients should be hospitalized with appropriate psychiatric evaluation and treatment.
3. Involve family members in the treatment; insist that they accompany the patient on office visits. The family may be very helpful in assessing the efficacy of the drug and may notice improvement in the patient's

TABLE 9-1
Symptomatology of Depressive Illness

Physiologic (biologic, vegetative)	Psychologic (behavioral)

Sleep disturbance
  Delayed insomnia
  Frequent awakening
	Dysphoric mood, unhappiness, sadness, crying spells

Somatic complaints
  Headaches
  Abdominal pain
  Dizziness
  Vague aches and pains
  Blurred vision
	Cognitive negatives
	  Negative feelings about self (low self-esteem, self-deprecation)
	  Negative feelings about relationships or friendships (or paranoia)
	  Negative feelings about the future (pessimism, hopelessness)

Alimentary tract disturbance
  Eating disorder (increase in or loss of appetite)
  Constipation
	Irritability, anger, poor frustration tolerance, temper outbursts

Weight change (loss or gain)	Social withdrawal
Fatigue	Guilt
	Loss of interest or pleasure in usual activities (including loss of interest in school)

Diminished sexual function (loss of libido)
Psychomotor disturbance
  Increased body activity (agitation or hyperactivity) or decreased body activity (retardation)
  Increased or decreased mental activity (including impaired concentration and confusion)
	Preoccupation with death, suicidal thoughts, threats, or attempts

Nonreactivity to surrounding events (including inconsolability or nonreactivity to cheering efforts)	
Diurnal variation in mood and symptoms (usually worse in the morning)	

condition before the patient does. Families are an excellent source of information with regard to compliance, side effects, and suicidal thoughts.

4. Be familiar with the side effects of tricyclic antidepressant medications. Patients may experience a dry mouth, drowsiness (especially in the mornings) and some constipation. Orthostatic hypotension, blurring of vision, tachycardia, and minor memory difficulties may also be trou-

blesome. Tell the patient that the side effects often subside with time.
5. There are three classes of drugs generally used to treat depression: selective serotonin reuptake inhibitors (SSRIs), tricyclic antidepressants (TCAs), and novel drugs, which do not fall into either class. These medications are listed in Table 9-2 and include the usual starting dose as well as the usual effective dose and side effects. Generally SSRIs are the drugs of choice. The drugs should be selected on the basis of their side effect profile, although individual patients may not have such severe side effects as listed. In patients with agitation and depression, a drug with high sedating properties would be the drug of choice. Monoamine oxidase inhibitors (MAOIs) are also reasonably effective antidepressants but are rarely used.

Caveat: Severely depressed patients are most apt to commit suicide as they improve; in such patients, hospital admission for medication administration and careful monitoring is preferable.

6. Encourage the patient to continue with usual activities but to make as few important decisions as possible while in the depressed state. Irretrievable steps such as resigning from a job, divorcing a spouse, or selling property should be expressively discouraged while the patient is depressed.
7. Discontinue prescribing the antidepressant medication gradually over a period of several weeks after the patient has been asymptomatic for at least 6 months.
8. Recognize anticholinergic psychosis characterized by restless agitation, confusion, disorientation, and perhaps seizures. The patient may have dry and sometimes flushed skin, tachycardia, dilated pupils, constipation, and urinary retention. This occurs especially in elderly patients who are taking other drugs such as benzodiazepines, antihistamines, and phenothiazines in addition to tricyclic antidepressants.

Drug-Induced Depression
In otherwise normal people (as well as people susceptible to depression), the following drugs may induce depression: alcohol, reserpine, propranolol (Inderal), α-methyldopa, benzodiazepines (such as diazepam [Valium]), barbiturates, clonidine, corticosteroids, and oral contraceptives.
Treatment: Withdrawal of the aforementioned drugs will often, but not always, result in remission of the depression. Concomitant pharmacotherapy for major depression is sometimes necessary.

Depression with Neurologic Disorders
The following neurologic diseases are commonly accompanied by depression:
1. Huntington's disease
2. Parkinson's disease
3. Multiple sclerosis
4. Stroke syndrome (especially involving the right hemisphere or bilateral frontal lobes)

TABLE 9-2
Antidepressant Medications

Generic name	U.S. brand name	Daily dose (mg)		Side effects			Cost
		Usual starting	Usual effective	Sedation	Anticholinergic	Nausea	
SELECTIVE SEROTONIN REUPTAKE INHIBITORS							
Fluoxetine	Prozac	20	20-80	L	L	M	20-mg tablets, 30 tablets $68.87
Paroxetine	Paxil	20	20-60	M	M	M	20-mg tablets, 30 tablets $68.25
Sertraline	Zoloft	50	50-200	L	L	M	50-mg tablets, 30 tablets $61.12
Citalopram	Celexa	20	20-60	L	L	M	20-mg tablets, 30 tablets $58.84
TRICYCLICS							
Amitriptyline	Elavil	50-75	100-300	VH	VH	L	25-mg tablets, 30 tablets $5.49
Desipramine	Norpramin	50	100-300	L	M	L	25-mg tablets, 60 tablets $7.09
Imipramine	Tofranil	75	100-300	H	H	L	50-mg tablets, 30 tablets $31.61
NOVEL							
Bupropion	Wellbutrin	100	200-450	L	L	M	100-mg tablets, 61 tablets $126.36
Nefazodone	Serzone	100	300-600	M	L	M	200-mg tablets, 60 tablets $69.29
Trazodone	Desyrel	50-100	150-300	VH	L	M	100-mg tablets, 30 tablets $8.78
Venlafaxine	Effexor	75	75-300	L	L	M	75-mg tablets, 61 tablets $76.96

L, low; *M,* medium; *H,* high; *VH,* very high.

5. Myotonic dystrophy

Treatment: Physicians often identify the depressed patient with neurologic disease ("I'd be depressed too, if I were that disabled"). However, if such patients have symptoms of major depression, a therapeutic drug trial is indicated and will often be successful. Antidepressant pharmacotherapy usually makes the neurologic disease more amenable to treatment.

Organic Disease Disguised as Depression

1. *Dementia:* especially in elderly patients, depression (depression-related dementia, depressive pseudodementia) may be virtually indistinguishable from dementia (see Chapter 6). Clinical clues for distinguishing these two entities are shown in Table 9-3.
2. *"Silent" brain tumor:* with severe frontal or right parietal lobe involvement, the patient may have only an alteration in mood. Paresis and alteration in reflexes may be subtle or absent. Such patients usually do not have a history of mood fluctuation; differentiation from dementia and depression may be made by the following:
   a. Focal neurologic findings
   b. Abnormal neuropsychologic test results
   c. Magnetic resonance imaging (MRI) or computed tomographic (CT) scan abnormality
3. *Pseudobulbar palsy:* such patients will cry easily with minimal provocation but will deny a feeling of sadness or emptiness. They have bilaterally increased deep tendon reflexes and an active jaw reflex. This is most frequently seen in elderly patients with hypertension and multi-infarct state (see Chapter 6).

Bipolar Disorder ("Manic Depressive" Illness)

Manic depressive patients have depressive episodes that alternate with periods of excessive activity. They are usually very talkative, have grandiose plans, and sleep very little. These cases are best managed by a psychiatric referral, and they are usually treated with either lithium (Eskalith) 300 mg by mouth twice a day or divalproex (Depakote) sodium 250 mg by mouth 3 times a day. Serum lithium levels are usually in the range of 0.8 to 1.2 mEq/L. Common side effects are tremors, ataxia, dysarthria, weight gain, diarrhea, hypothyroidism, and diabetes insipidus.

TABLE 9-3
Features Distinguishing Depression and Dementia

Feature	Dementia	Depression
Onset	Gradual	History of mood fluctuation
Appetite	Normal	Decreased
Constipation	Rare	Frequent
Motor activity	Relatively normal	Often decreased (may be agitated)
Mental status	Errors frequent	Tasks performed slowly but accurately

ANXIETY

Anxiety commonly accompanies many illnesses but sometimes may be the underlying illness itself. When an anxious patient walks into the office, the following features may be observed:
1. A hesitant or inappropriately hurried gait
2. Rigid posture, often fidgeting
3. Poor eye contact
4. Excessive decoy activity (e.g., lighting a cigarette)

The history will often include the following:
1. Gastrointestinal disturbances (anorexia, nausea, vomiting, abdominal cramps, diarrhea, constipation)
2. Genitourinary dysfunction (urgency, frequency, dysmenorrhea, impotence)
3. Insomnia
4. Cardiovascular symptoms (chest pain, palpitations)

On examination, the following may be noted:
1. Dilated pupils and tremulousness
2. Excessive sweating
3. Elevated blood pressure and rapid pulse

Recognition of anxiety symptoms is important in the following conditions or situations:
1. Headache: especially important with muscle contraction headache (see Chapter 3).
2. Low back pain (see Chapter 17).
3. Alcohol and drug abuse: anxiety may be an early symptom of alcohol withdrawal (see Chapter 8) or amphetamine or cocaine abuse.
4. Excessive use of coffee, caffeine-containing soft drinks, and tobacco.
5. Vertigo: especially the hyperventilation syndrome (see Chapter 4).
6. Possible presenting symptom of a serious depression.

Caveat: Benzodiazepines, such as alprazolam (Xanax), aggravate depression; this is one of the more common medication errors.

7. Patients receiving neuroleptic medication (such as haloperidol): such patients may develop an inward restlessness and fidgety legs and hands (akathisia). This is not a symptom of anxiety but a movement disorder as a manifestation of neuroleptic toxicity; an increase in the neuroleptic dosage will only increase this toxicity.
8. Hypoglycemia, thyroid disorders, and pheochromocytoma (Box 9-1): symptoms resembling anxiety may be seen in these medical conditions.

Treatment:
1. Identify the cause of anxiety (e.g. stressful occupation or home situation, phobias). A supportive physician-patient relationship is often sufficient treatment; occasionally psychologic or psychiatric counseling is indicated.
2. Withdraw all drugs or toxic substances that may be related to anxiety and diagnose and treat any underlying medical condition.

BOX 9-1
Medical Causes of Anxiety-Like Symptoms

CARDIOVASCULAR SYSTEM
Angina pectoris
Acute myocardial infarction, arrhythmia, congestive heart failure, shock

RESPIRATORY SYSTEM
Asthma, emphysema, pulmonary embolism

NEUROLOGIC SYSTEM
Encephalopathy, seizure disorder, familial tremor, vertigo

HEMATOLOGIC (BLOOD AND IMMUNE SYSTEM)
Anemia, anaphylactic shock

ENDOCRINE SYSTEM
Diabetes mellitus
Hyperthyroidism
Parathyroid disease
Cushing's disease
Pheochromocytoma

---

3. Pharmacologic treatment of anxiety.
   a. Avoid pharmacologic treatment if possible. Never use drugs as a substitute for a supportive physician-patient relationship.
   b. Never prescribe barbiturates for patients in anxiety states. The risk of dependency is too great, and overdosing is more lethal than with other drugs.
   c. Benzodiazepines are sometimes recommended in the treatment of anxiety, but a paradoxical reaction may worsen the anxiety in some patients and may cause drowsiness or ataxia. If benzodiazepines are used, monitor the patient closely and limit the length of treatment. Although alprazolam is commonly prescribed, we do not recommend it because of its highly addictive potential and a propensity to result in seizures on withdrawal and an increased depressive state.
   d. Never combine antianxiety drugs, and be sure to obtain a drug history before prescribing any medications. Patients with a history of heavy use of alcohol, tobacco, and nicotine should be given antianxiety agents with caution. The risk of dependency in such patients is high.
   e. The largest dose of an antianxiety drug may be given at bedtime to exploit its sedative properties. Diazepam is the most frequently prescribed antianxiety drug; the dosage is 5 to 10 mg by mouth 3 times a day.

f. Buspirone (BuSpar) hydrochloride is an antianxiety drug unrelated to the benzodiazepines; the usual dosage is 5 mg by mouth 3 times a day.

g. Propranolol 10 mg by mouth 4 times a day will alleviate many symptoms but should be prescribed with caution because it may induce or exacerbate a depression.

h. Paroxetine (Paxil) 20 mg by mouth at bedtime is an effective SSRI that will alleviate many symptoms of anxiety and depression. Others include venlafaxine (Effexor) 50 mg every day and citalopram (Celexa) 20 mg every day.

CONVERSION DISORDERS

There are two major categories of conversion disorders: (1) patients with factitious illnesses such as malingering or Munchausen's syndrome and (2) patients with signs and symptoms that have no organic basis; however, the patient is not deliberately attempting to mislead the physician.

Caveat: The diagnosis of conversion disorder should be established on the basis of positive evidence, not on the fact that all tests are negative. It is not a diagnosis of exclusion. Also, even if the patient has an obvious conversion disorder, a serious medical illness may still be present (remember that even hysterics become ill). However, many medical diagnostic tests carry serious risks, and patients with conversion disorder should never be subjected to unnecessary tests.

Factitious Disorders

1. The patient with a factitious disorder (malingering, conscious, non-physiologic disorder) consciously feigns an illness to obtain something perceived as valuable.

2. Often the examination is inconsistent with the complaint; for example, weakness of an extremity or side of the body will not be associated with any change (increased, decreased, or pathologic) in tone or reflexes. When testing muscle strength, the patient may give way with a ratchetlike quality.

3. Some patients make malingering a lifelong occupation. These individuals feign illness with remarkably clever and complex histories, inflicting self-injury or administering drugs to produce abnormal signs consistent with the reported disease process. For example, such a patient will instill atropine into one eye to produce a fixed, dilated pupil and then go to the physician's office with neurologic symptoms suggesting intracranial disease.

Treatment:

1. The physician should attempt to determine the nature of the underlying gratification the patient obtains from the illness. Occasionally the patient will have had an organic disability that has resolved; however, because of the adverse social or legal repercussions of improvement, the patient maintains the appearance of illness.

2. Confrontation is usually of no benefit. A cure most frequently occurs when legal matters are settled or when the patient realizes that a secondary gain is not obtainable.

Conversion Disorders

1. Conversion symptoms (subconscious, nonphysiologic disorder with apparent neurologic dysfunction) have no physiologic or pathologic substrate. *Remember* that the patient is asking for help, but in an inappropriate way.
2. Conversion symptoms often occur in mentally defective individuals or in adolescents as a way of coping with the environment (albeit inadequately).
3. Common reactions include blindness, deafness, paresis, sensory disturbances, ataxia, seizures, and unconsciousness.
4. The following is a list of some conversion reactions with suggestions on how they may be recognized during the neurologic examination:
   a. *Bilateral blindness:* the patient will commonly avoid injury when walking and will blink to unexpected threat. Pupillary reactions are normal, and optokinetic nystagmus (nystagmus induced by rotating a striped drum in front of the patient's eyes) is normal. In organic blindness, pupillary reflexes and opticokinetic nystagmus are frequently abnormal. A hysterical visual field defect, when plotted out on a tangent screen, will not change with varying distance between the patient and the screen.
   b. *Unilateral blindness:* if there is an organic basis, the lesion must be anterior to the optic chiasm, and the pupillary reaction is usually abnormal. Marcus Gunn's phenomenon is especially useful in evaluating unilateral blindness (see Chapter 10).
   c. *Paralysis of the legs:* reflexes are normal, and there is no atrophy. A useful test is as follows:
      1) With the patient supine, the examiner places both palms beneath the heels of the patient.
      2) The patient is then asked to lift the nonparalyzed leg. The patient will unconsciously increase the pressure in the palm of the hand under the paralyzed leg.
      3) The patient is then asked to press down with both heels. If pressure is not applied as it was when the patient lifted the nonparalyzed leg, a conversion reaction can be suspected (Fig. 9-1).
   d. *Hemiparesis:* a patient with a paralyzed leg and arm may incorrectly assume that there will also be difficulty in turning the head toward the paralyzed side (Fig. 9-2). Pronator drift and hemiplegic posturing are also absent on station and gait.
   e. *Reduced level of consciousness:* in a conversion reaction the pupillary and corneal reflexes and plantar responses will be normal. Often, when the patient's hand is held and dropped over the face, it will swerve to avoid striking the face. A patient with an organically caused reduced level of consciousness will usually have pupillary abnormalities and other positive neurologic signs (Fig. 9-3).

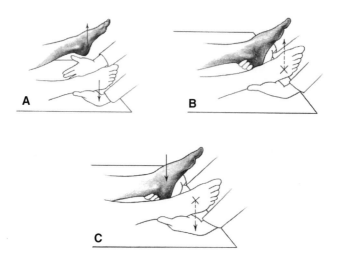

FIG. 9-1 Distinguishing true paralysis from hysterical paralysis of the leg. Place both hands under the heels and ask the patient to raise the *good* leg. **A,** The examiner will feel increased downward pressure by the "paralyzed" leg. **B,** Ask the patient to lift the paralyzed leg; there is little or no response. **C,** Then ask the patient to bear down with both heels; if the same pressure noted in maneuver **A** cannot be exerted, "something is rotten in the state of Denmark."

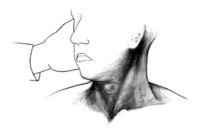

FIG. 9-2 The *left* sternocleidomastoid muscle turns the head to the *right*. Patients with a psychogenic *left*-sided weakness will often show weakness when turning toward the *left* (or vice versa).

    f. *Deafness:* the patient with a conversion reaction may startle to loud noise and can be awakened from a sound sleep by a loud noise.

    g. *Sensory disturbance:* conversion reactions that involve only the sensory systems are difficult to prove. Organic sensory losses make anatomic sense, whereas conversion reaction sensory disturbances will follow the patient's perception of body anatomy.

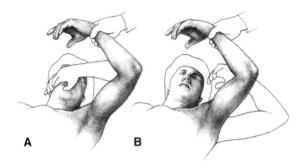

FIG. 9-3 A, A hand dropped over the face of a comatose patient will strike the face. **B,** In psychogenic coma, a hand held over the face and then dropped often swerves to the side.

1) Patients with organic sensory disturbances are able to appreciate a vibrating tuning fork placed on either side of the head and on either side of the sternum because of the conduction of the vibration through the bone. In a conversion reaction, the sternum or head is split (i.e., vibration is perceived on one side of the midline of the forehead or sternum but not on the other) (Fig. 9-4).
2) If anesthesia is present, instruct patients to close their eyes, and then instruct them to answer "yes" if they feel a pinprick or "no" if they do not. Obviously, the only appropriate answer is silence when the supposedly anesthetic area is touched. *Remember* that many of these patients have limited intelligence.
3) If a sensory disturbance involves the hands, have the patient make a fist as illustrated in Fig. 9-5, and then quickly touch the fingers for differences in sensation. In this position, most hysterical patients cannot tell the difference between their right and left hands.

h. *Pain syndrome:* the patient with a conversion reaction has a vivid description of the pain, but the pain usually does not interfere with the "pleasures of life." Analgesics, even narcotics, have little effect on the pain. Often the patient is addicted to narcotics. The patient with pain from an organic disorder will usually receive some relief from narcotics, and the pain will interfere with such pleasures of life as sleeping.

Treatment:
1. Confronting the patient is usually not helpful, since the patient often will develop other symptoms and "doctor-shop." Such patients usually find psychiatrists very threatening and often will refuse a psychiatric interview.
2. Rather than confront such a patient, emphasize that the symptoms are not medically serious (e.g., "I'm so happy to be able to tell you that you do not have cancer or a brain tumor"). From that point on, try to substitute a discussion of life problems and interpersonal relations. It

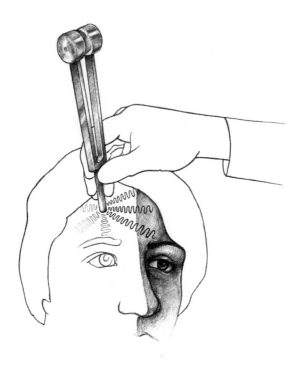

FIG. 9-4 Even with an anesthetic face, the vibrations from a tuning fork will be transmitted via bone to the opposite side.

is important to not reject or become angry with the patient. Limited, precisely scheduled visits and telephone calls on a regular basis are often helpful. With time, you may learn what goal or conflict is producing the conversion reaction. Administration of the Minnesota Multiphasic Personality Inventory (MMPI) and hypnosis in the hands of a skilled specialist may be helpful in this regard.
3. Once the diagnosis is made, the major goal is to avoid unnecessary hospitalization and surgery.
4. Avoid drugs of any kind in conversion states.

SCHIZOPHRENIA

Schizophrenia and the following neurologic problems occasionally cause diagnostic confusion:
1. *Basal ganglia disease:* as a side effect of therapy with neuroleptics (phenothiazines and major tranquilizers), the schizophrenic patient

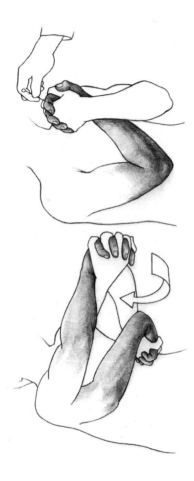

FIG. 9-5 After having first demonstrated a sensory deficit in one hand, have the patient perform this maneuver and then quickly test sensation in the fingers again. This maneuver seriously distorts a person's sense of which hand is which, and accurate responses are extremely difficult unless sensation is truly disturbed.

may develop a restlessness, especially in the legs (akathisia). These patients are usually more "inwardly" restless than is immediately apparent. Neuroleptics may also produce a parkinsonian syndrome (see Chapter 7).

2. *Dementia* (see Chapter 6): patients with catatonic schizophrenia may appear to be demented. However, schizophrenia causes a disorder to thought and spares memory.

3. *Aphasia* (see Chapter 12): the patient with parietal or temporal lobe damage (from tumor, infarct, hemorrhage, or trauma) may have a speech disturbance in which speech melody is normal but the words make little sense. Specific testing for aphasia will distinguish aphasia from schizophrenia.

4. *Complex partial seizures* (see Chapter 11): with seizures, the onset of symptoms may begin and end abruptly. An electroencephalogram (EEG) using sphenoidal electrodes may reveal an epileptic focus in the temporal lobe. Patients with complex partial seizures have a distinctive personality profile, perhaps because of a disturbed limbic system; this profile may be confused with schizophrenic personality profiles.

5. *Illicit drugs:* illicit drugs such as lysergic acid diethylamide (LSD), amphetamines, and phencyclidine (PCP) may produce states closely resembling schizophrenia. A history of drug abuse and a subacute onset are usually distinguishing features. Prescribed medications such as thiazides, steroids, and disulfiram (Antabuse) may also cause a disturbance of thinking that resembles schizophrenia.

6. *Delirium tremens:* delirium tremens may produce hallucinations and an agitated state (see Chapter 8). The hallucinations with delirium tremens are usually visual, whereas those of schizophrenia are generally auditory.

7. *Wernicke-Korsakoff syndrome* (see Chapter 8): Wernicke-Korsakoff syndrome is an acute or subacute onset of extraocular muscle paralysis, ataxia, and mental status changes that may resemble schizophrenia. When this syndrome is suspected, immediately give thiamine 100 mg intravenously (IV). Schizophrenic patients do not have abnormal eye movements and ataxia.

8. *Diffuse CNS vascular disease:* diffuse CNS vascular disease, such as that seen in hypertensive encephalopathy, tertiary syphilis (meningovascular syphilis), or collagen-vascular disease, may produce acute or chronic disturbances in thought processes that resemble schizophrenia.

9. *Endocrine dysfunctions:* endocrine dysfunctions, especially those associated with thyroid and adrenal disorders, produce changes in mentation on occasion.

10. *Hereditary neurologic disease:* hereditary neurologic disease, especially Huntington's disease, may produce schizophrenic symptoms years before the movement disorder becomes obvious.

To differentiate true schizophrenia from the preceding schizophrenic-like states, it is essential to take a careful history with special regard to the following signs:

1. Mode of onset (acute, subacute, or chronic)
2. Past history of similar disturbances

3. Drugs (licit and illicit)
4. Alcohol intake
5. Head trauma, seizures, or headache
6. Temperature intolerance or weight change
7. Family history
8. History of viral encephalitis, especially herpes simplex encephalitis

On a screening neurologic examination, pay particular attention to focal neurologic signs, abnormal movements, and posture.

Minimal laboratory tests that should be performed include the following:

1. Complete blood count (CBC) with erythrocyte sedimentation rate (ESR)
2. Serum electrolyte levels and renal function tests
3. Serum test for syphilis
4. Thyroid function tests
5. Consider the following tests:
   a. Lumbar puncture (LP)
   b. CT scan or MRI
   c. EEG

The following points may help the primary care physician recognize a schizophrenic patient. Florid schizophrenia is seldom seen, but borderline or subclinical schizophrenia, schizophrenia in remission, and schizophrenic patients being treated with neuroleptics are relatively common.

1. Schizophrenic patients may be described as having "sunburned minds," meaning they are extremely sensitive to criticism, emotional closeness, and rejection.
2. Onset of symptoms is usually before 40 years of age.
3. The patient has a disorder of thought processes with an inappropriate rate, flow, or content of thinking, but the sensorium is clear and memory is normal. When a patient has delusions or hallucinations, there is no disorientation or memory disturbance.

Caveat: The presence of delusions, hallucinations, paranoid ideation, or catatonia (disturbed psychomotor activity) should not automatically lead to the diagnosis of schizophrenia. These symptoms are also common among bipolar patients.

4. Often there is a blunted, shallow, inappropriate affect or bizarre motor behavior, or both. Unfortunately, physicians often have little sympathy for emotional reactions in schizophrenic patients.
5. Patients are often single and have poor premorbid social adjustments or work history.
6. Frequently there is a family history of schizophrenia.

Treatment:

1. Acutely disturbed schizophrenic patients are usually best treated with antipsychotic medications at inpatient mental health facilities.
2. When the primary care physician is following a schizophrenic patient in remission on neuroleptics (phenothiazines or other major tranquilizers), it is important to recognize that akathisia may be a symptom of

TABLE 9-4
Characteristics of Common Personality Types

Personality type	Description	Practical suggestions
Passive-dependent	Has a chronic inability to adjust to life demands, is completely dependent on others; commonly has long-term hospitalization or institutionalization	"I'll take care of you."
Passive-aggressive	Is a stubborn obstructionist who makes intentional errors; follows directions poorly; is intolerant of authority; blames others for any bad outcomes	"I know you are tough enough to do it."
Antisocial	Is selfish and callous, and has no loyalty or trustworthiness; has no sense of guilt; has low frustration tolerance with frequent interpersonal difficulties; exhibits antisocial behavior	These are extremely difficult patients to treat (see Cleckley's *The Mask of Sanity*).
Obsessive-compulsive	Has excessive concern about standards, morals, image; has excessive inhibitions; is frequently isolated and usually chronically unhappy	The patient should be given orders, lists, and schedules.
Paranoid	Is suspicious, blames others for all problems; is frequently involved in lawsuits; feels self-important and entitled to better	All procedures should be explained in a simple, straightforward manner.
Hysterical	Exhibits immature behavior; is sexually seductive in most interactions; is dependent but avoids meaningful interpersonal relationships	The physician should avoid seduction and recognize dependency needs and should not become angry and punitive towards these patients.
Schizoid	Is isolated, secretive, eccentric; avoids interpersonal relationships of all kinds	These patients are threatened by the natural warmth and closeness of many physicians; on the other hand, the door to communication must be left open because these patients are also very sensitive to rejection.

neuroleptic toxicity. The symptoms of akathisia are often mistakenly interpreted as anxiety, and the dose of the neuroleptic may be increased, when the proper treatment is to decrease the dose or discontinue the medication.

RECOGNIZING PERSONALITY TYPES AS AN AID TO PATIENT MANAGEMENT

The primary care physician should be able to recognize the common personality types and disorders to avoid letting his or her own emotional reactions interfere with the physician-patient relationship. Recognizing personality types will aid the primary care physician in ensuring better compliance to treatment (Table 9-4).

BIBLIOGRAPHY

Barrett JE, Williams JW Jr, Oxman TE et al: The treatment effectiveness project: a comparison of the effectiveness of paroxetine, problem-solving therapy, and placebo in the treatment of minor depression and dysthymia in primary care patients: background and research plan, *Gen Hosp Psychiatry* 21(4):260-273, 1999.

Binzer M, Eisemann M: Childhood experiences and personality traits in patients with motor conversion symptoms, *Acta Psychiatr Scand* 98(4):288-295, 1998.

Brown C, Schulberg HC: Diagnosis and treatment of depression in primary medical care practice: the application of research findings to clinical practice, *J Clin Psychol* 54(3):303-314, 1998.

Carr VJ: The role of the general practitioner in the treatment of schizophrenia: specific issues, *Med J Aust* 166(3):117-118, 1997.

Cleckley H: *The mask of sanity,* St Louis, 1976, Mosby.

Ettinger AB, Devinsky O, Weisbrot DM et al: A comprehensive profile of clinical, psychiatric, and psychosocial characteristics of patients with psychogenic nonepileptic seizures, *Epilepsia* 40(9):1292-1298, 1999.

Halligan PW, Bass C, Wade DT: New approaches to conversion hysteria, *Br Med J* 320(7248):1488-1489, 2000 (editorial).

Keeley R, Smith M, Miller J: Somatoform symptoms and treatment nonadherence in depressed family medicine outpatients, *Arch Fam Med* 9(1):46-54, 2000.

Kennedy SH, Eisfeld BS: Clinical aspects of depression, *Clin Cornerstone* 1(4):1-16, 1999.

Pingitore D, Sansone RA: Using DMS-IV primary care version: a guide to psychiatric diagnosis in primary care, *Am Fam Physician* 58(6):1347-1352, 1998.

Rakel RE: Depression, *Prim Care* 26(2):211-224, 1999.

Sahr N: Assessment and diagnosis of elderly depression, *Clin Excell Nurse Pract* 3(3):158-164, 1999.

Unutzer J, Katon W, Sullivan M, Miranda J: Treating depressed older adults in primary care: narrowing the gap between efficacy and effectiveness, *Milbank Q* 77(2):225-256, 1999.

10

Multiple Sclerosis

Modern technology, particularly the invention of magnetic resonance imaging (MRI), has greatly improved the accuracy of diagnosing multiple sclerosis (MS). Because the disease is common and because it is emphasized in medical school neuroscience curricula, it is often mistakenly listed as a presenting symptom in primary care surveys. In fact, MS is a specific disease entity with protean manifestations. Accurate diagnosis is important because MS is now considered a treatable disease.

COMMON HISTORICAL EVENTS IN A PATIENT WITH MS

1. Transient blurring of vision in one eye (retrobulbar neuritis), which is very common (Vision is often normal by the time the patient is examined by a physician.)
2. Double vision
3. Transient clumsiness of one arm (cerebellar involvement)
4. Urinary urgency or frequency and male impotence (spinal cord involvement)
5. Excessive fatigue unrelated to focal symptoms
6. Paralysis of a leg or arm
7. Symptoms that usually begin in the third decade of life (but cases have been reported in children and in the sixth decade)
8. More severe symptoms when patients are overheated (e.g., hot shower, fever)

Caution: Most patients with MS have repeated exacerbations and remissions of symptoms, but 10% of MS patients may have a gradually progressive course without readily apparent exacerbation or remissions.

Examination
Because any central nervous system (CNS) white matter may become demyelinated, almost any neurologic abnormality is possible. The following are common findings in MS patients:

1. The optic nerve often shows temporal pallor as a residuum of retrobulbar neuritis. A Marcus Gunn pupil, which indicates damage to the

optic nerve anterior to the chiasm from any cause, is frequently present (Fig. 10-1).

2. Internuclear ophthalmoplegia, especially if bilateral (Fig. 10-2). There are incomplete forms such as pronounced nystagmus in the abducting eye and minimal nystagmus in the adducting eye. Rare causes of internuclear ophthalmoplegia include brainstem infarcts or tumors.

3. Intention tremor and incoordinated rapid alternating movements are common because of cerebellar peduncle involvement.

4. Tingling or electric shocklike paresthesias travel down the spine when the neck is flexed (Lhermitte's sign).

5. There is impaired recognition of objects by touch alone (astereognosis).

6. There is motor involvement, as shown by increased or asymmetrical reflexes, or a Babinski's reflex.

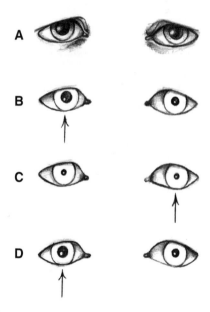

FIG. 10-1 Marcus Gunn pupil. The pupil that paradoxically dilates with direct light. **A,** Body pupils initially are equal. **B,** Direct light into the affected eye *(arrow)* causes minimal constriction; the opposite pupil constricts equally because of consensual reflex. **C,** Direct light into the normal eye causes significant constriction of both pupils, direct and consensual. **D,** Swinging the flashlight back to the affected eye causes it "paradoxically" to dilate as a result of removal of strong consensual reflex.

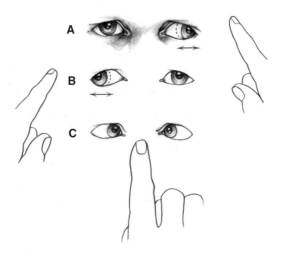

FIG. 10-2 Bilateral internuclear ophthalmoplegia. When looking to either side, the adducting eye does not go beyond the midline, the abducting eye shows nystagmus (**A** and **B**). This looks somewhat like a bilateral medial rectus palsy; however, the patient is able to converge and focus on a near object (**C**).

Caution: Multiple sclerosis affects *only* the CNS; absent reflexes, muscle atrophy, and sensory loss in the distribution of a peripheral nerve make the diagnosis unlikely. The presence of significant dementia, papilledema, or symmetric proximal muscle weakness also makes the diagnosis unlikely.

Laboratory Studies

The diagnosis of MS is confirmed by the following laboratory studies:

1. *MRI:* the presence of multiple, predominantly periventricular plaques in a young patient with exacerbations and remissions of neurologic symptoms strongly supports the diagnosis of MS, and further tests probably need not be done. If no plaques are seen on MRI, the diagnosis of MS is unlikely. Lesions that enhance suggest an active disease process.

2. *Evoked responses:* visual, somatosensory, and brainstem auditory-evoked responses are abnormal in a majority of patients but are nonspecific. They are not necessary in a patient with an MR image highly suggestive of MS.

3. *Lumbar puncture* (LP) (see Chapter 2): An LP should be performed if MRI is not diagnostic. Acute disseminated encephalomyelopathy, Lyme disease, and hypertensive white matter changes may mimic the

abnormalities of MS seen on MRI. Routine studies show a normal or slightly increased cell count, normal or slightly increased protein level, and an increased immunoglobulin G (IgG) level. More specific tests for MS include the following:

a. IgG synthesis calculated by the formula:

$$\frac{CSF\ IgG/Serum\ IgG}{CS\ albumin/Serum\ albumin} = [normal <0.7]$$

b. Oligoclonal bands

c. Myelin basic protein (normal <1.0 ng/ml)

These tests establish the diagnosis with more than 90% accuracy. Computed tomographic (CT) scans, electroencephalography (EEG), electromyography (EMG), myelography, and radionuclide scans are of little or no use in establishing a firm diagnosis of MS.

Specific Treatment

Experts agree that MS is associated with an altered immune response. The cause is unknown, but the disease might be triggered by an unspecified viral agent. Three agents are currently approved by the Food and Drug Administration (FDA) as specific immunomodulators in the treatment of MS: interferon beta-1b (Betaseron, 0.25 mg subcutaneous every other day), interferon beta-1a (Avonex, 30 mg intramuscularly [IM] weekly), and glatiramer acetate (Copaxone, 20 mg subcutaneous every day). Efficacy has been demonstrated in clinical trials, including serial MRI scans to demonstrate active lesions. There have been no head-to-head trials of these agents, but Avonex and Betaseron are composed of very similar molecules. A major difference between these two agents is dosage. The dose of Avonex is half that of Betaseron, and efficacy is dose-related. The strategy with these drugs is to prevent new attacks, not to repair brain damage caused by old attacks. These drugs are approved for relapsing-remitting MS (patients are relatively normal between attacks) and secondarily progressive MS (most relapsing-remitting MS patients sooner or later become gradually progressive). They are not approved for MS progressive from the onset; this generally is a much more severe disease. The efficacy of these drugs may not be apparent for 6 months. The authors prefer Betaseron as the initial treatment, but this is unsupported by appropriate clinical studies.

Caveat: Needle phobias can be minimized with an autojector, a device that spring-loads the syringe.

Note: The aforementioned three drugs cost approximately $12,000 per year and thus should be prescribed by a physician experienced in the diagnosis and care of MS patients. The pharmaceutical firm sometimes will supply the drug free-of-charge to low income patients.

Mitoxantrone (Novantrone) has recently been approved for secondarily progressive MS, but the agent has significant toxic side effects, namely cardiotoxicity and hepatotoxicity.

Physician Advice

1. Advise patients to use only FDA-approved medications or to participate in drug trials sponsored only by respectable scientific agencies.
2. Most patients are initially upset with their diagnosis. Emphasize the positive features of the disease: one third of patients have a relatively benign course, the recovery rate from individual attacks is 80% or more, and specific treatment is available.
3. Explain that stress is generally recognized as a precipitating factor for attacks. This includes infections such as influenza or pneumonia.
4. Advise patients to avoid situations that raise the body temperature (e.g., hot baths, saunas, and prolonged exposure to the hot sun) because this may cause a temporary exacerbation of old symptoms.
5. Emphasize bladder hygiene; patients with a significant bladder residuum should catheterize themselves several times daily.

Symptomatic Drug Therapy

1. Antispasticity agents
   a. Gabapentin (Neurontin) 400 mg in the evening. Gabapentin has no drug interactions and may be titrated up to 3600 mg a day. It is agonistic with benzodiazepines and codeine derivatives. The drug not only decreases spasticity but also treats leg cramps and, in some cases, tremor.
   b. Baclofen (Lioresal) at an initial dosage of 5 mg twice a day up to 20 mg 3 times a day. Dose should be slowly titrated for maximal benefit.
   c. Dantrolene (Dantrium): begin with 25 mg daily; every 3 or 4 days increase the dose by 25 mg until the therapeutic goal is obtained. Dosages as high as 100 mg 3 times a day occasionally are necessary. If this drug is used, liver function tests should be performed at regular intervals, since hepatitis and liver failure have been reported.
2. Fatigue
   a. Fatigue is a most bothersome symptom to MS patients; a few patients improve dramatically with 100 mg of amantadine (Symmetrel) hydrochloride once or twice a day.
   b. Pemoline (Cylert) 18.75 mg twice a day, gradually titrated to a maximum of 75 mg/day, may alleviate fatigability.
   c. Modanfinil (Provigil) is a new FDA-approved stimulant for the treatment of narcolepsy. Preliminary reports indicate its beneficial effect on MS-related fatigue.
   d. In MS patients with major depression or emotional lability, tricyclic antidepressants, specifically amitriptyline (Elavil) hydrochloride 50 to 150 mg/day, may ameliorate the symptoms.
3. Intravenous (IV) corticosteroids should never be used on a chronic basis. They may hasten recovery after an attack, but they do not change the outcome of MS as measured by disability.

Rehabilitation

1. Physical therapy is indicated for patients in remission with residual motor disability. Ideally, this is best carried out in a rehabilitation center.

2. Occupational therapy assists patients with a fixed disability in adjusting to the activities of daily living.

Patient Education

The National Multiple Sclerosis Society is a good source of information: National Multiple Sclerosis Society, 733 Third Ave., New York, NY 10017; (212)463-7787 or (800)344-4867; website: www.nat@nmss.org. In addition, most cities have a local MS society and support groups that are invaluable sources of education and emotional support.

BIBLIOGRAPHY

Fazekas F, Barkhof F, Filippi M et al: The contribution of magnetic resonance imaging to the diagnosis of multiple sclerosis, *Neurology* 53(3):448-456, 1999.

Noseworthy JH, Gold R, Hartung HP: Treatment of multiple sclerosis: recent trials and future perspectives, *Curr Opin Neurol* 12(3):279-293, 1999.

Noseworthy JH, Lucchinetti C, Rodriguez M, Weinshenker BG: Multiple sclerosis, *N Engl J Med* 343(13):938-952, 2000.

Olek MJ: Multiple sclerosis. I. Overview, pathophysiology, diagnostic evaluation, and clinical parameters, *J Am Osteopath Assoc* 99(11):574-588, 1999.

Paty DW, Oger JJ, Kastrukoff LF et al: MRI in the diagnosis of MS: a prospective study with comparison of clinical evaluation, evoked potentials, oligoclonal banding, and CT, *Neurology* 38:180-185, 1988.

Petersen RC, Kokmen E: Cognitive and psychiatric abnormalities in multiple sclerosis, *Mayo Clin Proc* 64:657-663, 1989.

Tselis AC, Lisak RP: Multiple sclerosis: therapeutic update, *Arch Neurol* 56(3):277-280, 1999.

Walther EU, Hohlfeld R: Multiple sclerosis: side effects of interferon beta therapy and their management, *Neurology* 53(8):1622-1627, 1999.

Weinstock-Guttman B, Jacobs LD: What is new in the treatment of multiple sclerosis? *Drugs* 59(3):401-410, 2000.

11

Seizures and Epilepsy

A seizure is a sudden change in functioning resulting from abnormal, excessive electrical discharges of neurons in the brain. Epilepsy is a symptom complex with a tendency to have repeated seizures. Not everyone who has seizures has epilepsy, but everyone who has epilepsy has seizures. Neither seizures nor epilepsy is a final diagnosis but is a symptom complex requiring a search for underlying causes.

Frequently, only generalized tonic-clonic or other repetitive motor movements are recognized as seizures, but consideration of seizures should arise whenever a patient has a loss of consciousness or any sudden, brief change in functioning with or without loss of consciousness. Paroxysmal changes in consciousness, sensation, emotion, or thought processes may all be manifestations of a seizure disorder. A diagnosis of a seizure disorder is especially likely if such changes are repetitive, stereotyped, and preceded by a premonition or warning (aura) or followed by (postictal) confusion, exhaustion, or headache.

The physician's initial task when a patient has what might be a seizure is to determine whether the episode was a seizure or some other episodic, periodic, or recurrent paroxysmal event that is nonepileptic, such as syncope, migraine, sleep parasomnias, nonepileptic seizures, paroxysmal dyskinesia or dystonia, transient ischemic attacks (TIAs), or narcolepsy. When the diagnosis of a seizure is made, the patient should be evaluated for common toxic-metabolic or structural abnormalities. These abnormalities commonly include hypoglycemia, hypoxia, infection, alcohol or drug withdrawal, stroke, and tumor.

Patients with recurrent seizures over a long time (epilepsy syndrome) most likely have either no structural abnormality or a static abnormality such as a glial scar. Recurrent seizures with neurologic deterioration require evaluation for inborn errors of metabolism, chronic infection, or another progressive neurologic disease.

Patients with recurrent seizures and an anatomically normal brain or a nonprogressive lesion require only symptomatic treatment with antiepileptic drugs (AEDs). If the seizures are secondary to a generalized systemic medical condition or a progressive brain lesion, then the patient requires etiologic treatment in addition to symptomatic treatment with AEDs.

Summary of Diagnostic/Management Approach:

1. Seizure or nonseizure?
2. If seizure, what type?
3. Acute medical or neurologic condition or epilepsy?
4. If epilepsy, which epilepsy syndrome?
5. Symptomatic, syndrome-specific, or etiologic treatment?

   In the primary epilepsies, no focal brain lesions are found, there is often a family history of epilepsy, and the findings of a neurologic examination are normal. Epilepsies often begin in childhood, and the response to anticonvulsants is usually very good. In the secondary epilepsies, neurologic abnormalities may be present, a family history of epilepsy is usually lacking, and the response to anticonvulsants is variable to poor.

HISTORY

The patient's history is the single most important part of the diagnostic evaluation and management of seizures. It should include the following:

1. An accurate description of the onset of seizures. (If the patient cannot give a history, interview an eyewitness.)
   a. A bilaterally symmetric onset without warning (primary generalized seizure) versus focal, partial, or unilateral onset. For example, an arm jerking on one side suggests a lesion in the frontal lobe of the opposite hemisphere.
   b. The dynamic character (symptoms) of seizures (march of movement, focal movement becoming generalized, etc.).
   ▶ c. Drowsiness or confusion that follows the seizure event, which is *an important diagnostic clue*. This does not occur after other episodic phenomena such as TIAs, noncomplicated migraine, and syncope.

Caveat: An episodic, stereotyped event followed by sleepiness is likely to be a seizure.

   d. Postictal lateralizing symptoms, such as aphasia, hemiparesis, or hemianopsia. The symptoms indicate the focal, rather than generalized, onset of seizures.
2. A review of symptoms suggesting seizures: loss of memory; strange, unexplained smells or other sensations; visual hallucinations; distortions in visual, auditory, or time sensation; a feeling of having experienced events before; previous staring episodes (absences); previous undiagnosed nocturnal seizures with bed-wetting or rolling out of bed; and awakening exhausted with muscle aches and pain.
3. A family history of seizures (what type, what age at onset, what course). (In primary generalized epilepsies the familial incidence is as high as 25%.)
4. Previous head trauma or other central nervous system (CNS) brain-damaging illnesses, such as meningitis, encephalitis, and stroke.
5. A consideration of the patient's age. Epilepsy syndromes tend to occur with the highest frequency at certain ages (Table 11-1).

TABLE 11-1
Age Correlation with Seizures and Epilepsy Syndromes

Age	Seizures and syndromes	Etiologic factors	Outcome
Newborn (up to 3 wk)	Subtle seizures; generalized tonic, focal tonic-clonic and multifocal clonic, myoclonus Benign, familial neonatal convulsions	Hypoxia, hemorrhage, congenital malformations, hypoglycemia, hypocalcemia, infection Autosomal dominant	The outcome is dependent on etiologic factors.
Infants and toddlers (3 wk-3 yr)	Simple febrile seizures, infantile spasms, Lennox-Gastaut syndrome, myoclonic epilepsies Simple, complex partial seizures	Inborn errors of metabolism, no specific cause (as in febrile seizures), hypoxic brain damage, tuberous sclerosis Cortical dysplasia, meningitis, encephalitis	There is an excellent prognosis for febrile seizures; for infantile spasms here is 10%-20% mortality and 75%-90% morbidity (mental retardation, hypotonia, spasticity, epilepsy); 20% of cases developing into epilepsy evolve into Lennox-Gastaut syndrome.
Children (3-12 yr)	Primary generalized absence, benign centrotemporal epilepsy, benign occipital epilepsy	Genetic	Excellent

			Long-term prognosis for control of seizures with treatment is excellent in most generalized seizure types; 25% of partial-onset seizures achieve remission within 5 years of diagnosis with appropriate treatment. The outcome is dependent on etiologic factors.
Adolescents (13-20 yr)	Generalized tonic-clonic	Familial	
	Juvenile myoclonic epilepsy		
	Generalized convulsions on awakening		
	Juvenile absence epilepsy		
	Autosomal dominant nocturnal frontal lobe epilepsy	Genetic	
	Febrile seizures plus generalized convulsive epilepsy	Genetic	
	Progressive myoclonic epilepsies		
Adults (21-60 yr)	Complex (and simple) partial- or focal-onset secondarily generalized, localization-related epilepsy	Head trauma, tumor, vascular malformation	
Elderly (>60 yr)	Partial- or focal-onset secondarily generalized seizures, localization-related epilepsy	Postinfarction (vascular)	

MINIMAL LABORATORY STUDIES

The laboratory examination will be directly based on the clinical history and type of seizure and will be different for each type of seizure and each age group.

1. Electroencephalogram (EEG): An EEG measures the electrical activity of cortical surface neurons. It is a finite sample of activity in time. Remember that the recording is often done between seizures (interictal) and may not reveal epileptiform abnormalities. The reliability of the EEG also depends on the competence of the EEG technologist who is recording and the expertise of the electroencephalographer. Routine activation techniques such as hyperventilation, photic stimulation, and sleep deprivation and the use of sphenoid electrodes may add more information. In specialized referral centers, long-term monitoring by ambulatory, outpatient or inpatient video EEG, and ambulatory cassette recording are now available when refractory epilepsies are present or when diagnostic difficulties arise.

Caveat: A normal EEG does not rule out epilepsy; and patients rarely may have abnormal EEGs with no clinical symptoms. *Never* use an EEG to "rule out" a seizure disorder.

SEIZURES

Neonatal seizures: newborns, unlike older infants, do not have well-organized, symmetric tonic-clonic seizures. Seizures in premature infants are even less organized. Suspect seizures when there are unexplained autonomic, respiratory, or motor changes, including the following:

1. Subtle seizures: eye blinking, tonic eye deviation, sucking, lip-smacking, drooling, swimming movements, bicycling movements, or apnea.
2. Tonic seizures: usually an extension of all limbs (generalized tonic), but may involve only one limb (focal tonic).
3. Multifocal clonic seizures: brief, repetitive jerking of limbs and face irregularly and asynchronously, usually associated with perinatal asphyxia.
4. Focal clonic seizures: repetitive jerking of one limb, usually caused by hypocalcemia; focal brain contusion.
5. Myoclonic seizures: multiple or single flexion jerks of the upper or lower extremities.
6. An underlying cause: generally there is an underlying cause, such as neonatal hypoxia-ischemia, trauma, intracranial hemorrhage, meningitis, hypocalcemia, or rarely, inborn errors of metabolism (pyridoxine dependency, biotin deficiency, maple syrup urine disease, or disorders of neurotransmitter metabolism). Ultrasound imaging or a computed tomographic (CT) scan of the head may demonstrate anatomic abnormalities (hemorrhage, hydrocephalus, developmental brain anomalies). Routine chemistries, blood for amino acids, urine for organic acid analysis, and blood for tandem mass spectroscopy

may detect metabolic disturbances. A rare genetic cause of neonatal seizures is benign, familial neonatal convulsions, which are autosomal dominant.

Generally, the best prognosis is seen with focal clonic jerking, and the worst prognosis is with fragmentary multifocal clonic seizures. The prognosis for normal neurologic development and recurrent seizures relates ultimately to the cause and response to treatment of the underlying cause. Reversible metabolic disorders (hypocalcemia and pyridoxine dependency) have the best prognosis.

Treatment:

1. Prevention or early detection with adequate etiologic treatment of the underlying disorder or disorders is the best approach to neonatal seizures.
2. If seizures occur frequently, do the following:
   a. Draw blood for glucose, calcium, magnesium, and electrolyte testing, and leave the needle in place for an intravenous (IV) line.
   b. Inject the following solutions (if there is an immediate response, the cause of the seizures will have been determined):
      1) 50% glucose 1 to 2 ml/kg
      2) Calcium gluconate 200 mg/kg
      3) Pyridoxine 50 mg
3. If the seizures still do not stop, infuse phenobarbital 20 mg/kg IV slowly over 10 minutes. Order subsequent IV phenobarbital doses according to serial serum phenobarbital levels, and attempt to keep the blood level between 25 and 30 μg/ml. If seizures continue, you can also use fosphenytoin 20 mg/kg IV. Phenobarbital can be continued orally for long-term maintenance, but oral phenytoin (Dilantin) in infants usually cannot be maintained in the therapeutic reference range and is not recommended for long-term maintenance.
4. If seizures stop in the neonatal period, it is accepted practice to continue AEDs for 3 months. If no seizures occur after the neonatal period, and EEG findings at 3 months of age are normal, phenobarbital can be weaned.

Simple Febrile Seizures

1. Simple febrile seizures are the most common type of seizures in infants and toddlers; the greatest incidence is between 18 and 36 months of age.
2. In the relationship between fever and a seizure: the temperature may be rapidly rising or falling and may not be detected until after the seizure occurs.
3. They are brief (less than 10 minutes), generalized seizures; the seizure has almost always stopped by the time the patient arrives at the physician's office. Occasionally, patients do have febrile status epilepticus (convulsions lasting longer than 20 minutes).
4. An EEG is normal by 2 weeks after the seizure.
5. A family history of simple febrile seizures in early childhood supports the diagnosis of simple febrile seizures.

Caution: If the seizure is focal, recurrent, or prolonged or if the neurologic examination shows focal abnormalities, it is *not* a simple febrile seizure, and a search must be made for underlying pathologic factors, especially infection. It is also unusual for the *first* simple febrile seizure to occur before 6 months or after 3 years of age.

Treatment:
1. If a CNS infection is suspected, patients should have a lumbar puncture (LP) and a cerebrospinal fluid (CSF) examination.
2. Parents should be reassured that the condition is benign (not associated with brain damage and highly unlikely to develop into epilepsy). The first incidence with febrile status epilepticus carries no higher risk for development of epilepsy than short, simple febrile seizures.
3. For the physician who may find it difficult to resist pressure from parents to treat a child, giving the parents a prescription for a rectal suppository of diazepam (Diastat 5 or 10 mg) with instructions to insert it for frequent repetitive seizures or prolonged (greater than 10 minutes) seizures may calm their fears, give them a sense of control if seizures recur, and prevent recurrent emergency room visits.
4. If the aim is to prevent future febrile convulsions, anticonvulsants are *not* beneficial if given intermittently (i.e., with fever). Phenobarbital is effective (*phenytoin* is not) prophylactically, but enough must be given to produce therapeutic blood levels (15 to 30 μg/ml). The usual dosage of 3 to 5 mg/kg/day can be given as a single evening dose. However, it is rarely necessary to give prophylactic AEDs.
5. Valproic acid is the only other effective prophylactic anticonvulsant for simple febrile seizures but is not recommended because of possible hepatotoxicity, particularly in patients under 2 years of age.

Complex Febrile Seizures
1. Fever lowers the seizure threshold. Fever of any cause may trigger seizures in individuals with underlying epilepsy, or fever and seizures may be associated with a CNS infection such as meningitis or encephalitis.
2. These seizures occur in all age groups but are a diagnostic problem, especially in children under 5 years of age.
3. Thorough neurologic evaluation is necessary if it is the patient's first seizure. The risk of febrile seizures developing into epilepsy is increased by neurologic abnormalities, developmental delay, focality or long duration of the seizure, multiple seizures with each febrile episode, multiple prolonged seizures (longer than 15 minutes), family history of epilepsy, or epileptiform abnormalities in the EEG.
4. Severe myoclonic epilepsy (SME) syndrome often begins with febrile status epilepticus. A family history of febrile seizures and generalized convulsions should engender suspicion of a recently described genetic epilepsy syndrome—febrile seizures and generalized convulsions.

Treatment:
1. A diagnostic LP and appropriate antibiotic or antiviral treatment are necessary for meningitis or encephalitis (see Chapter 14).

2. Reduce or prevent the fever with antipyretics (acetaminophen or ibuprofen) to reduce the likelihood of seizures.

Caution: Although its role is still undetermined, aspirin has been associated with Reye's syndrome, particularly when the underlying cause of fever has been influenza or chickenpox.

3. A rectal suppository diazepam (5 or 10 mg) with the same instructions as in simple febrile seizures is recommended. If seizures subsequently occur without fever, consider prophylactic AEDs.

EPILEPTIC DISORDERS
Infantile Spasms

Infantile spasms (called *West's syndrome*) is an epileptic syndrome consisting of massive myoclonic seizures in the first year of life, developmental arrest, and a hypsarrhythmic EEG. It is the most devastating seizure syndrome and should be considered an emergency.

1. Massive myoclonic seizures are usually flexor and last a second or more. They consist of a sudden bending forward at the waist and extending the arms and legs, with the patient simulating a jackknife position. A lesser number are extensor spasms, with the patient arching the back and extending the neck. Rarely there are hemispasms involving only one half of the body.
2. The spasms occur in flurries many times daily, usually on awakening.
3. The spasms are often misdiagnosed as "colic," particularly if they appear during feeding times.
4. The usual onset is between 3 and 12 months of age.
5. They are associated with developmental arrest and subsequent moderate to severe mental retardation in more than 90% of these children.
6. The EEG shows a hypsarrhythmic pattern consisting of disorganized background activity and multiconfigurational and multifocal discharges during the awakening state. Sleep tracings may mimic "burst-suppression" patterns. Prehypsarrhythmic patterns are quantitatively less severe and precede the full expression of the syndrome. If a spasm is recorded, the EEG shows a decremental pattern.
7. Causes follow:
   a. Symptomatic: previous static encephalopathies or (rarely) progressive CNS disease, or neurocutaneous syndromes, particularly tuberous sclerosis
   b. Cryptogenic: normally developing babies who suddenly have the syndrome and in whom no CNS disease is found
8. The seizures may be difficult to control and may evolve into complex partial seizures in other seizure syndromes (see the section on Lennox-Gastaut syndrome in this chapter).

Treatment:
1. Early treatment of the seizures is not sufficient. Search for an underlying cause with a urine neurometabolic screen or urine organic acid

and blood amino acid tests and a CT scan or magnetic resonance imaging (MRI) (for developmental brain malformations such as agenesis of the corpus callosum or cortical tubers). Functional neuroimaging studies such as single photon emission computed tomography (SPECT) or positron emission tomography (PET), should be considered if seizures have a focal signature (hemispasms, or development of complex partial seizures) and the brain MRI findings are normal.

2. After obtaining baseline EEGs, treat with adrenocorticotropic hormone (ACTH) 100 to 150 units/m^2/day for 2 weeks followed by a taper to 0 over the next 2 weeks. At present, ACTH has to be obtained through the National Organization for Rare Diseases (NORD); www.rarediseases.org. Monitor for steroid toxic side effects, the most important of which is hypertension. Clinical improvement usually does not occur before 10 to 14 days and may be preceded by EEG improvement.

3. The most effective drug for symptomatic infantile spasms from tuberous sclerosis is vigabatrin. It has not been approved by the Food and Drug Administration (FDA) because of visual field defects reported in human trials. It is not available in the United States, but can be imported through foreign pharmacies in a 3-month supply.

4. Genetic counseling is necessary if a genetic syndrome can be identified.

5. Families should be offered assistance in managing a mentally retarded child (see Chapter 16).

Lennox-Gastaut Syndrome

Lennox-Gastaut syndrome consists of astatic/akinetic seizures, developmental arrest, and an EEG showing multifocal and generalized slow (<2.5 cycles/sec) spike-wave discharges.

1. The syndrome usually affects children between 2 and 5 years of age. Akinetic and astatic seizures *(drop spells)*, absences, and generalized convulsions occur, often many times daily. Tonic seizures occur in sleep. Rarely, there are myoclonic seizures in the astatic-myoclonic loose variant.

2. Developmental arrest evolves into mild to moderate mental retardation, hyperactivity, and behavior disturbances. As with the infantile spasms syndrome, causes are either symptomatic (previously known static encephalopathy) or cryptogenic (previously developmentally and neurologically normal but assumed to have an as yet undiagnosed cause).

3. Characteristic EEG changes consist of poorly developed background activity and multifocal, slow, atypical (less than 3 Hz) spike-and-wave complexes.

4. Since both the infantile spasms and Lennox-Gastaut syndromes are clinically devastating, initial management is probably best handled by someone experienced with these disorders such as a pediatric neurologist, an epileptologist, or a pediatrician with specialized training and experience with epilepsies.

Treatment:
1. Total control of seizures is difficult to achieve. Protective helmets (football or hockey type) help prevent head injury from drop spells.
2. If the subsequent course shows persistent myoclonic seizures and persistent developmental arrest or developmental regression, suspect a progressive CNS disease (such as a ganglioside storage disease) and refer the patient to a pediatric neurologist.
3. AED drugs are used (Table 11-2). The initial mainstays are usually divalproex sodium and clonazepam (Klonopin). Felbamate has been shown to be very effective, but caution must be used because of hepatotoxicity and bone marrow depression. Lamotrigine (Lamictal) and topiramate have been shown to be effective. The ketogenic diet and the vagus nerve stimulator have been reported to work. Corpus callosotomy stops the drop spells.

Benign Rolandic Epilepsy

Benign rolandic epilepsy (benign centrotemporal epilepsy, sylvian syndrome, and lingual seizures) is a relatively common, but often unrec-

TABLE 11-2
Drugs Used in Treatment of Seizures

Drug	Dosage		Plasma* half-life (hr)	Cost
	Adults (mg)	Children (mg/kg)		
Phenobarbital	100-180	3-5	72-96	100 mg (100 tablets): $8.95
Phenytoin (Dilantin)	300-400	4-7	12-24	100 mg (90 capsules): $22.70
Primidone (Mysoline) (partially metabolized to phenobarbital)	750-1500	10-25	3-12	250 mg (90 tablets): $90.33
Carbamazepine (Tegretol)	800-1600	20-30	7-18	200 mg (60 tablets): $29.82
Ethosuximide (Zarontin)	750-2000	20-30	24-48	250 mg (60 capsules): $56.24 250 mg/5 ml (1 bottle, 300 ml): $61.44
Clonazepam (Klonopin)	1.5-20	0.01-0.2	18-50	1 mg (30 tablets): $27.37
Valproic acid (Depakene)	1000-3000	15-30	7-15	250 mg (60 tablets): $52.74

*Values vary depending on whether or not the patient is on polytherapy.

Continued

TABLE 11-2
Drugs Used in Treatment of Seizures—cont'd

| | Dosage | | Plasma* | |
Drug	Adults (mg)	Children (mg/kg)	half-life (hr)	Cost
NEWER DRUGS				
Gabapentin (Neurontin)	300-1200	NA	5-7	400 mg (90 capsules): $113.18
Lamotrigine (Lamictal)	150-250 mg twice a day	0.15 mg/ kg/day up to 1-5 mg/ kg/day	15-60	100 mg (60 capsules): $131
Oxcarbazepine (Trileptal)	600-2400	8-10 mg/ kg/day	10	300 mg (60 tablets): $98.36
Tiagabine (Gabitril)	56 mg/day	NA	7-9	20 mg (30 tablets): $79.58
Topiramate (Topamax)	200 mg/day	5-9 mg/ kg/day divided twice a day	19-23	100 mg (60 tablets): $164.15
Levetiracetam (Keppra)	500-3000	NA	6-8	NA
Zonisamide (Zonegran)	100-600	NA	25-70	NA
Felbamate (Felbatol)	400 mg 3 times a day	NA	14-24	400 mg (90 tablets): $108.28

NA, Not available.

ognized or misdiagnosed epileptic disorder. Making the correct diagnosis is important because of the benign prognosis—an excellent response to antiepileptics and "outgrowing" the disorder by middle or late adolescence.
1. This is a focal or partial seizure syndrome not associated with focal structural CNS lesion that will probably prove to be a genetic epilepsy.
2. It often presents as nocturnal (secondarily) generalized convulsions in children of school age.
3. The partial onset, seen easily after the institution of antiepileptics and incomplete control of the seizures, consists of localized tongue or oral paresthesias, dysarthria, drooling, and facial twitching, with the preservation of consciousness. A careful history for this initial onset of the seizures will give the diagnosis.

4. The EEG shows characteristic central and midtemporal spikes or sharp waves. These may be seen in an EEG performed while the patient is awake but are activated by sleep. Therefore order a sleep-deprived, an awake and an asleep EEG.

Treatment:

1. Usually any AED is effective. However, the seizures usually occur rarely, and only in sleep, so many neurologists do not treat with prophylactic AEDs.
2. If seizures occur in the daytime, are generalized convulsions, or occur frequently, which rarely happens, the most effective AEDs are gabapentin and sulthiame (which is not available in the United States).

PRIMARY GENERALIZED SEIZURES AND EPILEPSIES

The most common clinical types of primary generalized seizures are tonic-clonic or clonic convulsions, absence, and myoclonic. The following features apply to all generalized seizures:

1. The onset is almost always in childhood or adolescence.
2. From the onset the seizures are generalized with immediate alteration of consciousness. Motor manifestations are symmetric and bilateral.
3. EEG discharges are generalized and bilaterally synchronous from the start of a recorded seizure.
4. Findings from a neurologic examination and a CT scan or an MRI of the brain are normal during the interictal period.
5. Findings from an EEG background activity are normal, interrupted by generalized, bilaterally synchronous, symmetric spike-and-wave (absence) or many spike-and-wave complexes (myoclonic). These occur spontaneously or are activated by hyperventilation (absence), intermittent photic stimulation (myoclonic), or sleep (generalized convulsions).
6. There is no previous history of brain injury.
7. A family history of epilepsy is often positive.
8. There is a good response to appropriate AEDs.
9. There is a relatively good prognosis. Next to the primary partial epilepsies just described (benign rolandic), the primary generalized epilepsies (particularly absence epilepsy) have the best long-term prognosis for seizure control, as well as for intellectual, cognitive, and emotional functioning.
10. Previous terms commonly used that are synonymous with primary generalized epilepsy are *idiopathic* or *centrencephalic epilepsy.*

Primarily Generalized Absence Epilepsy

The term *petit mal* is probably the most misused term applied to seizures by the general physician. It does *not* denote any minor seizure that falls short of being a generalized convulsion. Staring spells as an expression of absence epilepsy are a *specific* clinical and EEG syndrome (referred to as *petit mal epilepsy*) with a *specific* therapy.

1. The usual onset is between 3 and 10 years of age.
2. Absences last 2 to 20 seconds, and are associated with a characteristic EEG abnormality (3-Hz spike-and-wave discharges activated by hyperventilation).
3. Absences clinically appear as staring spells during which the patient is momentarily unresponsive; usually with eyelid fluttering. Sometimes, the eyes roll upward or, rarely, there may be automatisms of lip-smacking, chewing, or other purposeless repetitive mouth or hand movements.
4. Absences occur frequently in flurries during the day; the child may be called a *day dreamer, absent-minded,* or *inattentive.* Absences may be recognized as transient pauses during eating, speaking, or any other activity.
5. Primary generalized absence seizures are distinguished from complex partial seizures by a lack of aura, a brief duration, and a lack of postictal confusion, drowsiness, or headache. Complex partial absences may be preceded by an aura, usually lasting longer than 30 seconds, and are followed by postictal confusion, which may be relatively brief.
6. Primary generalized absences can be brought out by hyperventilation that can be done as an office test: have the patient hyperventilate for 3 minutes under observation. During an absence, the hyperventilation will stop while the typical features of an absence seizure are observed, and then hyperventilation will resume immediately.
7. Absences may be complicated by other seizure phenomena: myoclonic jerks (a sudden increase in muscle tone, *throwing* the patient forward or backward) and atonic-akinetic seizures (dropping or *slumping* of the head or body because of a sudden decrease in muscle tone). If these symptoms occur in a patient younger than 3 years of age, they are termed *atypical absences* and are often part of another epilepsy syndrome such as Lennox-Gastaut syndrome or a myoclonic epilepsy. When absences occur initially after 10 years of age, they are part of another epilepsy syndrome—juvenile absence epilepsy—which many feel is a subset of or develops into juvenile myoclonic epilepsy.
8. Absences respond readily to treatment unless they are complicated by other seizure phenomena (see preceding paragraph); there is a risk for later development of generalized convulsions.
9. Absence status epilepticus consists of continuous absence seizures and may appear as a confusional state. The EEG shows continuous, bilateral 3-Hz spike-and-wave activity. It usually occurs:
   a. As a withdrawal syndrome (a sudden cessation of AEDs).
   b. As previously undiagnosed and untreated petit mal epilepsy occurring in adolescence or early adulthood.
   c. As incorrectly treated petit mal (e.g., using phenobarbital or phenytoin, rather than valproate or ethosuximide).

Treatment:

1. The drug of choice is ethosuximide (Zarontin) 20 to 30 mg/kg/day in 2 to 3 divided doses to maintain a blood level of 40 to 100 μg/ml.

2. Valproic acid in dosages of 10 to 30 mg/kg/day to maintain a therapeutic blood level of 50 to 100 μg/ml is also effective. Valproate is preferable as a single drug when absences are complicated by astatic or myoclonic seizures or if generalized convulsions occur concomitantly with absences. Other AEDs shown to be effective in absence seizures are lamotrigine and topiramate.

Generalized Convulsive Epilepsies

1. The onset is most frequent during childhood and adolescence.
2. Seizures, usually tonic-clonic, are bilaterally symmetric from the onset. Typically the patient loses consciousness and the body becomes rigid (a tonic phase) followed by jerky movements (a clonic phase) and postictal confusion or prolonged sleep.
3. An interictal EEG may be normal in as many as one third of patients.
4. Mental retardation and psychiatric disturbances are *not* usually associated with this disorder.
5. A family history of seizures is often elicited.
6. Findings from a neurologic examination and a CT scan or an MR image are normal. What was formerly termed *grand mal epilepsy,* referring to primarily generalized convulsions, now encompasses several epilepsy syndromes, including the following:
   a. Juvenile myoclonic epilepsy (JME): adolescents usually have generalized convulsions, but history uncovers early morning myoclonic jerks after awakening that had been occurring previously. Juvenile absences may also occur, and the EEG shows multiple spike–slow wave complexes activated by photic stimulation and drowsiness.
   b. Generalized tonic-clonic seizures on awakening: these seizures are usually found in adolescents who wake up in the morning with convulsions.
   c. Autosomal dominant nocturnal frontal lobe epilepsy: this is an inherited epilepsy in which seizures occur in sleep, with typical manifestations of frontal lobe origin; seizures are brief, or adversive (head or body turning contralateral to seizure focus), tonic postures. There may be few postical symptoms, or they may secondarily generalize into convulsions.
   d. Febrile seizures–generalized convulsions: this is another genetic syndrome, in which simple or complex febrile seizures in early childhood are followed years later by primary generalized convulsions.

Treatment: See comments concerning AEDs later in this chapter.

SEIZURES OF FOCAL ORIGIN (Partial seizures, localization-related epilepsies)

1. The onset is at any age. In early to middle adulthood the most common site of origin is the temporal lobe (mesial temporal sclerosis). In

infancy and childhood, extratemporal origin of focal seizures is more common.

2. The features of these partial seizures depend on the site and side of the lesion (and epileptogenic foci that result from the lesion) and the pattern of spread of the ictal electric discharge. A partial seizure with impairment of consciousness is categorized as a complex partial type; if consciousness is preserved, it is a simple partial type. Simple partial seizures may be sensory, psychosensory, or motor.

3. Partial seizures, simple or complex, may spread to both hemispheres, resulting in a secondarily generalized convulsion. Therefore an initial convulsion must always provoke the question: was it primarily, or secondarily, generalized?

4. A localized ictal EEG discharge is present at seizure onset, whereas the interictal EEG may show localized spikes or spike-and-wave activity with possible abnormalities of background activity focally or regionally. In secondarily generalized convulsions, the EEG findings may show bilaterally synchronous epileptiform discharges but a predominance of unilateral discharges at the same focus, called *secondary bilateral synchrony.*

5. MRI and a neurologic examination are mandatory in all cases and should include coronal cuts through the anterior temporal lobe and hippocampus, with appropriate sequences.

Focal Motor Seizures

Focal motor seizures manifest as clonic movements usually involving the arms or the legs. Sometimes the seizure may start in the thumb or the big toe and spread to involve the more proximal parts (a jacksonian seizure). A new-onset focal motor seizure suggests a structural lesion in frontoparietal lobes.

Complex Partial Seizures

1. Complex partial seizures are the most common form of seizures in adults.

2. These seizures consist of various automatisms—complex, coordinated but purposeless motor movements (e.g., lip-smacking or walking in a circle) with a blank stare or stereotyped verbal responses with impairment of consciousness. Any repeated stereotyped behavior may be a complex partial seizure.

3. The seizures are preceded by auras. (These may be only some type of difficult-to-describe feeling of strangeness.) Typical auras include the following:

   a. Déjà vu—the feeling of having experienced an event previously
   b. Jamais vu—the feeling of strangeness in familiar surroundings
   c. Fugue state—lapses in time (e.g., shopping in one store and then finding oneself without explanation of how or when one got there)
   d. Abdominal or epigastric sensations (often a rising sensation)
   e. An unexplained sudden fear with an urge to run, which may mimic panic attacks

    f. Visual, auditory, or olfactory hallucinations, which are usually complex, vivid, and unpleasant

    g. Distorted auditory or visual perceptions (macropsia, micropsia, macracusia, micracusia)

Note: Unpleasant olfactory hallucinations (called *uncinate auras*) are commonly associated with brain tumor.

    h. Distortions of time (desynchronization)—the feeling of being in slow motion (or in excessively rapid motion) compared to one's surroundings

4. Seizures last about 1 minute with a postictal state of confusion, headache, and exhaustion. Combativeness and violent behavior may occur during this period (especially if well-meaning observers attempt to help or restrain the individual).

5. Seizures may generalize secondarily with a loss of consciousness and tonic-clonic convulsive activity.

6. A routine awake EEG shows abnormality in less than 50% of patients; optimal records (about 65% showing temporal lobe spike discharge) are obtained with sphenoidal electrodes (during sleep) performed after 12 hours of sleep deprivation. EEG-activating procedures and long-term monitoring further increase the yield of positive tracings.

7. Personality, behavior, and cognitive disorders frequently complicate the picture and may produce severe psychosocial disability.

8. Complex partial status epilepticus may present as a state of confusion, altered behavior, or stupor. The EEG shows continuous 5- to 6-Hz high-voltage, rhythmic theta waves or spikes in temporal areas.

9. Complex partial seizures may also originate from the frontal lobe. The bizarre automatisms and postures are often diagnosed as pseudo-seizures. (See the section on generalized convulsive epilepsies [6c] in this chapter.)

Treatment: See comments regarding AEDs later in this chapter.

LATE-ONSET EPILEPSY

Up to 30 years of age in patients, primary generalized epilepsies may still present de novo. After that, seizures appearing for the *first time* are overwhelmingly caused by either acute or slowly progressive or acquired static lesions of the brain. Acute lesions include meningitis, encephalitis, cortical contusions from head injury, arterial or venous infarction, or tumors. The acute disturbance may also be a functional, potentially reversible encephalopathy. These include hypoglycemia, hepatic or uremic encephalopathy, hypertensive encephalopathy, or withdrawal syndromes from drugs or alcohol. Seizures starting after 60 years of age are often caused by underlying cerebrovascular disease.

    Old static lesions are most commonly a result of mesial temporal sclerosis, head injury (posttraumatic epilepsy), or stroke (postinfarction epilepsy) or are rarely caused by congenital hamartomas or mesial temporal sclerosis. Slowly progressive tumors may mimic old static lesions.

The most common seizures are partial seizures, which often generalize secondarily and usually result from lesions of the temporal lobe (complex partial seizures). Secondary generalized convulsions begin focally and then spread to involve both sides of the body rather than involving the body bilaterally and symmetrically from the onset.

Minimal studies in adults with a first seizure should include an EEG (preferably sleep deprived) and an imaging study, such as a CT scan if the presentation is emergent (with and without contrast enhancement), but preferably, an MRI or magnetic resonance angiography/venography (MRA)/(MRV) if a vascular formation, other vascular lesions, or neoplastic lesions are suspected. CSF studies may be needed when an infective metabolic or autoimmune cause is suspected. Besides routine CSF analyses, supplemental determinations are: polymerase chain reactions (PCR) for herpes simplex; Epstein-Barr cytomegalic inclusion virus and other viruses for encephalitis; elevated serum lactate to pyruvate ratio, elevated CSF lactate, or elevated lactate on brain MR spectroscopy for mitochondrial diseases; or GLUTR3 antibodies for Rassmussen's encephalitis, anti-GM1 ganglioside antibodies and antineuronal antibodies for autoimmune encephalitides. Therapy should be directed toward management of the underlying cause as well as symptomatic treatment of seizures.

ANTIEPILEPTIC DRUGS

1. The majority of patients should be treated with only *one* drug. Once a particular drug at a maximum tolerated dosage clearly does not completely control the seizures, another drug should be added. If this drug controls seizures, the first drug should be gradually weaned.
2. Trough serum levels should be obtained when there is a poor response to the dosage regimen, when there is intermittent illness, and when noncompliance is suspected. The correct dosage is one that renders the patient seizure free with no side effects; in some individuals, this dosage may be above or below the reference range of the laboratory.
3. Knowledge of the elementary clinical pharmacokinetics of the AEDs will make the physician a more skilled therapist. After a maintenance dosage regimen is started, it takes about five half-lives of the drug before a steady state is reached. Therefore the first blood levels for monitoring purposes should not be taken before that time (see Table 11-2 for half-lives). Trough levels (blood drawn just before a scheduled dose, preferably the first morning dose) should be assessed if seizure control or compliance is in question. If toxicity is the concern, a peak level (blood drawn 2 hours or more after a scheduled dose) should be assessed. Drugs with long half-lives (phenobarbital and phenytoin) can be given once a day, making compliance easier. Drugs with shorter half-lives (carbamazepine [Tegretol] and valproic acid) usually need to be given in three divided doses daily, but can be given as their sustained-release preparations twice a day or less.

4. Generic carbamazepine and phenytoins, made by different pharmaceutical companies, have different bioavailability. Switching from a brand name to a generic drug may lower AED blood levels and precipitate seizures. It is virtually impossible to get the same generic drug from the same pharmacist month after month.

Phenytoin

1. The usual dosage is 5 to 7 mg/kg/day (up to about 400 mg/day).
2. Phenytoin should be administered once daily, since the average serum half-life is 24 hours.
3. Dose-related side effects are:

Blood level (μg/ml)	Side effect
1-10	Undertreatment
10-20	Laboratory-defined therapeutic range (nystagmus in some patients)
20-30	Nystagmus
30-40	Diplopia, dysarthria, ataxia
>40	Drowsiness

Toxic effects—phenytoin has nonlinear pharmacokinetics so that at a critical point, a slight increase in dosage will cause a large increase in serum concentration, pushing the patient from therapeutic to toxic concentrations.

4. Side effects that are *not* dose-related include gum hypertrophy in about 40% of patients, coarsening of features over time, hirsutism in approximately 40% of patients, and exacerbation of acne. These side effects are especially noticeable in adolescents and may lead to noncompliance in women. Prevention of complications of gum hypertrophy (periodontal disease) requires habitual dental hygiene—toothbrushing and flossing twice daily.
5. Phenytoin rarely may cause a delayed hypersensitivity reaction consisting of fever and pruritic mucocutaneous maculopapular rash with subsequent desquamation that can be serious or fatal (Stevens-Johnson syndrome). Patients may cross-react to the other, older established AEDs (phenobarbitol, carbamazepine, valproic acid). This is called the AED hypersensitivity syndrome, and would cause the clinician to use the newer AEDs (such as gabapentin).
6. Oral dosage forms are 30- and 100-mg capsules and 50-mg chewable scored tablets.

Note: Oral suspensions with concentrations of either 25 or 6 mg/ml are available, but use of the oral suspension should be avoided, since it provides uneven doses because of the difficulty in achieving uniform mixing of the suspension.

7. Therapeutic phenytoin levels are hardly ever achieved by oral administration in the neonatal and toddler age group. Therefore chronic and prophylactic therapy should be avoided in this group. However, ther-

apeutic levels can be achieved quickly by parenteral administration (see 9 in this list) for its use in status epilepticus.

8. The parenteral dosage form is a solution of 50 mg/ml. The solution is highly alkaline and will precipitate if mixed with most other parenteral solutions. The solution should be injected, as much as possible, directly into the vein; saline may be used to flush the IV tubing. IV injection of phenytoin must be at a slow rate (no more than 50 mg/min in adults; no more than 1 mg/kg/min in infants) to prevent cardiac arrhythmias.

Caution: IM injection should *never* be used, since the phenytoin precipitates in muscle, producing necrosis and sterile abscesses, along with unpredictable serum levels of the drug.

9. All these considerations can be discarded by using fosphenytoin instead at equivalent doses that can be given IM (with rapid absorption and no local irritation) as well as IV in the usual parenteral solutions.

Carbamazepine

1. Carbamazepine is effective in partial seizures, simple and complex partial seizures, and secondarily generalized convulsions.
2. It is related structurally to the tricyclic antidepressants (TCAs), and is often effective in ameliorating the behavioral and emotional disturbances that accompany some complex partial seizure disorders.
3. This drug has been known to produce bone marrow suppression; all patients have a transient fall in white blood cell (WBC) count on initiation of the drug. Aplastic anemia and agranulocytosis are extremely rare (and have not been reported when the drug is used alone), but serial blood studies are recommended by the manufacturer.
4. Common initial side effects of the drug include ataxia, diplopia, and clouding of consciousness. The epoxide intermediary metabolite can be measured when toxic symptoms appear at reference range values.
5. The usual starting dosage of carbamazepine in adults is 200 mg 3 times a day (20 to 30 mg/kg/day in children). Since carbamazepine is an auto-inducer, a trough serum level should be done sometime after establishing the dosage, since one more adjustment may be necessary.
6. The drug is available in 200-mg scored tablets and 100-mg scored chewable tablets. A suspension (20 mg/ml) is also available.
7. Two sustained-release formulations of carbamazepine are available (Carbatrol and Tegretol XR). Their advantage is twice-a-day administration (increasing compliance), less toxic reactions, and usually more stable blood levels.
8. A new alternative is oxcarbazepine (Trileptal), which can be directly substituted for carbamazepine at equivalent doses. The advantages are less adverse side effects and twice-a-day administration, but the drug should be started by a neurologist.
9. This drug is useful if a depressive affect or depression accompanies epilepsy, presumably because of its "mood-stabilizing" effect. It is also sometimes effective if aggressive behavior is comorbid with the epilepsy.

Sodium Valproate, Valproic Acid, Divalproex Sodium

1. Valproate (Depakene, Depakote, Depacon) is a broad-spectrum AED that is highly effective in absence seizures, both typical and atypical; the myoclonic epilepsies; and primary or secondarily generalized convulsions. It is the first drug of choice when there is a combination of primary generalized convulsions and absence, myoclonus, or akinetic seizures.
2. Valproate is the only drug, besides phenobarbital, proven to be effective in prophylaxis of simple febrile seizures.
3. Periodic monitoring with a complete blood count (CBC) and liver function tests for the rare occurrence of bone marrow or hepatic toxicity, especially in children under 2 years of age, is recommended, although they probably are not cost-effective in older children and adults. What is probably more effective is explaining to the parents the symptoms of liver or bone marrow toxicity. If the symptoms appear, levels can then be checked.

Caution: Fatal hepatotoxicity has been reported in infants receiving multiple AEDs, including valproic acid. Valproic acid may precipitate underlying neurometabolic and neurodegenerative disease (organic acidurias or Alpers' disease) and should probably be avoided if these conditions are under diagnostic consideration.

4. Gastrointestinal upset with valproate is frequent in infants and toddlers, especially at the initiation of therapy. A mild tremor may appear. An abnormal platelet count and function may occur; hence platelet count and coagulation parameters should be checked before planned surgery. A skin rash may be benign but may also lead to Stevens-Johnson syndrome particularly if lamotrigine is also being given or is added on as polytherapy. Pancreatitis, which should be suspected when there is unexplained abdominal pain, is a serious complication and can be diagnosed by measuring serum lipase and amylase levels. Polycystic ovary disease is a possibility, particularly in obese women. It should be avoided, if possible, in women who are contemplating conception and pregnancy.
5. The usual dosage is 250 mg 3 times a day in school children (usually 20 to 30 mg/kg/day in younger children).
6. This drug is useful if "mood swings" or bipolar symptoms are comorbid with the epilepsy, presumably because of its action as a "mood stabilizer." Divalproex sodium is also useful for migraine prophylaxis, and comes in an extended-release preparation (Depakote 500 ER) that can be given once daily.
7. Valproate is available as enteric-coated divalproex sodium tablets (125, 250, and 500 mg) and also as sprinkle capsules (125 mg).
8. Depacon, the IV preparation of valproate, is useful for status epilepticus; for parenteral administration when the patient is taking nothing by mouth (NPO), as during surgery; or for rapid restoration of serum levels when patients have withdrawal seizures in the emergency room (noncompliance, low serum valproic acid levels). It has been reported effective in status migrainosus.

Phenobarbital

1. The usual dosage is 3 to 5 mg/kg/day (up to about 100 to 180 mg/day for men).
2. This drug may be administered as a single daily dose, since the average serum half-life is about 100 hours.
3. Phenobarbital in neonates and infants is still the drug of choice in the initial management of epilepsy but should be used with caution in older children or adolescents because of possible long-term cognitive side effects, though this is controversial.
4. It will produce hyperactivity in many children, particularly if the child has a previous tendency to be hyperactive or is neurodevelopmentally disabled. Methylated phenobarbital (mephobarbital or Mebaral) often eliminates the hyperactivity side effect, while maintaining the therapeutic effect.
5. It can exacerbate depression (affective disorder) in susceptible individuals and may be used in overdosage in suicide attempts.
6. This drug rarely may cause a delayed hypersensitivity reaction consisting of fever and pruritic mucocutaneous maculopapular rash with subsequent desquamation, which can be serious or fatal (Stevens-Johnson syndrome).
7. The oral dosage form is tablets of 15, 30, 60, or 100 mg and syrup of 4 mg/ml; in general, crushed tablets are preferred over the syrup in children, since an accurate measurement of the dose is difficult with the syrup and its taste is not pleasing to most children. There are compounding pharmacies in many locales that will mix any AED into a preparation that is pleasing to the taste and can be swallowed easily.

Ethosuximide

1. Ethosuximide is the drug of choice for typical primary generalized absence epilepsy.
2. It is less effective when absences are accompanied by myoclonic seizures or primary generalized convulsions; it is not effective in complex partial absences.
3. Gastrointestinal upset is the most frequent initial side effect of the drug.
4. Periodic monitoring with CBC and liver function tests for possible bone marrow and hepatic toxicity has traditionally been recommended but is probably not necessary or cost-effective.
5. The starting dosage of the drug is usually 250 mg 3 times a day.
6. The available dosage forms are 250-mg capsules and a syrup containing 50 mg/ml.

Clonazepam

1. Clonazepam is a diazepam derivative indicated primarily for myoclonic seizures, as in the JME syndrome or the benign, severe, or progressive myoclonic epilepsies.
2. This drug can be used as an adjunct in other primary generalized seizures, such as atonic-astatic seizures in the Lennox-Gastaut syndrome.

3. Drowsiness is a frequent initial side effect, so begin with a low dose at night, and build up slowly, using 0.5-mg tablets to 3 times a day. Drooling, particularly in infants and young children, is also a frequent side effect but can be relieved by glycopyrrolate (Robinul).

Caution: When used in combination with valproic acid, clonazepam may result in absence status ("electrical status" or "spike-wave stupor").

4. This drug is available as scored tablets of 0.5, 1.0, and 2.0 mg. An alternative with less drowsy side effects is clobazam, available in Canada and outside the United States, but it should be prescribed by a neurologist.

Newer Antiepileptic Medications
Gabapentin (Neurontin)

1. Gabapentin has no active metabolites. It is excreted unchanged by the kidneys. It is not protein bound and not a hepatic enzyme inducer.
2. The mechanism of the antiepileptic effect of gabapentin is unknown.
3. There are no known drug interactions with this drug.
4. Dosages ranging from 900 to 1800 mg/day have been used in clinical trials; however, dosages up to 3600 mg/day or greater may be used.
5. Side effects of this drug are usually minimal and include somnolence, dizziness, and fatigue.
6. Gabapentin is the drug of choice in patients with acute intermittent porphyria, since it has no effect on the liver.
7. It is the drug of choice in elderly patients on polypharmacy because of its lack of interactions.
8. Gabapentin would be the first AED to try in a patient with AED hypersensitivity syndrome.
9. It is the drug of choice in a typical benign rolandic epilepsy in which seizures may occur more frequently in daytime and in sleep, and when they generalize into convulsions.

Lamotrigine

1. Lamotrigine is a broad spectrum AED, showing efficacy in patients with partial seizures with or without secondary generalization, and also in the primary generalized epilepsies, such as absence seizures and in juvenile myoclonic epilepsy.
2. The most common side effects of this drug are dizziness, headache, diplopia, ataxia, and somnolence. A skin rash is seen in approximately 10% of patients. The incidence of rash is higher in patients taking valproic acid.
3. Lamotrigine is started at 25 mg/day for 1 week, then the daily dose is increased by 25 mg every week up to 100 mg twice a day. Dosages up to 500 mg/day have been used. The starting dose and rate of dose escalation should be halved in patients taking valproic acid to minimize the possibility of Stevens-Johnson syndrome.

Oxcarbazepine

1. Oxcarbazepine is the 10-keto analogue of carbamazepine. The absence of the oxidative step in its metabolism eliminates the occurrence of an

epoxide intermediate (and its toxicity) and minimizes the induction of cytochrome P-450 enzymes.

2. The indications for this drug are identical to those of carbamazepine.

3. Allergic skin reactions to this drug are rare, and cross-reactivity in carbamazepine-sensitive patients is only 25%.

   Topiramate (Topamax)

1. Topiramate is also a broad spectrum AED, indicated as an adjunctive AED for partial seizures with or without secondary generalization, but also effective in absence seizures.

2. It is started at 25 mg/day for 1 week, then the daily dose is increased by 25 mg/day every week. Dosages up to 1600 mg/day have been used.

3. Side effects of this drug include drowsiness, fatigue, cognitive changes, word-finding difficulties, renal stones, and weight loss.

   Levetiracetam (Keppra)

1. Levetiracetam is an adjunctive AED for partial seizures. In adults, it is usually started at 500 mg twice a day. In children, start at 125 mg twice a day and titrate upwards slowly.

2. Levetiracetam is eliminated primarily (66%) through the kidneys; it has a half-life between 6 and 8 hours.

3. The side effects of this drug include somnolence, asthenia, nervousness, dizziness, and headache.

   Zonisamide (Zonegran)

1. Zonisamide is a broad spectrum AED that is effective against partial, tonic, and myoclonic seizures. In adults, start the drug at 100 mg daily for 2 weeks, then increase every 2 weeks by 100 mg/day in twice-a-day doses. In children, start at 2 to 4 mg/kg/day. Maintenance in adults usually ranges from 200 to 600 mg/day; in children, maintenance ranges from 4 to 8 mg/kg/day.

2. Zonisamide is a sulfonamide and therefore is contraindicated in patients allergic to sulfa drugs. Patients will need adequate fluid intake to prevent renal stones.

3. Side effects of the drug include anorexia, somnolence, dizziness, difficulty concentrating, headache, weight loss, and renal stones.

Initiating AEDs

When the diagnosis of epilepsy is established, AED treatment should be instituted promptly. The appropriate drug should be chosen based on the type of seizure (Table 11-3).

1. Only *one* drug should be started at a time and given to its maximum therapeutic effect.

2. The medication should be initiated at about one half the suggested therapeutic dosage for 1 week. If no adverse side effects have appeared by that time and the patient has tolerated it well, the full therapeutic dosage may be given. Patients who experience adverse side effects from an excessive initial dose are likely to be poorly compliant in the future. Since it takes four or five half-lives to obtain a steady state, after approximately that elapsed time (see Table 11-2 for half-lives), obtain a serum drug level.

TABLE 11-3
Drugs of Choice in Treatment of Epilepsy

Seizure type	Drugs of choice
Generalized tonic-clonic seizures	Phenytoin, valproic acid
Simple and complex partial	Carbamazepine, oxcarbazepine
	Lamotrigine
	Primidone
	Phenobarbital, levetiracetam, zonisamide
	Gabapentin
	Ethosuximide
Absence	Valproic acid
Benign centrotemporal epilepsy	Phenytoin, gabapentin
	Phenobarbital
Neonatal seizures	Phenobarbital
Febrile seizures	Phenobarbital
	Valproic acid
Infantile spasms	Adrenocorticotropic hormone, vigabatrin
Lennox-Gastaut syndrome	Felbamate
	Clonazepam, lamotrigine, topiramate
NEWER DRUGS	
Generalized tonic-clonic seizures	Phenytoin, Valproic acid
Simple partial and complex partial	Carbamazepine, Oxcarbazepine
	Lamotrigine
	Primidone
	Phenobarbital
	Levetiracetam
	Gabapentin
Absence	Ethosuximide
Benign centrotemporal epilepsy	Gabapentin
Neonatal seizures	Phenobarbital
Febrile seizures	Diazepam (rectal Diastat)
Infantile spasms	Adrenocorticotropic hormone
Lennox-Gastaut syndrome	Felbamate

Drugs are listed in order of preference.

3. The process of instituting AED therapy is essentially a clinical titration. Serum levels are titrated against desired therapeutic effects (lessening or abolition of seizures), keeping in mind that undesirable side effects may limit attainment of the end point. The physician therefore needs accurate observations on the kinds, frequency, and duration of seizures from the patient. The physician can help the patient make these observations by requiring the patient to mail monthly calendars and progress reports in which seizures are charted. The patient should be encouraged to write down a descrip-

tion of the seizure from eyewitness observers as soon as possible after its occurrence.

4. Monotherapy: patients should be treated as far as possible with a single AED to avoid drug interactions that may affect efficacy and toxicity. If a single drug is ineffective or only partially effective, a second drug should be added. Then five half-lives later, if the blood level is within the therapeutic range and the seizures are controlled, the first drug should be withdrawn by one dose every five half-lives.

5. The general aim of the primary care physician is to aggressively control seizures within the first few months. If this is not achieved, prompt referral to a neurologist is indicated. Nowadays, if a general neurologist cannot control seizures after trying at least three or four established and new AEDs, this is termed *medication refractory epilepsy*. Referral to a level 3 or 4 epilepsy center is then made to determine whether the patient is a candidate for further drug trials, the ketogenic diet, epilepsy surgery, or the vagus nerve stimulator. In partial seizures, particularly temporal lobe epilepsy, if seizures are not controlled within 2 years, the patient should be referred to a level 3 or 4 epilepsy center to be considered for a temporal lobectomy.

Weaning from AEDs

A decision regarding drug weaning from AEDs depends on the duration of the seizure-free period, seizure type, epilepsy syndrome, age at onset, and the presence or absence of EEG abnormalities.

Neonates

The best data regarding neonatal seizures indicate that if seizures have stopped in the neonatal period, the AEDs can be withdrawn at 3 months of age. Whether seizures will recur later depends on the degree of cortical damage and underlying cause for neonatal seizures. Severe CNS damage suggests a high risk for developing the infantile spasms syndrome later in the first year of life.

Childhood and adolescence

1. Recent data indicate that in childhood epilepsy (exclusive of neonatal seizures, infantile spasms, the Lennox-Gastaut syndrome, or the severe myoclonic epilepsies), if a 2-year seizure-free period is obtained and EEG results show no epileptiform abnormalities, approximately 70% of children will remain seizure free for at least a 5-year follow-up period.

2. The EEG is a good predictor; patients with no slowing and no spikes are most likely to remain seizure free. Seizures of patients with both slowing and spikes are most likely to recur, whereas those of patients with either slowing or spikes are intermediate in likelihood of recurrence.

3. The particular epilepsy syndrome is also a factor for prognosis regarding recurrence of seizures after drug withdrawal. The primary partial epilepsies (benign centrotemporal epilepsy and benign occipital epilepsy) probably have the best prognosis and are likely to be "outgrown" (successful weaning of anticonvulsants with no recurrence) in adolescence. The same outcome occurs in approximately half of chil-

dren with primary generalized absence epilepsy by early adolescence and in most of the other half by the end of adolescence.

Late-onset (adult-onset) epilepsy

It is unclear whether the 2-year seizure-free criterion, or any other criterion, is applicable in adult-onset epilepsies. It is likely that in the majority of these patients, lifelong prophylactic AED therapy is a necessity. Even though the medical indications for continuing drugs after "good control" are hazy, many social factors conspire to adhere to anticonvulsants, such as the necessity to not have seizures to keep a driver's license and the fear of losing jobs if the individual has seizure recurrences. Finally, many patients prefer to feel "safe" rather than "sorry" and do not want to risk the possibility of status epilepticus if seizures recur when off AEDs.

When a decision is reached to withdraw AEDs, one drug at a time should be withdrawn. AEDs should be withdrawn slowly, at a rate of no more than one dose every five half-lives.

Compliance

1. Simple is best. A complex schema of drug administration may be scientifically optimal but will be difficult for a patient to follow. A minimal number of daily doses should be used; for phenobarbital and phenytoin, a single daily dose is effective. Adverse side effects resulting from large initial doses will lead to poor compliance later, so single doses are best given at bedtime.

2. The physician must encourage prescription renewal when at least 1 to 2 weeks' supply remains so that the patient will not run out of medication. Prescriptions should be written for 6 months to minimize risk of running out of medication.

3. The patient should be encouraged to always carry an extra full day's supply of AEDs to not be stranded without medication.

4. When traveling, the patient should carry a letter or card from the physician stating diagnosis and medications to obtain an emergency supply of medicines or treatment. This is particularly true when traveling in foreign countries, where strict drug enforcement laws may require confiscation of legitimate AED medication if it is not identified and justified.

5. Compliance can be assessed with the aid of serum AED levels.

6. *First impressions count.* The first several months after the diagnosis is made are the most important in establishing a pattern of patient compliance in both medication and follow-up treatment. *Physician availability* is important. When patients first begin taking AEDs, compliance can be fostered by the physician being available for telephone calls or for short, more frequent visits (every 3 to 6 weeks) to allay the patient's fears about side effects or toxic effects, to explain what to do if a seizure occurs, and generally to demystify epilepsy.

7. Appropriate patient, parent, and sibling education is necessary to ensure compliance. The more a patient knows about epilepsy and the more responsibility he or she takes for the management of this disorder, the more likely compliance will occur (see following paragraphs on patient education).

Patient Education

1. Initial patient reaction: when a patient receives the diagnosis of "seizure disorder" or "epilepsy," there is usually initial denial, followed by anger and perhaps depression, before final acceptance. Therefore the patient and physician should discuss the diagnosis in terms the patient can understand. No information should be released to employers or outside agencies without the patient's consent. Adolescents in particular are the group most likely to have difficulty accepting, "I am an epileptic."

2. Automobile driver's license: the patient should be seizure free for a period of time determined by law, which varies from state to state. In some states the physician is obligated to report to the state bureau of motor vehicles. It is important to note in the patient's chart that he or she has been advised of state law regarding driving.

3. School
   a. If seizures are frequent, a telephone discussion or a personal meeting between the physician and teacher or school nurse is helpful.
   b. The local chapter of the Epilepsy Foundation of America provides information useful for both the patient and family in dealing with the community and school and will sponsor in-service training for teachers and school officials on how to manage individuals with seizures.
   c. If seizures are rare, it is not necessary to inform the school.
   d. Learning disabilities and behavior problems can also occur in patients with seizures. These can relate to the seizures, the medications, a common underlying brain dysfunction or lesion, or may coexist independently.
   e. The physician must encourage vocational planning for patients with frequent seizures *early* in high school or even in junior high school.

4. Employment
   a. Unfortunately, discrimination against individuals with seizures still occurs. State agencies (generally in divisions of vocational rehabilitation) may be helpful in assisting the individual with seizures in finding employment or minimizing discrimination.
   b. Individuals with seizures should be encouraged to avoid occupations in which a seizure would be hazardous to themselves or coworkers.

5. Alcoholic beverages
   a. Consumption of alcoholic beverages in moderation will rarely increase the incidence of seizures, but alcohol and AEDs have additive effects, usually resulting in lowered alcohol tolerance.
   b. An alcoholic with seizures who continues to consume alcoholic beverages should probably not be given AEDs, since compliance is often poor and seizures from medication withdrawal alone may occur. Drinking must stop before AED prophylaxis can be effective.

6. Other drugs: reassure patients that they do not become addicted to AEDs. Warn them about drug interactions (Table 11-4), although the most commonly used over-the-counter medications, such as aspirin,

have no significant drug interactions. Warn that drug abuse with "speed," "uppers," or "downers" will result in significant drug interactions and probably exacerbate the epilepsy.

7. Birth control pills: although it is commonly believed that seizures are exacerbated by oral contraceptives, in reality this is unpredictable in any single patient. Other methods of birth control are available if seizures are exacerbated. Generally, the higher-progesterone, lower-estrogen oral contraceptives are less likely to exacerbate seizures.

8. Pregnancy: the risks of teratogenic effects of anticonvulsants on the fetus must be weighed against the risk of seizures occurring during pregnancy, with attendant effects on the pregnancy. Cleft lip, cleft palate, congenital heart defects, mental retardation, and neural tube defects have been reported to result in babies born of mothers taking AEDs during pregnancy but can be prevented if the mother takes

TABLE 11-4
Antiepileptic Drug Interactions

Drug	Serum level increased	Serum level decreased
Phenytoin	Chloramphenicol	Carbamazepine
	Disulfiram	
	Isoniazid	
	Dicumarol	
	Salicylates	
	Felbamate	
	Ethosuximide	
Carbamazepine	Erythromycin	Phenytoin
		Phenobarbital
		Primidone
Valproic acid	Felbamate	Carbamazepine
Phenobarbital	Valproic acid	
	Phenytoin	
Primidone	Valproic acid	Phenytoin
Felbamate	—	Phenytoin
		Carbamazepine
NEWER DRUGS		
Gabapentin	—	Intake with antacids
Lamotrigine	Valproic acid	—
Oxcarbazepine	—	Barbiturates
		Phenytoin
Levetiracetam	No significant interactions	
Zonisamide	—	Carbamazepine
		Phenobarbital
		Phenytoin
		Primidone

folic acid when thinking of conceiving. If at all possible, attempts should be made to keep mothers off AEDs when they are thinking of conceiving and through the first trimester of pregnancy. Fetal ultrasound studies and amniocentesis are recommended if there has been exposure to such drugs in early pregnancy. There is a risk for a bleeding tendency in babies born of mothers taking phenytoin. Giving vitamin K orally to the mother in the last month of pregnancy prevents this.

9. Genetics: several epilepsy syndromes follow mendelian inheritance, and the chromosomal location or gene itself are known. Most epilepsies, however, do not follow mendelian rules and have complex genetics. The primary generalized epilepsies are the most heritable of the epilepsies. There is a genetic component even in the acquired epilepsies. The risk of a child having epilepsy when one parent has either petit mal or grand mal is estimated to be as high as 12%. The genetics of the primary partial epilepsies is unclear. Although the secondary partial epilepsies, simple or complex, are caused by acquired lesions, whether these be demonstrable or not, there is some relationship to previous family history of epilepsy. Patients with severe head injury, for example, are more likely to develop posttraumatic epilepsy if there is a previous family history of epilepsy. However, it is not yet possible to predict the likelihood of epilepsy developing in the offspring of parents, one of whom has an acquired partial epilepsy.

10. Safety: AEDs should always be stored in locked cabinets to prevent the possibility of theft or accidental ingestion by children.

11. Dentists and dental hygiene: reassure dentists that there is no great danger of exacerbating seizures in the dentist's chair by giving local anesthetics and that there is no great danger of anesthetics interacting with anticonvulsants. Do instruct patients receiving phenytoin to visit their dentists at least twice a year and to brush their teeth at least twice daily. In addition, they should floss at least once daily.

12. Surgical operations: phenobarbital, phenytoin, and valproate can be given parenterally at equivalent doses during preoperative and postoperative phases when the patient is NPO. Phenytoin should *not* be given IM, since it is poorly absorbed through that route, but fosphenytoin can be given IV or IM. Because the period of NPO after surgery is usually less than 24 hours, parenteral administration of AEDs is usually not necessary. If seizures occur, IV diazepam or lorazepam, preferably, can tide the patient over until AEDs can again be taken orally.

13. Physical limitations: patients should be allowed to participate in physical and recreational activities that maintain physical fitness. Perhaps the only activities that require some limitations are swimming (in which the caution of never swimming alone should be scrupulously observed); contact sports, such as American football and ice hockey, in which serious injury could be sustained if a seizure occurs on the field or rink; and extreme sports, such as bungee jumping, skydiving, and hang gliding. (However there is wide room for individual physician judgment here.)

14. Resources
   a. For information about services to epileptics, low-cost prescription services, group life insurance, and general programs, the patient should contact the Epilepsy Foundation of America, 4351 Garden City Drive, Suite 406, Landover, MD 20785; (301)459-3700 or (800)332-1000; website: www.epilepsyfoundation.org. (See the bibliography for some reading materials that can be suggested for the individual with seizures.)

TREATMENT OF CONVULSIVE STATUS EPILEPTICUS
(see Chapter 20)

Convulsive status epilepticus is the state of continual seizures or, more commonly, recurrent convulsive seizures in which the patient does not fully regain consciousness between seizures. Status epilepticus most commonly occurs in known epileptics who stop taking medication. Rarely, status epilepticus is the first presentation of a seizure disorder, CNS infection (abscess or cerebral meningitis or encephalitis), metabolic disorder (hypoglycemia, hyponatremia, or hypocalcemia, inborn error of metabolism in young infants), or cerebrovascular disease (acute infantile hemiplegia, cortical venous thrombosis). It can occur in preschool children subject to febrile seizures as in febrile status epilepticus.

1. *Do not panic.* Treat the patient promptly but carefully.
2. Establish an adequate airway, then do the following:
   a. Remove false teeth.
   b. Turn the patient or his or her head to one side so that secretions can drain out of the mouth.
   c. Extend the neck (Fig. 11-1).
   d. Loosen tight clothing.
   e. Suction mouth as necessary.

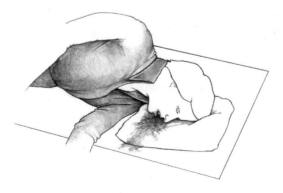

FIG. 11-1 Positioning the patient in convulsive status epilepticus.

    f. Place a padded object between the patient's teeth if the mouth is open. *(Do not force an object into a tonic, clenched jaw.)*

    g. Oxygen is not necessary immediately, as long as the airway is adequate.

3. Insert a needle into the patient's vein and draw blood for glucose, electrolyte, and calcium determinations; through the same needle instill 50% glucose 1 to 2 ml/kg (50 ml in an adult) and then begin continuous IV infusion with 5% dextrose in water solution.

4. Initially give lorazepam 0.1 mg/kg (up to 10 mg); you may give diazepam 0.37 mg/kg (up to 10 mg). *You must be prepared to support respiration with an Ambu bag, since brief respiratory arrest may occur after benzodiazepine (diazepam or lorazepam) administration. If you are unable or unprepared to provide respiratory support, do not give a benzodiazepine.*

5. After diazepam or lorazepam administration, whether or not seizures stop, or if a benzodiazepine is not administered, administer fosphenytoin 20 mg/kg.

6. If seizures do not stop within 10 minutes after administration of fosphenytoin (the drug takes about 10 minutes to reach a sufficient level in the brain to stop seizures), administer phenobarbital IV at a dose of 20 mg/kg. *At this point the patient's airway should be intubated.*

7. Continued seizures despite the previous medications are usually the result of a metabolic disturbance (such as hyponatremia or hypocalcemia) or a serious intracranial lesion (such as abscess, meningoencephalitis, or neoplasm), and the seizures will not stop until the underlying disorder is treated. General anesthesia, such as pentobarbital, propofol, or midazolam drip) coma, is a last resort and should be administered under EEG monitoring to titrate the burst-suppression pattern, preferably in an intensive care unit.

8. Maintenance doses of AEDs should be started immediately and administered IV (*never* IM) until oral doses can be started. These AEDs follow:

    a. Fosphenytoin 5 to 7 mg/kg/day (300 to 400 mg/day in adults) IV divided every 8 hours

    b. Phenobarbital 3 to 5 mg/kg/day (120 mg/day in adults) IV every 6 hours

    c. Valproate 20 mg/kg/day in children every 8 hours

TREATMENT OF NONCONVULSIVE STATUS EPILEPTICUS

Seizures other than generalized convulsions can occur continuously, and although not life threatening (because they do not derange respiratory function), they are disabling and must be recognized and treated.

1. *Absence status:* absence seizures occur either continuously or with only a few seconds break between seizures. The patient appears dazed, blank, or confused and may intermittently answer questions, usually slowly and irrelevantly. The EEG shows continual bilateral, generalized 3-Hz spike-and-wave complexes.

2. *Complex partial status:* the patient may appear similar to the patient with absence status, except that there may be automatisms continuously. The EEG concomitant is continual 5- to 6-Hz theta waves in one or both temporal lobes.
3. *"Subtle status":* patients, particularly the elderly, who may appear obtunded, usually because of an acute acquired lesion, may show on EEG negative focal low-to-moderate voltage sharp waves, or slow waves from areas of the brain other than the temporal lobes.
4. IV diazepam or lorazepam should immediately stop the status and confirm the diagnosis. In subtle status a return to the previously normal mental state may not be immediate and dramatic. The loading dose of the appropriate long-term AED should then be started.

BIBLIOGRAPHY

Arunkumar G, Morris H: Epilepsy update: new medical and surgical treatment options, *Cleve Clin J Med* 65(10):527-532, 534-537, 1998.

Bazil CW, Pedley TA: Advances in the medical treatment of epilepsy, *Annu Rev Med* 49:135-162, 1998.

Berkovic SF, Scheffer IE: Febrile seizures: genetics and relationship to other epilepsy syndromes, *Curr Opin Neurol* 11(2):129-134, 1998.

Berkovic, SF, Steinlein OK: Genetics of partial epilepsies, *Adv Neurol* 79:375-381, 1999.

Bowman ES: Pseudoseizures, *Psychiatr Clin North Am* 21(3):649-657, 1998.

Bowman ES: Nonepileptic seizures: psychiatric framework, treatment and outcome, *Neurology* 53(5 Suppl 2):S84-S88, 1999.

Bradford JC, Kyriakedes CG: Evaluation of the patient with seizures: an evidence based approach, *Emerg Med Clin North Am* 17(1):203-220, 1999.

Browne, TR, Hohnes GL: *Handbook of epilepsy,* Philadelphia, 1997, Lippincott-Raven.

Chokroverty S: *Management of epilepsy,* Woburn, Mass, 1996, Butterworth-Heinemann.

Cole AJ: Is epilepsy a progressive disease? The neurobiological consequences of epilepsy, *Epilepsia* 41(Suppl 2):S13-S22, 2000.

Delanty N, Vaughan CJ, French JA: Medical causes of seizures, *Lancet* 352:383-390, 1998.

Devinsky, O: *A guide to understanding and living with epilepsy,* Philadelphia, 1994, FA Davis.

Eisenschenk S, Gilmore R: Strategies for successful management of older patients with seizures, *Geriatrics* 54(12):31, 34, 39-40, 1999.

Freeman JM, Vining EPG, Pillas DJ: *Seizures and epilepsy in childhood: a guide for parents,* Baltimore, 1990, Johns Hopkins University Press.

Hart YM, Andermann F: Migraine aura, seizures, and temporal lobe epilepsy, *Adv Neurol* 81:145-152, 1999.

Hermann BP, Seidenberg M, Bell B: Psychiatric comorbidity in chronic epilepsy: identification, consequences, and treatment of major depression, *Epilepsia* 41(Suppl 2):S31-S41, 2000.

Jones MW: Consequences of epilepsy: why do we treat seizures? *Can J Neurol Sci* 25(4):S24-S26, 1998.

Krumholz A: Nonepileptic seizures: diagnosis and management, *Neurology* 53(5 Suppl 2):S76-S83, 1999.

Marks WJ Jr, Garcia PA: Management of seizures and epilepsy, *Am Fam Physician* 57(7):1589-1600, 1603-1604, 1998.

Mattson RH: Medical management of epilepsy in adults, *Neurology* 51(5 Suppl 4):S15-S20, 1998.

McLaughlin D: Epilepsy: key management issues, *Aust Fam Physician* 28(9):889-891, 896, 1999.

McNamara JO: Emerging insights into the genesis of epilepsy, *Nature* 399(6738 Suppl):A15-A22, 1999.

Pellock JM: Treatment of seizures and epilepsy in children and adolescents, *Neurology* 51(5 Suppl 4):S8-S14, 1998.

Ramsay RE, Pryor F: Epilepsy in the elderly, *Neurology* 55(5 Suppl 1):S9-S14 (discussion S54-S58, 2000.

Roth HL, Drislane FW: Seizures, *Neurol Clin* 16(2):257-284, 1998.

Sander JW: New drugs for epilepsy, *Curr Opin Neurol* 11(2):141-148, 1998.

Schachter SC, Montouris GD, Pellock JM: *The Brainstorms family, epilepsy on our terms: stories by children with seizures and their parents,* Philadelphia, 1996, Lippincott-Raven.

Schachter SC, Schomer DL: *The comprehensive evaluation and treatment of epilepsy, a practical guide,* San Diego, 1997, Academic Press.

Scheffer IE, Berkovic SF: Genetics of the epilepsies, *Curr Opin Pediatr* 12(6):536-542, 2000.

Schwartz JM, Marsh L: The psychiatric perspectives of epilepsy, *Psychosomatics* 41(1):31-38, 2000.

Shafer PO: New therapies in the management of acute or cluster seizures and seizure emergencies, *J Neurosci Nurs* 31(4):224-230, 1999.

Sirven JJ: Epilepsy in older adults: causes, consequences, and treatment, *J Am Geriatr Soc* 46(10):1291-1301, 1998.

Stephen LJ, Brodie MJ: Epilepsy in elderly people, *Lancet* 355(0213):1441-1446, 2000.

Sundaram M, Sadler RM, Young GB, Pillay N: EEG in epilepsy: current perspectives, *Can J Neurol Sci* 26(4):255-262, 1999.

Tomson T: Mortality in epilepsy, *J Neurol* 247(1):15-21, 2000.

Toone BK: The psychoses of epilepsy, *J Neurol Neurosurg Psychiatry* 69(1):1-3, 2000.

Torta R, Keller R: Behavioral, psychotic, and anxiety disorders in epilepsy: etiology, clinical features, and therapeutic implications, *Epilepsia* 40(Suppl 10):S2-S20, 1999.

Wiebe S, Blume WT, Girvin JP, Eliaszew M: A randomized, controlled trial of surgery, *N Engl J Med* 345:311-318, 2001.

Wiebe S, Derry PA: Measuring quality of life in epilepsy surgery patients, *Can J Neurol Sci* 27(Suppl 1):S111-S115 (discussion S121-S125), 2000.

WEBSITES

American Epilepsy Society: www.aesnet.org

Epilepsy Foundation of America: www.efa.org

Febrile seizures fact sheet: www.ninds.nih.gov/health_and_medical/disorders/febrile_seizures.htm

National Institute of Neurological Disorders and Stroke (NINDS): www.ninds.nih.org

Seizure disorders in childhood: www.meddean.luc.edu/lumen/MedEd/pedneuro/epilepsy.htm

12

The Stroke Syndrome

CLINICAL EVALUATION
Stroke, in Neurologic Terms
Stroke, in neurologic terms, refers to the sudden onset of a focal neurologic deficit caused by a central nervous system (CNS) vascular event. A transient ischemic attack (TIA) is an ischemic event, the symptoms of which last less than 24 hours and usually less than 1 hour. Stroke is the third leading cause of death and the leading cause of long-term disability in the United States, with 4 million stroke survivors and 750,000 new stroke cases annually. From an economic standpoint strokes cost more than $43 billion annually, with more than $28 billion in direct costs.

Stroke Classification
Strokes are generally classified as *ischemic* (approximately 85%) or *hemorrhagic* (approximately 15%). It is impossible to differentiate the two types of strokes based solely on the clinical examination.

Ischemic stroke is the result of vascular occlusion from thrombosis or embolus. The majority of ischemic strokes are a result of small vessel lacunar disease. Other causes of thromboembolic strokes are large vessel atherosclerotic disease and cardioembolic disease (atrial fibrillation, prosthetic valve disease, rheumatic heart disease, bacterial endocarditis, atrial myxoma, or dilated cardiomyopathy). The remainder of large vessel ischemic strokes are caused by arterial dissection, hypercoagulable states, hypotension, vasculitis, or cryptogenic causes. Small vessel ischemic strokes are caused by chronic hypertension.

Hemorrhagic strokes are the result of hypertension (subcortical hemorrhages in the basal ganglia, thalamus, pons and cerebellum), a ruptured berry aneurysm, bleeding, an arteriovenous malformation (AVM), or amyloid angiopathy (lobar hemorrhages in older patients).

Conditions That Mimic Stroke
Conditions that mimic stroke include seizures with postictal paralysis, migraine, drug intoxication (e.g., hypoglycemia/hyperglycemia, hypothyroidism), and hyperventilation. Occasionally, other CNS diseases appear with abrupt onset of focal neurologic symptoms, such as brain neoplasm, multiple sclerosis (MS), brain abscesses, and subdural hematoma.

TABLE 12-1
Clinical Features and Localization of Stroke

Symptoms	Signs	Location
Weakness: limb (arm or leg) and face on one side	Contralateral limb and facial weakness (arm greater than leg), spasticity, increased reflexes (not acutely)	Hemispheric/cortical
Associated sensory loss, visual loss, and speech and language disturbances	Sensory loss aphasia, apraxia, neglect, hemianopia	
Weakness: face, arm, and leg on one side	Contralateral limbs and facial weakness, arm and leg (often equally affected) spasticity, increased reflexes, sensory loss	Subcortical/internal capsule
Sensory loss in same areas as weakness		
Speech disturbance (no language disturbance)	No aphasia, apraxia, neglect, or hemianopia	
Weakness: face on one side with limbs on the opposite side	—	Brainstem
Incoordination	—	Cerebellum

HISTORY

The patient's history may be helpful in determining the cause of the stroke syndrome. It is important to have the patient's story corroborated by a family member or witness. In some cases, such as in comatose patients or patients with aphasia, family members may be the only source of history.

1. Onset
   a. An abrupt onset followed by a gradual improvement suggests embolus. ("While I was washing dishes, my right arm suddenly became paralyzed and I dropped a cup.")
   b. An acute onset with a progression to maximal deficit over minutes to hours suggests thrombosis.
   c. A stepwise development or an onset during sleep usually suggests thrombosis.
   d. Focal neurologic symptoms usually lasting minutes but no longer than 24 hours suggest a TIA.
   e. An onset associated with a severe headache or alteration in consciousness suggests intracerebral hemorrhage.
2. Questions should be directed to the following symptoms (also see Table 12-1):
   a. An alteration of consciousness
   b. Severe headache

c. Neck stiffness

d. Visual disturbances (Amaurosis fugax—a monocular blindness of short duration—usually indicates carotid artery disease with embolism to the ophthalmic artery, which is the first branch of the internal carotid artery.)

e. A disturbance of equilibrium (common in posterior fossa disorders)

f. Motor or sensory disturbances (Fig. 12-1)

g. The time of symptom onset (the last time the patient was known to be without symptoms)

h. Head trauma

i. A seizure at onset

j. Chest pain or palpitations (suggesting concurrent myocardial infarction)

k. Precipitating factors and risk factors, including the following:

1) Hypertension
2) Diabetes mellitus
3) Atherosclerosis
4) Cardiovascular disease, especially atrial fibrillation in the patient or family members
5) Hypercholesterolemia or hyperlipidemia

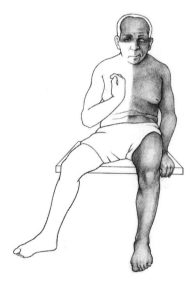

FIG. 12-1 Spastic hemiparesis and lower facial weakness sparing the forehead suggest contralateral cerebral hemisphere damage, often a result of medically or surgically treatable carotid artery disease. Other symptoms are described in Table 12-1.

6) Cigarette smoking
7) Obesity and sedentary lifestyle
8) Excessive alcohol intake
9) Illicit drug use, especially cocaine use
10) A hypercoagulable state
11) Male gender, age, family history, and race
12) A TIA

Note: A TIA is an independent risk factor with a 28% risk of stroke within 5 years after a TIA. Always admit patients with TIAs to the hospital and work them up urgently for treatable causes. Do not investigate acute stroke or TIAs on an outpatient basis.

3. The patient may have a past medical history, especially of cardiovascular disease, hypertension, diabetes, head trauma, warfarin (Coumadin) use, or a recent infection.
4. The patient's family may have a history of atherosclerotic cardiovascular disease or cerebral aneurysm.

EXAMINATION

In addition to the routine examination of the patient, the following steps are especially important:
1. Check for fever or a stiff neck (often associated with intracranial hemorrhage or infections).
2. If possible, take the blood pressure in both arms with the patient in the lying and standing positions (subclavian steal, postural hypotension).
3. Record the level of consciousness using the Glasgow Coma Scale (see Chapter 13).
4. Check the heart for arrhythmias, murmurs, and enlargement; check the lungs for congestion and friction rubs.
5. Check all peripheral pulses. (A cardiac mural thrombus may fragment and occlude arteries of the limbs.)
6. Evaluate carotid artery blood flow by listening for carotid bruits. The classic carotid bruit of carotid stenosis is harsh and systolic, emanates from the carotid bifurcation, and radiates to the angle of the jaw. A bruit on the same side as the brain lesion is especially important. Diminished carotid pulse is of no value because an occluded carotid may appear to pulsate normally. (The pulsations are transmitted directly from the aorta.) A bruit over the supraclavicular fossa suggests stenosis of the vertebral or subclavian arteries (Fig. 12-2).
7. Examine the optic fundi for the following:
   a. Early signs of papilledema (e.g., loss of venous pulsations and wet-appearing retinas), indicating subarachnoid hemorrhage or mass lesions
   b. Retinal infarction or cholesterol embolus (a small, bright-yellow fragment in an artery), suggesting carotid artery ulceration

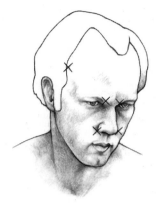

FIG. 12-2 Palpation of temporal, nasal, and supraorbital pulses (*X* marks) may provide evidence of collateral circulation following a carotid occlusion.

   c. Signs of subacute bacterial endocarditis (SBE), such as petechial conjunctival hemorrhages or hemorrhages beneath the fingernails

LABORATORY EVALUATION

The following studies are available in all hospitals and should be performed in every stroke patient in the first hour of presentation:

1. A computed tomographic (CT) scan of the head without contrast, the single most important emergency diagnostic test. It is not currently possible to care for a stroke patient without access to CT scans 24 hours a day, 7 days a week. The scans should be done *without* contrast to differentiate ischemia from hemorrhage (hemorrhage and contrast are both white on CT scan images).
2. An electrocardiogram (ECG) to evaluate for arrhythmias and concurrent myocardial infarction.
3. A glucose test (hypoglycemia appears with focal neurologic deficits); an immediate fingerstick glucose for a more rapid result.
4. A complete blood count (CBC), platelet count, type, and screen.
5. The erythrocyte sedimentation rate (ESR). (An elevated ESR may be related to an infection or an autoimmune process such as lupus erythematosus or temporal arteritis.)
6. The prothrombin time/international normalized ratio (PT/INR) and partial thromboplastin time (PTT).
7. Liver and renal panels.
8. Serum and urine toxicology tests.
9. If myocardial infarction is suspected, serum for cardiac enzymes.

10. Test arterial blood gases if respiratory compromise is suspected.
11. Other laboratory tests to consider:

> Antinuclear antibody (ANA) levels
> Lipid profile
> Urinalysis
> Thyroid stimulating hormone (TSH) levels
> Venereal Disease Research Laboratory test (VDRL)

The following laboratory tests should be considered in select patients:

Laboratory tests	Indications
Human chorionic gonadotropin (hCG) β levels	Female
Antiphospholipid antibody levels	Prior miscarriages
Protein C and S levels	Hypercoagulable state
Antithrombin III levels	Hypercoagulable state
Factor V Leiden levels	Hypercoagulable state
Lupus anticoagulant levels	Hypercoagulable state
Anticardiolipin antibody levels	Hypercoagulable state
Prothrombin gene mutation assay	Hypercoagulable state
Homocysteine level	Hypercoagulable state
Human immunodeficiency virus (HIV) tests	Clinical suspicion
Lyme titer	White matter lesion
Serum protein electrophoresis	Vasculitis

The following imaging studies are included in stroke evaluation:
1. A CT scan: a CT scan of the head without contrast can rule out hemorrhage. The five possible CT scan findings include the following:
   a. An intracerebral hemorrhage (hyperdense or white matter on a noncontrast CT scan)
   b. A subarachnoid hemorrhage (hyperdense or white matter in the cisterns of subarachnoid areas)
   c. A cerebral infarction (hypodense or dark matter on a noncontrast CT scan), not seen in the first 3 hours after symptom onset
   d. Normal findings (a CT scan may not show any abnormalities for up to 12 hours after a stroke)
   e. Lesions other than stroke (tumor, abscess, AVM, subdural hematoma, or epidural hematoma)
2. Magnetic resonance imaging (MRI): an MR image can identify many abnormalities not evident on a CT scan, such as lacunar infarct, MS plaques, or tumors. MRI diffusion-weighted imaging (DWI) becomes positive for ischemia within 30 minutes of symptom onset. Therefore DWI is used to define the extent of an acute stroke. MRI perfusion-weighted imaging (PWI), a relatively new imaging technique, is used to define the area of the brain with reduced perfusion. This allows the clinician to determine the tissue at risk for stroke. When a mismatch between DWI and PWI exists, thrombolysis or neuroprotective agents can reduce the risk of stroke extension (see Management of Acute Stroke in this chapter).

Note: An MR scanner may not be available in all hospitals or available 24 hours a day, 7 days a week. When such a study is needed to determine stroke management, the patient should be transported to a designated stroke center.

3. Magnetic resonance angiography (MRA): MRA is used to screen the patency of major arteries of the brain. Magnetic resonance venography (MRV) can evaluate for venous thrombosis.
4. Four-vessel cerebral angiography: if the patient is suspected of having a subarachnoid hemorrhage, whether or not a CT scan is confirmatory, an angiogram is required to identify an aneurysm or AVM. If the patient is a candidate for intraarterial thrombolysis, an angiogram is required. If a carotid stenosis is seen on an ultrasound or MRA and a carotid endarterectomy is being considered, an angiogram is recommended to define the vasculature. Angiography carries a 1% risk of complications, including stroke and death, so the procedure should be ordered with caution.
5. Carotid ultrasound: this ultrasound technique is a useful and accurate method of noninvasive assessment of the carotid arteries in the neck. Stenosis and plaques are identified through high resolution B-mode imaging, and the flow velocity is assessed by Doppler signals. This technique is also ideal for serial studies to assess the progression of plaques and degree of stenosis.
6. Transcranial ultrasound: this ultrasound technique allows assessment of intracranial vessel patency.
7. Transesophageal echocardiogram: this study identifies cardiac mural thrombi, heart valve vegetations, and fibrin strands that can be sources of emboli.
8. Electroencephalography (EEG): this study is most useful in patients suspected of having a seizure disorder associated with stroke or in the identification of an underlying toxic-metabolic disorder. It is also useful in supporting the diagnosis of a superficial hemispheric lesion.
9. Lumbar puncture (LP): An immediate LP is indicated in the following situations:
   a. In suspected cases of a CNS infection without evidence of increased intracranial pressure.
   b. When xanthochromic CSF would be a contraindication to anticoagulation. A normal LP sample (often found with ischemic infarcts) decreases the probability that the deficit is caused by intracranial hemorrhage, tumor, or subdural hematoma.

MANAGEMENT OF ACUTE STROKE

Ideally a stroke team of a neurologist and an interventional neuroradiologist will manage a case of acute stroke.

After Stabilization of the Patient

After stabilization of the patient, and if the CT scan is normal, candidacy for thrombolysis should be considered. If the onset of symptoms was

---

BOX 12-1
Protocol for IV rt-PA for Acute Stroke

INCLUSION CRITERIA

- Acute ischemic brain infarction with onset, clearly defined, less than 2 hours before rt-PA will be given
- A significant neurologic deficit expected to result in major long-term disability
- A noncontrast CT scan showing no hemorrhage or well-established infarct
- No exclusions (see below)

ABSOLUTE EXCLUSION CRITERIA

- Mild or rapidly improved deficits
- Hemorrhage on a CT scan; well-established acute infarct on a CT scan; any other CT diagnosis that contraindicates treatment (e.g., tumor, abscess)
- Known CNS vascular malformation or tumor
- Bacterial endocarditis

RELATIVE CONTRAINDICATIONS*

- Significant trauma within 3 months (includes CPR with chest compressions within the past 10 days)
- Stroke within 3 months
- A history of intracranial hemorrhage; or symptoms suspicious for subarachnoid hemorrhage
- Major surgery within past 14 days
- Minor surgery within past 10 days, including liver or kidney biopsy, thoracentesis, lumbar puncture
- Arterial puncture at a noncompressible site within past 14 days
- Pregnant (up to 10 days postpartum) or nursing woman

---

rt-PA, Recombinant tissue plasminogen activator; *CT,* computed tomography; *CNS,* central nervous system; *CPR,* cardiopulmonary resuscitation.
*Also consideration should be given to the increased risk of hemorrhage in patients with severe deficits (National Institute of Health stroke scale [NIHSS]>20), age 75 or early edema with mass effect on a CT scan.

Continued

within 3 hours, the patient may be a candidate for intravenous (IV) thrombolysis using alteplase (recombinant tissue plasminogen activator [rt-PA]). rt-PA is administered in a hospital with a stroke service that has the capability of diagnosis and management of neuro critical care patients (Box 12-1).

Symptom Onset

If the symptom onset was within 6 hours, the patient may be a candidate for intraarterial thrombolysis. A certified interventional neuroradiologist should be consulted to perform this procedure.

BOX 12-1
Protocol for IV rt-PA for Acute Stroke—cont'd

RELATIVE CONTRAINDICATIONS—cont'd

- Gastrointestinal, urologic, or respiratory hemorrhage within past 21 days
- Known bleeding diathesis (includes renal and hepatic insufficiency)
- Peritoneal dialysis or hemodialysis
- PTT>40 sec; PT>15 sec; (INR>1.7 sec); platelet count <100,000
- SBP>180 mm Hg or DBP >110 mm Hg, despite basic measures to lower it acutely (see treatment recommendations below)
- Seizure at onset of stroke (This relative contraindication is intended to prevent treatment of patients with a deficit caused by postictal Todd's paralysis or with seizure caused by some other CNS lesion that precludes rt-PA therapy. If a rapid diagnosis of vascular occlusion can be made, treatment may be given in some cases.)
- Glucose <50 mg/dl or >400 mg/dl (This relative contraindication is intended to prevent treatment of patients with focal deficits caused by hypoglycemia or hyperglycemia. If the deficit persists after correction of the serum glucose or if a rapid diagnosis of vascular occlusion can be made, treatment may be given in some cases.)

PRETREATMENT WORK-UP

- Temperature, pulse, blood pressure, respirations
- Physical examination/neurologic examination
- Electrocardiogram
- CBC with platelets, basic metabolic and hepatic function panel, PT/INR, PTT, ESR, fibrinogen level
- Urine hCG in women of child-bearing potential
- Consider hypercoagulable panel in young patients without apparent stroke risk factors
- Blood for type and cross-match
- A noncontrast head CT scan

PTT, Partial thromboplastin time; *PT,* prothrombin time; *INR,* international normalized ratio; *SBP,* systolic blood pressure; *DBP,* diastolic blood pressure; *CBC,* complete blood count; *ESR,* erythrocyte sedimentation rate; *hCG,* human chorionic gonadotropin.

Antiplatelet Agents

Antiplatelet agents for secondary prevention of atherothrombotic strokes and TIAs include aspirin (50 mg to 325 mg/day), clopidogrel (75 mg/day at approximately $80/month), and a combination of aspirin and extended-release dipyridamole (25 mg/200 mg twice a day at approximately $80/month). The risks, benefits, and cost should be considered when choosing an agent. Aspirin has been found to have a stroke risk reduction that is equivalent to clopidogrel but with more gastrointestinal (GI) adverse effects. Extended-release dipyridamole combined with aspirin has been shown to be more effective than aspirin alone and has a similar side effect profile as clopidogrel.

Anticoagulation with Warfarin

Anticoagulation with warfarin for the prevention of stroke in patients with atrial fibrillation or in patients with other high-risk cardiac conditions who have had a stroke or a TIA is recommended. A target INR of 2.5 seconds is beneficial.

Supportive Therapy for Stroke Victims

1. Nursing orders to monitor neurologic status. During the first 24 hours after a stroke, the patient should be evaluated hourly. In addition to the Glasgow Coma Scale (see Chapter 13), and monitoring of blood pressure, pulse, temperature (rectal), and respirations, the nursing staff should be taught to evaluate pupillary size, equality, and reaction to light.

2. Nursing management. The following precautions may be beneficial:

a. Use above-the-knee elastic stockings to minimize the development of phlebothrombosis or thrombophlebitis.

b. Use dorsiflexion splints or a footboard and sandbags to maintain the foot of the paralyzed leg in dorsiflexion.

c. Roll towels or other soft objects in the patient's hand to maintain the hand's function.

d. Be aware of and apprise the nursing staff of hemianopia and hemineglect and position the patient approximately to accommodate these phenomena.

e. Frequently turn the patient to prevent bedsores.

f. If the patient cannot close the eyelids, instill artificial tears to prevent corneal ulcers.

g. In the patient with diplopia, alternate patching of the eyes to improve vision and make the patient comfortable.

h. In the alert patient with speech difficulty, provide a communication board that contains common requests.

i. Use stool softeners early to prevent fecal impaction.

j. As soon as possible, place the patient in an upright or sitting position intermittently to prevent postural hypotension.

k. Especially in the case of the aphasic patient, explain to the family that speech difficulty does not mean dementia. A simple explanation of the problem will relieve family anxiety.

3. Blood pressure management. Most stroke victims will have transient hypertension. A moderately elevated blood pressure is the body's protective mechanism to ensure adequate cerebral perfusion. (Even in hemorrhage, vasospasm is common.) A recommended target blood pressure in ischemic stroke is 160 to 180 mm Hg/80 to 90 mm Hg. A recommended target systolic blood pressure in hemorrhagic stroke is 140 to 160 mm Hg.

Note: Avoid treating blood pressure aggressively in a patient with acute ischemic stroke. If the systolic blood pressure rises above 220 mm Hg and the diastolic blood pressure rises above 120 mm Hg, consider using IV labetalol drip. Never prescribe oral antihypertensives in this case.

   4. Nutritional support. Nutritional support should include the following:
   a. IV fluids should contain multivitamins, including thiamine, to prevent Wernicke's encephalopathy.
   b. Syndrome of inappropriate antidiuretic hormone (SIADH) can occur with stroke. Recording of fluid intake and output is important.
   c. Nitrogen and electrolyte balance is best accomplished with nasogastric feedings. The patient should receive nutrition via this route (rather than IV) as soon as possible.

   5. Bladder care. Urinary retention in the acute phase is common, but an indwelling catheter should be used cautiously. If an indwelling catheter is used, intermittent clamping should be done to avoid loss of bladder tone. Bladder function returns quicker in patients who have intermittent rather than continuous catheterization. Patients with indwelling catheters tend to have severe urinary tract infections and bladder dysfunction caused by chronic scarring.

   6. Pulmonary care. Frequent suctioning of excess secretions, frequent turning, induced coughing, and deep breathing will help prevent atelectasis. Oxygen should be administered only when arterial oxygen pressure is low.

   7. Cardiac care. Because there is such a high correlation between cerebral infarction and cardiac abnormalities, continuous cardiac monitoring should (whenever possible) be instituted.

   8. Physical therapy. Patients who remain bedridden for any length of time are at risk for developing serious complications, such as pulmonary embolism or orthostatic hypotension. With the exception of patients who suffer from subarachnoid hemorrhage, stroke victims who are encouraged to sit or stand as soon as possible improve more rapidly and have fewer complications. If the patient is bedridden for any length of time, passive physical therapy can reduce the risk of pulmonary embolism. Physical therapy is also important in preventing contractures, since significant contractures may develop in the shoulder girdle within 24 hours.

   9. Treatment of cerebral edema. Treatment should include the following:
   a. Approximately 48 to 72 hours after infarction, cerebral edema can develop, causing the patient's condition to deteriorate. Corticosteroids have little effect on this edema and may have detrimental side effects in a stroke patient (as opposed to the dramatic effect of corticosteroids on the edema surrounding a tumor).
   b. Mannitol (in a 10% to 20% solution), at a dose of 1 g/kg in extreme cases, will aid in dehydration. Daily weighing of the patient and monitoring of electrolytes and osomolarity are mandatory with this type of therapy.

   10. Speech and language therapy. If communication is disturbed by the stroke, speech and language therapy may be helpful. The speech (language) pathologist specifically evaluates auditory processing; retention, reading, and writing abilities; and speaking abilities. From this evaluation, a treatment program is designed using the patient's strengths to improve weakness. The speech therapist identifies the specific problems in communication, consults with the physician and hospital staff, and counsels and advises the family members. The speech therapist can assist the physician in educating the family regarding difficulties, such as those of aphasic patients, and can work with the family and patient on a home program. Thorough explanation of the patient's communication difficulties to the family alleviates embarrassment stemming from misunderstanding. The patient should be encouraged to participate in social situations as much as possible. Follow-up treatment is usually arranged for reevaluation and updating of therapy. Speech therapists may note minor changes in speech patterns, which may be subtle signs of recurring disease.

11. Occupational therapy. In the rehabilitation of stroke patients, the aim of occupational therapy overlaps those of speech and physical therapy with a strong emphasis on functional skills for the activities of daily living (ADLs). In cooperation with physical therapy, occupational therapy includes improving or maintaining the range of motion, strength, coordination, and balance and reducing spasticity. Therapists provide splints to prevent contracture and slings to prevent subluxation of the shoulder. Evaluation and training is available for patients with perceptual dysfunctions. In conjunction with speech therapy, occupational therapists improve coordination for speech and fine coordination for writing. Special attention is given to retraining or assistance in the ADLs, such as dressing and feeding. Adaptive equipment is provided, and patients are taught how to use it most effectively.

12. The rehabilitation hospital. There is increasing pressure on the physician to discharge patients from the acute care hospital as soon as possible. Rehabilitation hospitals offer an environment in which physical therapists, speech therapists, occupational therapists, and physicians specializing in neurorehabilitation work as a team to help the patient reach maximal functional capacity. A stroke victim will continue to improve for approximately 6 to 12 months. This alternative should be considered if the patient is moderately to severely disabled and rehabilitation efforts cannot be accomplished on an outpatient basis.

Educational materials and other information for patients and families may be obtained from the following resources:

National Rehabilitation Center: www.naric.com/naric/
National Stroke Association: www.stroke.org
Stroke support and information homepage: www.members.aol.com/scmmlm/main.htm
The American Heart Association: www.americanheart.org/

APHASIA

Aphasia is considered in this chapter because it so commonly occurs in stroke victims, but it must be remembered that aphasia is a *sign* (like a hemiparesis) and can occur in any disease process that injures the perisylvian dominant (usually left) hemisphere. It is defined as an acquired disorder of language, and in the absence of other obvious neurologic symptoms, it can easily be confused with dementia and psychiatric disorders.

Aphasia is a disturbance of *language* only and must be differentiated from the myriad disorders of *speech*. For example, a patient with cerebellar dysfunction may have hypophonia or a loss of speech melody with explosive, irregular vocalization; a patient with vocal cord or tongue paralysis will have a normal speech cadence but a marked change in clarity or tone; and a patient with bilateral upper motor neuron lesions will have slow, arduous speech. None of these patients would have any difficulty thinking of words or expressing thoughts appropriately and thus would *not* have a language disturbance (aphasia). Schizophrenic patients, on occasion, may have a senseless "word salad" in which there is apparently no connection between one word and the next; speech melody is normal, and when listened to closely, the patient's thought processes will fit into the patient's own private code. Thus the schizophrenic patient does not have aphasia. Aphasia must also be differentiated from dementia: aphasia is a disturbance of language only, whereas dementia is a disturbance of all cognitive processes, including language.

It must be stressed that a diagnosis of aphasia should not be a casual diagnosis, but one that requires the physician to examine the patient specifically for an aphasic syndrome. In general, the physician should be readily able to differentiate the following four basic types of aphasic phenomena (Table 12-2):

1. *Nonfluent* or *Broca's aphasia:* the patient understands language well but produces little spontaneous speech. The nonfluent patient (commonly referred to as a *motor aphasia, anterior aphasia, nonfluent aphasia, expressive aphasia,* or *Broca's aphasia*) may suffer from the following symptoms:

   a. In right-handed patients, the aphasia is almost always associated with damage to the left third frontal gyrus and is usually associated with some degree of paralysis of the right side of the body.

   b. The patient is aware of the speech difficulty and often becomes extremely frustrated and angry (a catastrophic reaction); secondary depression may frequently complicate the clinical picture.

   c. The patient's speech is effortful and ungrammatic with short telegraphic phrases that are poorly articulated. The speech melody and

TABLE 12-2
Simplified Summary of Language Problems in Aphasia

Language function	Type of aphasia			
	Broca's	Wernicke's	Global	Anomic
Fluency	−	+	−	+
Comprehension	+	−	−	+
Naming	+	−	−	−

rhythm are abnormal, and perseveration (repeating the same word) is common.

d. The patient's auditory comprehension is well preserved, and he or she can follow most directions.

e. In the severe form, the patient may only be able to utter automatic speech such as obscenities and social amenities ("hello"). In the milder form or during recovery, more complicated automatic speech can be observed, such as singing "Happy Birthday" or reciting the Lord's Prayer.

f. Reading silently for meaning is relatively preserved but slow for the patient; reading aloud is impaired, and writing is large, messy, and effortful, paralleling the verbal expression.

Caveat: A diagnosis of aphasia cannot be made if the patient has absolutely no speech production.

2. *Fluent* or *Wernicke's aphasia:* the patient is unable to understand the language but produces voluminous verbal production with meaningless content (commonly called *sensory aphasia, Wernicke's aphasia, posterior aphasia,* or *receptive aphasia*). The patient may suffer from the following symptoms:

a. In right-handed patients, damage is almost always confined to the left posterosuperior temporal area. This aphasia is usually not associated with a paralysis, although some patients can have a homonymous right visual field defect.

b. With the pure form of aphasia, the patient is unaware of the difficulty; usually the patient is pleasant and jovial but can become angry with the examiner's inability to understand his or her speech.

c. The patient's speech rhythm and melody are normal, but the content is incomprehensible. This is true in all languages; for example, the aphasic German appears to be speaking German and the aphasic Frenchman appears to be speaking French, but the language is incomprehensible.

d. In mild form or during recovery, paraphasias are common; for example, "Resident pea gun staked on the telegram" means "President Reagan talked on the television." Speech with frequent paraphasias is also called *jargon speech.*

e. The patient has very poor auditory comprehension but can respond to whole-body commands, such as "stand up," "walk backward," and "open your mouth."

f. Both reading aloud and reading silently for comprehension are defective for the patient; writing is well formed but contains the same errors and lack of meaning as verbal expression.

3. *Global aphasia:* the patient has nonfluent speech and poor comprehension. The patient may suffer from the following symptoms:

a. The patient has both frontal lobe and temporoparietal lobe damage; this is basically a combination of the fluent and nonfluent aphasias involving all aspects of language.

b. The patient is awake and alert but for the most part sits silently and is unresponsive.

   c. Global aphasia is almost always associated with right hemiparesis in right-handed patients; there is often a right homonymous hemianopia.

4. *Anomic aphasic:* the patient has good verbal output and a good understanding of the language but has difficulty with word finding in spontaneous speech and in naming objects. The patient may suffer from the following symptoms:

   a. In right-handed individuals anomic aphasia is usually caused by a lesion of the left angular gyrus (at the junction of the parietal, occipital, and temporal lobes).

   b. The patient's speech is fluent but may be hesitant because of word-finding difficulties (usually nouns).

   c. As in fluent or Wernicke's aphasia, paraphasias (sound or word substitutions) are common in the patient's spontaneous speech.

   d. Because of the word-finding difficulties, this syndrome is often confused with nonfluent or Broca's aphasia but can be differentiated from it because the anomic aphasic has fluent, nondysarthric, effortless speech, and in the pure form there is no accompanying hemiparesis.

   e. Verbal comprehension is intact.

   f. When presented with objects, the patient misnames them (often with paraphasic errors) or cannot produce the name, although the patient will select the correct name when given a multiple-choice format.

   g. Anomic aphasia is often accompanied by Gerstmann's syndrome (right-to-left disorientation, finger agnosia, acalculia, or agraphia).

The aphasic syndromes can be more discretely defined and subcategorized, but familiarity with and identification of these four basic types will allow the physician to describe most aphasic patients.

Treatment:

1. Specific language therapy may accelerate a patient's recovery. Treatment should also be directed at the underlying lesion.

2. Rehabilitation of the patient with aphasia is necessary. For patients with intact understanding, it is important to find mechanisms to assist the patient with communication. The speech and language therapist is helpful in this regard. Simple signboards, letter boards, and other signaling devices are sometimes helpful, but new advances in computer technology, in some areas, have superseded these devices. The family must be educated to the patient's expressive difficulties and provide a nonstressful environment for his or her expression. Appropriate reading materials or talking books should be provided for the patient. In the patient with impaired comprehension, supervised care may be necessary.

STROKE IN CHILDREN

The clinical evaluation of stroke in children follows that of adults. The causes, however, are different (since atherosclerosis and hypertension are not common risk factors) and tend to be age related. A prenatal stroke may be present in the first year of life as a porencephalic cyst. Hypoxic-ischemic encephalopathy is the most common reason perinatally, whereas in premature infants, intraventricular hemorrhage is the most common reason for stroke.

Cyanotic congenital heart disease, complications of meningitis, or "acute infantile hemiplegia" syndrome tend to occur in early childhood. In later childhood and adolescence, sickle cell anemia, coagulopathies, vasculitides, and rare causes such as mitochondrial encephalopathy, lacticacidosis, and strokelike episodes (MELAS) and moyamoya disease should be considered. (See Roach, Pavlakis et al, and Kirkham in bibliography.)

BIBLIOGRAPHY

Albers GW, Easton JD, Sacco RL et al: Antithrombotic and thrombolytic therapy for ischemic stroke, *Chest* 114:683S-698S, 1998.

Brott T, Bogousslavsky J: Treatment of acute ischemic stroke, *N Engl J Med* 343(10):710-722, 2000.

Bushnell CD, Goldstein LB: Diagnostic testing for coagulopathies in patients with ischemic stroke, *Stroke* 31(12):3067-3078, 2000.

Caplan, LR: *Stroke: a clinical approach,* Woburn, Mass, 1999, Butterworth-Heinemann.

Davenport R, Dennis M: Neurologic emergencies: stroke, *J Neurol Neurosurg Psychiatry* 68:277-288, 2000.

Hacke, W, editor: Advances in stroke management: update 1998, *Neurology* 53(7):1S-37S, 1999.

Kirkham FJ: Stroke in childhood, *Arch Dis Child* 81(1):85-89, 1999.

Miller, LP, editor: *Stroke therapy: basic, preclinical, and clinical directions* New York, 1999, John Wiley & Sons.

Pavlakis SG, Kingsley PB, Bialer MG: Stroke in children: genetic and metabolic issues, *J Child Neurol* 15(5):308-315, 2000.

Roach ES: Etiology of stroke in children, *Semin Pediatr Neurol* 7(4):44-60, 2000.

Tanner, DC: *The family guide to surviving stroke and communication disorders,* Toronto, 1999, Prentice Hall Trade.

WEBSITES

National Rehabilitation Center: www.naric.com/naric/

National Stroke Association: www.stroke.org

Stroke clinical trials database from the Washington University School of Medicine: www.neuro.wustl.edu/smart/stroke-research1.htm

Stroke support and information homepage: www.members.aol.com/scmmlm/main.htm

The American Heart Association: www.americanheart.org

13

The Comatose Patient

C oma is a medical emergency. The purposes of this chapter are to outline immediate measures to care for the comatose patient, establish criteria for deciding whether coma is secondary to a toxic-metabolic disorder (more than 80% of cases are) or a structural central nervous system (CNS) disorder, and provide guidelines for the management of coma secondary to a CNS disorder.

IMMEDIATE MEASURES

1. Establish and maintain a clear airway in the comatose patient. In many cases this requires insertion of an endotracheal tube with ventilatory assistance.
2. Check the patient's pulse, blood pressure, and temperature, and apply a cardiac monitor. If profound hypotension is present or if there are gross cardiac abnormalities, the cause of coma is evident and should be treated appropriately.
3. Insert an intravenous (IV) line and draw blood for glucose, electrolyte (Na^+, K^+, Cl^-, CO_2, Ca^{++}), complete blood count (CBC), blood urea nitrogen (BUN), and creatinine determinations. Samples for arterial blood gas tests, toxic screening, and thyroid and liver function tests are often also drawn at this time.
4. Administer thiamine 100 mg IV, then 50 ml of 50% glucose. Many authorities also suggest administration of naloxone (Narcan) hydrochloride 2 mg, especially if the patient has small pupils; however, if the patient does not respond to a total dose of 10 mg, a diagnosis of narcotic overdose is unlikely.
5. Catheterize the patient's bladder and monitor urinary output.
6. Determine the depth of coma:
   a. The Glasgow Coma Scale (Table 13-1) is commonly used to quantitate the severity of coma; it can be repeated at intervals to monitor the clinical course and effect of therapy.

Note: This scale is especially useful in determining the prognosis in coma from head injuries and cardiorespiratory arrest. Thus 87% of patients who have a coma score of 4 or less 24 hours after a head injury die or remain

TABLE 13-1
Glasgow Coma Scale
(Circle the Appropriate Number and Compute the Total)*

EYES OPEN	
Never	1
To pain	2
To verbal stimuli	3
Spontaneously	4
BEST VERBAL RESPONSE	
No response	1
Incomprehensible sounds	2
Inappropriate words	3
Disoriented and converses	4
Oriented and converses	5
BEST MOTOR RESPONSE	
No response	1
Extension (decerebrate rigidity)	2
Flexion abnormal (decorticate rigidity)	3
Flexion withdrawal	4
Localizes pain	5
Obeys	6
TOTAL (RANGE)	**3-15**

*The sum of the highest value in each category is the coma score: full mental capacity, 15; highest level of coma, 8; brain death, 3.

in a vegetative state. Of those who score greater than 11, 87% show good recovery with mild-to-moderate disability.

    b. Press the styloid processes to evaluate the patient's response to noxious stimuli (Figure 13-1). This is an extremely painful stimulus that should be performed with caution; however, it is preferable to rubbing the sternum, twisting the nipples, or squeezing the testicles, which give less information, may leave unsightly marks that the family later questions, and is downright uncivilized. Note the type of response (arousal, decerebrate posturing, decorticate posturing, or asymmetric).

    c. *Confused* patients respond to verbal stimuli but are drowsy, slow, and often disoriented.

    d. *Stuporous* patients respond transiently to vigorous stimuli only.

    e. *Comatose* patients are unarousable and unresponsive but may exhibit abnormal postures.

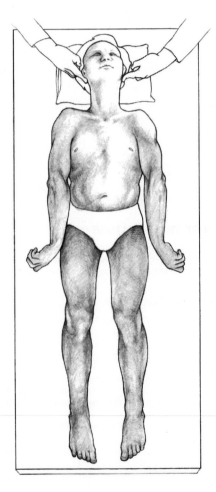

FIG. 13-1 The examiner is applying pressure on the styloid processes in the comatose patient and producing decerebrate posturing. This posture is seen in patients with brainstem dysfunction.

TABLE 13-2
Differentiation of Coma Caused by CNS Structural Lesion from Metabolic Coma

Examination	Suggestive of structural CNS coma	Suggestive of metabolic coma
Blood pressure	Increased	Decreased
Respiration	Ataxic	Regular or rhythmic
Temperature	Increased	Normal or decreased
Pupils	Asymmetric	Normal, usually reactive, even when brainstem function is suppressed
Oculocephalic and oculovestibular response	Asymmetric or absent	Usually intact
Posture	Asymmetric	Symmetric
Fundi	Possible papilledema	Usually normal
Reflexes	Asymmetric	Symmetric
Neck suppleness	Stiff or normal	Normal
Myoclonus	Rare	Frequent

EXAMINATION OF THE COMATOSE PATIENT

Table 13-2 lists the mandatory examinations that can be completed in a few minutes and allow the physician to make a tentative decision as to whether the coma resulted from a toxic-metabolic cause or a CNS lesion.

CNS VERSUS METABOLIC COMA

CNS coma is the term for coma secondary to CNS structural pathologic findings; however, *metabolic coma* is the term for coma from toxic-metabolic effects.

The mandatory examinations may reveal the following types of information:

1. *Blood pressure and pulse:* if the blood pressure is high and the pulse is low, severe increased intracranial pressure should be suspected. This finding is much more common in children than it is in adults. Most metabolic causes of coma cause hypotension.
2. *Breathing patterns* that may be seen in coma
   a. Normal respiration
   b. Hyperventilation—metabolic acidosis (e.g., uremia, diabetic ketoacidosis, exogenous toxins such as ethylene glycol) leads to hyperventilation; sustained, regular, rapid, deep hyperpnea is also seen in midbrain lesions (central neurogenic hyperventilation).
   c. Hypoventilation—a respiratory depression is seen both with medullary lesion and with drug overdose.
   d. Cheyne-Stokes respiration—this periodic smooth increase and decrease in respirations from apnea to hyperpnea occurs both in bi-

lateral lesions deep in the cerebral hemispheres and in metabolic coma.
   e. Ataxic respiration—a completely irregular pattern may be caused by a low brainstem lesion (such as with cerebellar or pontine hemorrhage, medullary infarction, or trauma), but this may also occur in cases of severe meningitis.

Caution: The use of sedatives in a patient with ataxic breathing may cause respiratory arrest.

3. *Temperature:* a significantly elevated temperature in the presence of an altered state of consciousness strongly suggests a CNS infection; unless signs of imminent cerebral herniation or gross papilledema are present, the cerebrospinal fluid (CSF) must be examined and cultured before antibiotics are started. Subarachnoid hemorrhage may give a mildly elevated temperature; heat stroke may give a markedly increased temperature.
4. *Pupils*
   a. A metabolic coma is suggested by symmetric pupils that react to light. Bilaterally fixed and dilated pupils are found in anoxia and in glutethimide, scopolamine, and atropine poisoning. The pinpoint pupils, which occur in narcotic overdose, dilate and become reactive with a small dose of a narcotic antagonist.
   b. A CNS coma is suggested by asymmetric pupils.

Caution: Pupillary inequalities of 1 mm or more may be seen in up to 10% of the normal population, and asymmetric pupils may also be the result of previous eye surgery or trauma.

5. *Oculocephalic response (doll's eye movement)* and *oculovestibular (caloric) test*

Caution: Do not perform an oculocephalic reflex test on a patient with trauma.

   a. *Oculocephalic response:* while holding the patient's eyelids open, passively rotate the head rapidly to both sides. In the comatose patient, the eyes remain as if fixed on an object in the foreground (Fig. 13-2). Awake patients have no oculocephalic response. A unilateral response suggests a brainstem lesion. The presence of a normal doll's eye response in both directions indicates that the brainstem between cranial nerve III (oculomotor nerve) and cranial nerve VIII (vestibuloacoustic nerve) is intact, which suggests that the cause of coma is not destruction of the brainstem. Absence of the response suggests a metabolic depression of the brainstem or severe brainstem dysfunction.
   b. *Caloric test:* if the doll's eye response is equivocal or if there is some reason the neck should not be rotated (such as head trauma or a cervical spine injury), caloric testing (oculovestibular reflex)

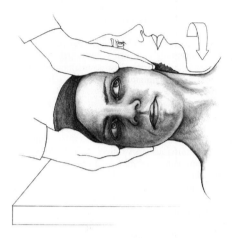

FIG. 13-2 Doll's eye movements. The eyes remain relatively stationary when the head is rapidly turned to one side.

may provide the same type of information. Check to see that the tympanic membrane is intact and that the external auditory canal is not blocked by wax or blood. Slowly inject at least 50 ml of ice water through a small polyethylene catheter into the external auditory canal. The head should be at approximately a 30-degree elevation with respect to the ground. In patients with suspected cervical spine fracture, elevate the head of the bed instead of bending the neck. Deviation of the eyes toward the ear being stimulated with nystagmus to the opposite side suggests an intact brainstem and a metabolic cause of the coma (Fig. 13-3).

6. *Pressure on the styloid process*
   a. Decerebrate posture (Fig. 13-1) is characterized by extended and internally rotated arms and extended legs with plantar flexion of the feet. Asymmetric posturing (e.g., one side moves, the other does not; or one side is decerebrate, the other is decorticate) suggests a structural CNS coma. Symmetric posturing is seen in brainstem and metabolic coma.
   b. Decorticate posture (Fig. 13-4) is characterized by flexion of the upper extremities, extension of the legs, and plantar flexion of the feet. Asymmetric posturing suggests a structural CNS coma; symmetric posturing is seen in bilateral hemisphere lesions.
7. *Fundoscopy:* look for early signs of papilledema, including loss of venous pulsations, enlargement of veins, a wet-appearing retina, and blurring of the margins of optic discs. This may be seen in both CNS mass lesions and in metabolic disturbances causing cerebral edema.

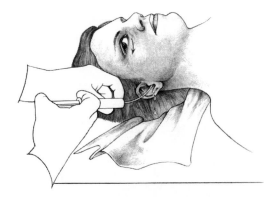

FIG. 13-3 Caloric test. In a patient with intact brainstem (cranial nerves III through VIII), cold water in the auditory canal will cause the eyes to deviate toward the cold ear.

8. *Reflexes:* asymmetric reflexes suggest a structural CNS coma; symmetric reflexes and a bilateral Babinski's reflex are seen in both CNS and metabolic disturbances. Suggested techniques for eliciting the patellar and Achilles reflexes are shown in Figs. 13-5 and 13-6.
9. *Neck suppleness:* a stiff neck suggests a subarachnoid hemorrhage or infection.

Caution: The neck should not be manipulated in the case of head trauma in which there is a possibility of a cervical spine fracture.

10. *Myoclonus:* this is manifested as uncoordinated generalized twitches and is more often seen in metabolic coma and after anoxic insults. Asterixis with flap tremor is another common finding in metabolic encephalopathy.

Note: Rarely, patients with metabolic coma may show focal CNS abnormalities. Asymmetric pupils may be congenital or a result of trauma. Fixed, pinpoint pupils may be secondary to the treatment of glaucoma.

HISTORY OF THE COMATOSE PATIENT

The patient's history, when obtainable, often eliminates the need for a number of diagnostic tests and points to a specific cause of the coma. The history may sometimes be obtained from relatives, friends, a family physician, or the police. It should include the following:
1. The onset: an abrupt onset of coma indicates intracranial hemorrhage or infarction; a gradual onset suggests a toxic or metabolic cause

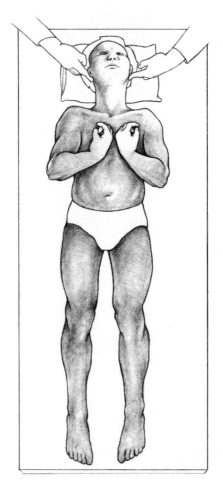

FIG. 13-4 Decorticate posturing seen in patients with bilateral hemisphere dysfunction. This may be spontaneous or produced by painful stimulus.

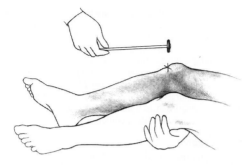

FIG. 13-5 Patellar reflex testing in a comatose patient. Place arm under the knees so that they are slightly flexed as illustrated; pay close attention to asymmetries.

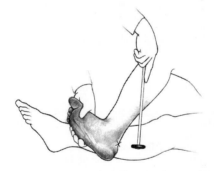

FIG. 13-6 Achilles reflex. Cross legs as illustrated and slightly dorsiflex the foot before tapping the Achilles tendon.

2. Preceding neurologic complaints: convulsions, confusion, hallucinations, headache, diplopia, vertigo, numbness, weakness, or ataxia
3. Recent trauma: trauma is suggestive of structural damage
4. Past medical history: psychiatric disturbances, diabetes, heart disease, hypertension, renal disease, epilepsy, alcoholism
5. Drug history: both prescribed and illicit drugs are important
6. Social history: pay particular attention to any traumatic event that might be linked to depression and suicide attempts

STRUCTURAL CNS LESIONS CAUSING COMA

A *unilateral* cerebral hemispheric lesion does not result in coma unless the lesion, for some reason (e.g., edema), causes damage to the other hemisphere as well. For coma to occur secondary to a CNS lesion, either both hemispheres must be severely damaged or the reticular activating system in the brainstem must be damaged directly or indirectly because of a shift (usually laterally) in the hemispheres. When both hemispheres are involved, the neurologic examination almost always shows asymmetries; in this situation the computed tomographic (CT) scan or magnetic resonance imaging (MRI) should readily lead the physician to the correct diagnosis (e.g., massive intracerebral hemorrhage, subdural hematoma large enough to cause herniation, multiple infarcts from emboli, or unilateral edema causing shifts in intracerebral contents).

Cerebral Herniation

The cerebral falx and the tentorium of the cerebellum are relatively rigid structures that separate the cranial contents into three major compartments. Displacement of brain tissue by mass lesions (blood, edema, or tumor) from one compartment to another is termed *herniation* (Fig. 13-7). The process is ominous because blood vessels may be compressed, causing additional damage by ischemia. Secondary hemorrhages (Duret hemorrhages) in the brainstem are also common. Cerebral herniation has the following characteristics:

1. Uncal herniation of the medial temporal lobe.
   a. Stretching of the third cranial nerve causes ipsilateral pupillary dilation.
   b. Pressure (from edema or mass effect) on the precentral motor cortex or the internal capsule causes contralateral hemiplegia. This is a false localizing sign.
   c. As the process progresses, the contralateral cerebral peduncle is pressed against the sharp edge of the tentorium of the cerebellum, causing ipsilateral paralysis.
2. Central herniation of the basal parts of both cerebral hemispheres through the incisura of the tentorium of the cerebellum. The clinical picture is not particularly distinctive.
   a. Early signs include a progressive loss of consciousness, small but reactive pupils, Cheyne-Stokes respiration, and bilateral motor signs with decorticate posturing.

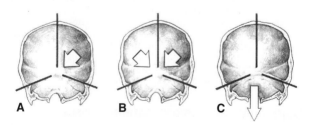

FIG. 13-7 Herniation. **A,** Beneath the cerebral falx. **B,** Through the incisura of the tentorium of the cerebellum. **C,** Through the foramen magnum.

b. Later signs include central hyperventilation, hyperthermia, pupils unreactive to light and in midposition, a loss of oculovestibular reflexes, and decerebrate posturing.

Treatment: Herniation may temporarily be halted or reversed by the following agents:

1. Mannitol 0.5 to 1 g/kg up to 50 g in a 20% solution IV administered over 20 minutes
2. Dexamethasone 0.3 mg/kg IV up to 12 mg IV followed by 0.06 mg/kg up to 6 mg every 4 hours

Posterior Fossa Mass

A posterior fossa mass (cerebellar hematoma, posterior fossa subdural hematoma, rapidly expanding posterior fossa tumor) has the following characteristics:

1. There is a subacute onset of symptoms.
2. There is usually a past history of hypertension or occipital trauma.

Note: Cerebellar hematomas are a complication of chronic hypertension; symptoms include rapidly accelerating hypertension, headache, weakness, and confusion.

3. A rapid progression of symptoms and signs, which may include the following:
   a. Early signs include occipital headache, repeated vomiting, dizziness, confusion, and marked "malignant" hypertension.
   b. Midstage signs include an inability to stand or walk, bilateral extensor plantar responses, urinary incontinence, dysarthria, tonic deviation of eyes away from the side of the lesion, miosis, and irregular respirations.
   c. Later signs include coma, absent doll's eye responses and caloric responses, respiratory failure, and flaccid limbs with diminished deep tendon reflexes.

Caution: A lumbar puncture (LP) in the presence of a posterior fossa mass carries an especially high risk of cerebellar herniation through the foramen magnum, and possibly death.

Treatment: This is a neurosurgical emergency. Immediate surgical decompression can be life saving. A definitive diagnosis is best established by a CT scan or an MRI.

Brainstem Infarction

A brainstem infarction has the following characteristics:

1. Acute symptoms with coma and other findings are maximal at the onset.
2. The lesion is often preceded by transient episodes consisting of diplopia, vertigo, dysarthria, dysphagia, motor weakness, and an episodic loss of consciousness.
3. A respiratory disturbance (periodic breathing, central hyperventilation, or ataxic breathing) is prominent from the onset.

4. There is a variable abnormality of the pupils, which often are small and react sluggishly to light in a pontine lesion.
5. A dysconjugate position of the eyes or dysconjugate eye movements (seen in doll's eye or caloric tests) suggest lesions of cranial nerves III, IV (trochlear nerve), or VI (abducens nerve); eye movements on doll's eye or caloric tests suggest brainstem involvement; facial paralysis is noted by asymmetric movement of the cheek during respirations.
6. Quadriparesis with a Babinski's reflex (extensor plantar response) and decerebrate posturing is often present. Cranial nerve abnormalities on one side with paralysis on the opposite side strongly suggest a brainstem lesion.

Treatment: Evaluation and treatment is discussed in Chapter 12.

Caution: Certain patients with upper pontine lesions may develop the locked-in syndrome (also referred to as *pseudocoma* or *deafferented state*) and have "a mind . . . clogged by a body rendered utterly incapable of obeying its impulses." Such an individual is awake but is unable to communicate except with eye movement ("a corpse with living eyes") such as the character Monsieur Noirtier de Villefort in *The Count of Monte Cristo*. These patients may be very much aware of their surroundings; therefore the physician must be cautious in making comments in the presence of the patient. The locked-in syndrome must be distinguished from the persistent neurovegetative state (imprecisely referred to as *coma vigil*) in which the patient appears awake (and may even have an awake electroencephalogram [EEG]) but is unable to communicate in any form (thought to be caused by a high midbrain lesion).

TREATMENT OF PATIENTS WITH COMA SECONDARY TO A CNS LESION

1. Ensure oxygenation with endotracheal suctioning, a cuffed endotracheal tube, and assisted ventilation with oxygen.
2. Maintain the circulation by replacing blood volume losses, administering vasoconstrictors, and maintaining cardiac rhythm.
3. Administer thiamine 100 mg IV then ensure adequate levels of blood glucose (the major substrate for brain metabolism) by administering 25 g of glucose IV in a 50% solution initially and by frequently monitoring blood glucose levels.
4. Lower the intracranial pressure if the patient is found to have a raised intracranial pressure. (Optimally the intracranial pressure should be determined by direct measurement with an intracranial pressure gauge inserted by a neurosurgeon.)
   a. Hyperventilate the patient's lungs to lower the carbon dioxide pressure to 25 to 30 mm Hg (thereby decreasing cerebral blood flow). This is only done initially to avoid injury from decreased perfusion.
   b. Mannitol 0.5 to 1 g/kg in a 20% solution is given IV over 20 to 30 minutes.
   c. Dexamethasone 10 mg IV is given and is repeated with 4 to 6 mg every 6 hours.

d. If a cerebral ventricular enlargement is evident on a CT scan as a result of obstruction of CSF pathways, ventricular drainage may be life saving.

Caveat: Hyperventilation should not be performed in patients with ischemia as a cause of coma. Mannitol is temporarily effective but may have a rebound effect. Steroids are most effective for edema caused by brain tumors. Steroids are not used for edema secondary to ischemia. Thus it is important to combine the history, the neurologic examinations, and the neuroimaging scan to obtain as accurate a diagnosis as possible.

5. Treat seizures, if present (see Chapter 11). An urgent EEG is indicated if subtle status epilepticus is a consideration.
6. Treat infection, if present. A patient with fever, a stiff neck, and coma should have an LP *immediately,* even if a CT scan is not available. The risk from herniation in this situation is much less than the adverse effect of failure to identify the cause of the meningitis.
7. Treat respiratory and metabolic alkalosis and acidosis; abnormalities may further depress respirations or worsen cardiovascular abnormalities.
8. Treat hyperthermia. An elevated body temperature may kill an already damaged brain and, if high enough, kill a normal brain. A cooling blanket is preferred.

METABOLIC COMA

Approximately 80% of comas in adults are caused by toxic-metabolic abnormalities; common causes include hypoxia (cardiac arrest, pulmonary insufficiency), drug overdose (barbiturates or other sedatives, alcohol), diabetes (insulin overdose, ketoacidosis), hyperosmolar nonketotic coma, uremia, hepatic failure, and heat stroke. Although coma in children is approached similarly as to adults, and CNS structural causes are often the same, the causes of metabolic comas (though encompassing similar causes as in adults) also include metabolic causes caused by genetic inborn errors of metabolism. (See reference materials on coma in children in bibliography.)

PSYCHOGENIC COMA

Even astute physicians are sometimes fooled by a physiologically awake patient who does not respond to the environment and thus appears comatose. The following tests may be of value in confirming psychogenic coma:
1. The pupils and deep tendon reflexes are normal.
2. In caloric tests, 10 ml of cold water causes *nystagmus with the fast component away* from the irrigated side.
3. Doll's eye movements are absent in an awake patient. Patients with absent doll's eye movement resulting from a brainstem infarct usually have other, obvious signs.

4. Hold the patient's hand over the face and drop it; the hand will hit the face of the comatose patient but will deviate to the side in an alert patient (see Fig. 9-3).
5. Press the styloid processes; this very painful stimulus will arouse most noncomatose patients.

BIBLIOGRAPHY

Arieff AI, Griggs RC: *Metabolic brain dysfunction in systemic disorders,* Boston, 1992, Little Brown & Co.

Brooks DN, Hosie J, Bond MR et al: Cognitive sequelae of severe head injury in relation to the Glasgow Outcome Scale, *J Neurol Neurosurg Psychiatry* 49:549-553, 1986.

Fitzgerald FT, Tierney LM, Wall SD: The comatose patient: a systematic diagnostic approach for you to follow, *Postgrad Med* 74:207-215, 1983.

Fraser CL, Arieff AI: Hepatic encephalopathy, *N Engl J Med* 313:865-873, 1985.

Gascon GG, Ozand PT: *Aminoacidopathies and organic acidopathies, mitochondrial enzyme defects, and other metabolic errors.* In Goetz CG, Pappert EJ, editors: *Textbook of clinical neurology,* Philadelphia, 1999, WB Saunders.

Gascon GG: *Encephalopathies in children.* In Elzouki AY, Harfi HA, Nazer H, editors: *Textbook of clinical pediatrics,* Philadelphia, 2001, Lippincott-Williams & Wilkins.

Levy DE, Caronna JJ, Singer BH et al: Predicting the outcome from hypoxic-ischemic coma, *JAMA* 253:1420-1426, 1985.

Maiesek K, Cuvonna JJ: Coma following cardiac arrest: a review of the clinical features, management, and prognosis, *J Intensive Care Med* 3:153-163, 1988.

Ozand PT, Alessa M: *Disorders of organic acid and amino acid metabolism.* In Elzouki AY, Harfi HA, Nazer H, editors: *Textbook of clinical pediatrics,* Philadelphia, 2001, Lippincott-Williams & Wilkins.

Plum F, Posner J: *The diagnosis of stupor and coma,* ed 3, Philadelphia, 1980, FA Davis.

Posner JB: The comatose patient, *JAMA* 233:1313-1314, 1975.

Ropper AH: Lateral displacement of the brain and level of consciousness in patients with acute hemispheral mass, *N Engl J Med* 314:953-958, 1986.

Ropper AH, Kennedy SK, Zervas N: *Neurobiological and neurosurgical intensive care,* Baltimore, 1983, University Park Press.

Schewman DA, DeGiogio CM: Early prognosis in anoxic coma: reliability and rationale, *Neurol Clin* 7:823-843, 1989.

Young GB, Ropper AH, Bolton CF: *Coma and impaired consciousness,* New York, McGraw-Hill, 1998.

14

Infections of the Central Nervous System

Most infections of the central nervous system (CNS) are life-threatening, the exception being the so-called aseptic or viral meningoencephalitis (other than that caused by herpes simplex). Immediate diagnosis and treatment may prevent death or brain damage. Signs and symptoms may mimic other neurologic disorders, so the clinician must have a high index of suspicion. After the initial history and examination, the clinician makes an educated guess as to the likely causative organisms and then selects appropriate antibiotics. Antibiotics and management are subsequently modified, depending on laboratory results.

HISTORY AND EXAMINATION SUGGESTING INFECTION

History

Historical points that direct the physician to consider a CNS infection in the patient with developing neurologic signs or symptoms include the following:

1. A *fever* may rise to 40° C (105° F) or higher in adults, whereas other infections seldom produce fever this high.

Caution: Fever often may be absent in neonates, elderly or immunosuppressed patients, and occasionally in all patients.

2. *Photophobia* is often a historical manifestation in patients with meningitis.
3. *Vomiting with or without nausea* is often seen in patients with a CNS infection and should not be misinterpreted as resulting from a gastrointestinal disturbance.
4. *There are alterations in sensorium, mentation, or behavior.*
5. A severe *headache* is worsened by movement of the head or neck, particularly flexion of the neck.

6. A known *blood-borne infection,* such as bacteremia or endocarditis, is present.

7. A *debilitating condition from another disease* (e.g., chronic renal failure or diabetes mellitus) or from reduced immunity (such as in leukemia or lymphoma, administration of immunosuppressant drugs, or in congenital or acquired immunodeficiency syndrome [AIDS]) is present.

8. An *infection of superficial or deep structures adjoining the nervous system* (such as paranasal sinuses, skin of the face, pilonidal sinus) is present, especially if there has been recent manipulation in the area or if the condition is chronic.

9. An *abnormality of the blood-brain barrier,* such as in a recent ischemic infarction or emboli from congenital heart disease, occurs.

10. There is *exposure of CNS structures secondary to trauma or surgery* (such as in compound or basilar skull fractures) or evidence of a fistula connecting with the subarachnoid space (such as through the nose, producing cerebrospinal fluid [CSF] rhinorrhea, or through developmental anomalies).

Physical Examination

Following are some aspects of the physical examination that suggest the presence of a CNS infection:

1. Fever, especially with an altered level of consciousness progressing, or fluctuating neurologic signs and symptoms.

2. Meningismus, including nuchal rigidity, a sign of meningeal irritation, a preference for lying in bed with the head extended and the back arched. Kernig's and Brudzinski's signs may be present (Figs. 14-1 and 14-2).

Caution: In infants and some elderly patients, fever and signs of meningeal irritation may be absent.

3. Neurologic findings that suggest multiple localizations of involvement of the nervous system, such as cranial nerve palsies, alterations of sensorium, convulsions, and papilledema.

4. Signs of acute or chronic middle ear or mastoid infection, particularly in children.

Cerebrospinal Fluid Examination (see Chapter 2)

1. CSF studies should be done in all patients *without delay* whenever meningitis or encephalitis is suspected. The indication for a lumbar puncture (LP) is if you *think* of it.

Caution: If there are focal neurologic abnormalities or papilledema, a computed tomographic (CT) scan or magnetic resonance imaging (MRI) is strongly recommended before an LP is performed.

2. A Gram's staining of CSF sediment will show organisms in 70% of untreated bacterial meningitis. India ink preparations for *Cryptococcus*

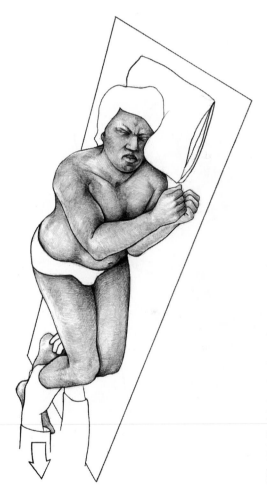

FIG. 14-1 Kernig's sign. A patient with meningitis may lie in bed with the knees and hips flexed. A positive sign (pain) is elicited when the legs are extended.

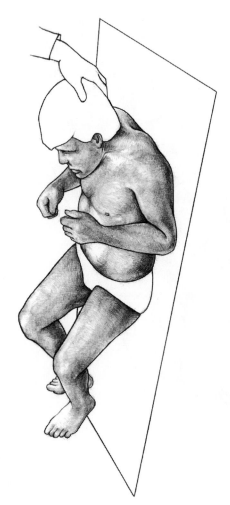

FIG. 14-2 Brudzinski's sign. Passive flexion of the neck causes spontaneous flexion of the lower limbs.

and acid-fast stains for tubercle bacilli are rarely positive but nonetheless should be performed.

3. Normally the CSF contains *no* polymorphonuclear leukocytes and no more than 5 lymphocytes/μl (mm^3). *More cells* than this suggest meningeal inflammation.

4. CSF glucose level less than 50% of the serum glucose level suggests a bacterial infection, tuberculosis (TB), fungal meningitis, or carcinomatous meningitis. The blood glucose level takes several hours to equilibrate with the CSF glucose level in patients with hypoglycemia or hyperglycemia.

5. The CSF protein level and pressure are commonly elevated.

6. CSF *culture* and sensitivity testing should always include bacteria (aerobic and anaerobic), TB, brucellosis, and fungi. Although the yield is very low, viral cultures should be obtained when viral meningoencephalitis is suspected and where facilities for viral culture are available.

7. Antigen-antibody studies include the following:
    a. Cryptococcal antigen (the latex particle agglutination test) determinations should be ordered when fungal meningitis is suspected and should be done routinely in all patients who are immunocompromised. Skin antigen testing is of no value. Serologic tests for coccidioidomycosis are also warranted in areas where this disease is endemic.
    b. CSF herpes simplex serologic testing is positive in herpes simplex meningitis or encephalitis.
    c. Routine countercurrent immunoelectrophoresis (CIE) or, more recently, latex agglutination tests may rapidly detect polysaccharide antigens associated with meningococcal, pneumococcal, and *Haemophilus influenzae* (type B) meningitis.
    d. Routine syphilis serologic tests, such as CSF, venereal disease research laboratory (VDRL), or rapid plasma reagin (RPR), test positive for neurosyphilis. A CSF fluorescent treponemal antibody absorption (FTA-ABS) test is neither sensitive or specific.
    e. CSF immunoglobulin G (IgG) and measles antibody titers must be obtained if subacute sclerosing panencephalitis (SSPE) is suspected.
    f. A dark-field examination and appropriate serologic tests should be obtained if leptospirosis is suspected.

8. Whenever possible, 2 to 3 ml of CSF should be stored frozen so that the physician can perform further studies if clinically indicated during the initial phase of the illness.

9. CSF cytologic studies and flow cytometry are warranted if lymphomatous or carcinomatous meningitis is suspected.

GENERAL PRINCIPLES OF ANTIBIOTIC TREATMENT

1. Antibiotics should be started empirically immediately after the LP is done, if there is evidence of a bacterial infection. Choose antibiotics that are bactericidal against known or presumed causative organisms.

2. Antibiotics should be started empirically *before* a CT scan or MRI is done when they may delay the performance of the LP.
3. Combinations of drugs should be avoided unless a synergistic effect is known to occur. Combinations of drugs may be necessary if the following statements are true:
   a. Sensitivities are initially unavailable.
   b. The organism is felt to be resistant (e.g., enteric gram-negative bacilli, a fungal infection, TB, or *Brucella* infection).
   c. The patient is immunosuppressed.
   d. A polymicrobial infection is suspected.
4. The antibiotics must be capable of penetrating into CSF in concentrations well above the mean bactericidal concentration for the infective organism.
5. Intrathecal antibiotic administration is unnecessary in the initial treatment of the patient with acute meningitis and is useful only in certain circumstances (such as resistant fungal meningitis). Select the best antibiotic at the correct daily dosage (Tables 14-1 to 14-3).
6. It should be certain that the patient is receiving what has been ordered. Renal function tests and serum level determinations can be done for aminoglycosides, and the dosage may be adjusted accordingly.
7. In children, administration of corticosteroids along with the antibiotics may reduce the incidence of complications.

BACTERIAL MENINGITIS IN NEONATES

Meningitis in the full-term and premature newborn has serious consequences.
1. Mortality rates are about 20% for *Escherichia coli* and group B streptococcal meningitis, which together account for 60% to 75% of cases.
2. Long-term sequelae range from blindness, deafness, seizures, and hydrocephalus to cognitive disorders, such as mental retardation, attention disorders, and learning disabilities.
3. A brain abscess may complicate meningitis in the neonate.
Diagnosis:
1. An early diagnosis is difficult because signs and symptoms may be nonspecific or minor (irritability, poor feeding, jitteriness, respiratory difficulty, and lethargy), and the index of suspicion must be high.
2. CSF changes are delayed, especially in the premature infant, and the relatively poor defense mechanisms of newborns allow rapid progression of the disease.
3. Neonates require treatment based on suspicion alone.
4. Pretreatment blood, urine, and CSF cultures are obtained, and treatment is discontinued if they do not provide evidence of a treatable infection.
5. Normal neonatal CSF protein may be as high as 150 mg/dl, cell counts could be up to 25 white blood cells (WBCs)/μl and 650 red blood cells (RBCs)/μl, and peripheral WBC counts may be as high as

TABLE 14-1
Antibiotic Dosages for Bacterial Meningitis*

Antibiotic	Dosage
Ampicillin	150-200 mg/kg/day IV q8h
Penicillin G	
<1 wk	150,000 units/kg/day IV q8h
1 wk-2 mo	150,000-250,000 units/kg/day IV q6h
Group B *Streptococcus*	250,000-400,000 units/kg/day IV q6h
Methicillin sodium	100 mg/kg/day IV q8h
Nafcillin sodium	100 mg/kg/day IV q8h
Carbenicillin	300 mg/kg/day IV q8h
Ticarcillin	200-300 mg/kg/day IV q8h
Piperacillin sodium	200 mg/kg/day IV q8h
Kanamycin sulfate	
<1 wk	20 mg/kg/day IM or IV q12h
1 wk-2 mo	30 mg/kg/day IM or IV q8h
Gentamicin sulfate	
<1 wk	5 mg/kg/day IM or IV q12h
1 wk-2 mo	7.5 mg/kg/day IM or IV q8h
Tobramycin	
<1 wk	5 mg/kg/day IM or IV q12h
1 wk-2 mo	7.5 mg/kg/day IM or IV q8h
Amikacin	
<1 wk	15 mg/kg/day IM or IV q12h
1 wk-2 mo	22.5 mg/kg/day IM or IV q8h
Moxalactam disodium	100-150 mg/kg/day IV q8h
Cefotaxime sodium	100-150 mg/kg/day IV q8h
Vancomycin hydrochloride	
Birth to 1 wk	30 mg/kg/day IV q12h
1 wk-2 mo	45 mg/kg/day IV q8h
Metronidazole	15 mg/kg/day IV q12h

IM, Intramuscularly; *IV,* intravenously; *q6h,* every 6 hours; *q8h,* every 8 hours; *q12h,* every 12 hours.
*Birth to 2 months.

$25,000/\mu l$. By 1 month of age in patients, these values decrease to adult values.

6. The CSF pressure is almost always greater than 180 mm/H_2O, but values greater than 400 mm/H_2O indicate impending herniation.

Treatment:

1. Care of the neonate with meningitis may be complicated by respiratory insufficiency, hypoglycemia, dehydration, shock, or convulsions and is best undertaken in a neonatal intensive care unit (ICU). Unless the primary care practitioner has considerable experi-

TABLE 14-2
Antibiotic Dosages for Bacterial Meningitis*

Antibiotic	Dosage
Ampicillin	300-400 mg/kg/day IV q4
Penicillin G	250,000 units/kg/day IV q4h
Methicillin sodium	200-300 mg/kg/day IV q4h
Nafcillin sodium	200 mg/kg/day IV q4h
Carbenicillin	400-600 mg/kg/day IV q4h
Ticarcillin	300-400 mg/kg/day IV q4h
Piperacillin sodium	300-400 mg/kg/day IV q4h
Gentamicin	4 mg/kg/day IM q8h
Tobramycin	4 mg/kg/day IM q8h
Amikacin	15 mg/kg/day IM q8h
Moxalactam disodium	150 mg/kg/day IV q4h
Cefotaxime sodium	150 mg/kg/day IV q4h
Cefoperazone sodium	300 mg/kg/day IV q8h
Ceftriaxone sodium	100 mg/kg/day IV q12h
Rifampin	20 mg/kg/day PO q8h (up to 600 mg)
Streptomycin sulfate	20-40 mg/kg/day IM q12h (not more than 1 g)
Vancomycin hydrochloride	60 mg/kg/day IV q6h
Sulfadiazine	150 mg/kg/day IV q8h
Metronidazole	40 mg/kg/day PO q8h
	30 mg/kg/day IV q6h

IM, Intramuscularly; *IV,* intravenously; *PO,* by mouth; *q4h,* every 4 hours; *q6h,* every 6 hours; *q8h,* every 8 hours; *q12h,* every 12 hours.
*Over 2 months of age and up to 50-kg body weight.

ence with neonates, it is best to refer the patient to a pediatrician or neonatologist.
2. Recommendations for initial therapy are third-generation cephalosporins combined with ampicillin (to ensure coverage for *Listeria monocytogenes*). Cefotaxime sodium, 50 mg/kg intravenously (IV) every 6 hours, or moxalactam disodium are preferred in combination with ampicillin until the pathogen is known. See Table 14-1 for other specific drug dosages.
3. Third-generation cephalosporins offer higher levels than the aminoglycosides.
4. All medication is given IV and is usually continued for 21 days after the CSF has been sterilized.

BACTERIAL MENINGITIS IN INFANTS AND CHILDREN

Bacterial meningitis is primarily a disease of early childhood.
1. Some 90% of cases occur from 1 month to 5 years of age.
2. The most common causes are pneumococci *(Streptococcus pneumoniae)* and meningococci *(Neisseria meningitidis).*

TABLE 14-3
Antibiotic Therapy for Bacterial Meningitis with a Known Etiologic Agent in Adults

Organism	Preferred therapy (antibiotic dosage/24 hr)	Alternative therapy (antibiotic dosage/24 hr)
GRAM POSITIVE		
Pneumococcus	Penicillin G 24 million units IV	Chloramphenicol 4 g IV
Multiply resistant	Vancomycin hydrochloride 2 g IV	Vancomycin 2 mg IV plus 2-5 mg intrathecally
Streptococcus		
Groups A and B	Penicillin G 24 million units IV	Chloramphenicol 4 g IV
Group D (enterococcus)	Penicillin G 24 million units IV + gentamicin sulfate 5 mg/kg IM or IV	Vancomycin 2 g IV + 2-5 mg intrathecally
Staphylococcus aureus	Nafcillin sodium 10-12 g IV	Vancomycin 2 g IV + 2-5 mg intrathecally
Listeria monocytogenes	Ampicillin 12 g IV	Tetracycline 1.5 g IV
GRAM NEGATIVE		
Haemophilus influenzae	Chloramphenicol 4 g IV	Ampicillin 12-14 g IV
Meningococcus ***Escherichia coli,*** **Klebsiella, Proteus, Pseudomonas, Serratia,** and similar organisms	Penicillin G 24 million units IV Carbenicillin 30-40 g IV + aminoglycoside IV	Chloramphenicol 4 g IV Aminoglycoside 2-5 mg intrathecally

IM, Intramusculary; IV, intravenously.

3. The incidence of *H. influenza* type B has dropped after the use of the vaccine.
4. All three of these organisms colonize the nasopharynx of healthy children, and most children with meningitis have a preceding or concurrent nasopharyngitis.

Diagnosis: Signs and symptoms pointing to a CNS invasion are more easily elicited in this group, compared to neonates.

1. Often, the main difficulty is distinguishing between acute viral and acute bacterial meningitis, since the early symptoms are similar.

2. Antibiotics frequently have already been administered to the child, so the differential diagnosis is often between partially treated bacterial meningitis and viral meningitis, both of which have a similar CSF profile.

3. Appropriate smears and cultures should be obtained, and countercurrent immunoelectrophoresis or latex precipitation on the CSF should be performed. Therapy should be continued in all cases of partially treated meningitis, but in other instances, if there is no evidence of bacterial infection, therapy can be discontinued.

Treatment:

1. *Initial therapy:* Ampicillin 300 to 400 mg/kg/day IV every 4 hours; maximum daily dose is 12 g to avoid cerebral irritability, plus chloramphenicol 75 mg/kg/day IV every 6 hours.

2. A single antibiotic should be used whenever possible once sensitivity patterns have been determined. See Table 14-2 for drug dosage and regimens.

3. A second LP should be obtained within 48 hours of starting antibiotic therapy, unless the patient's condition has become completely asymptomatic. By this time no organisms should be detectable on stained CSF smears, or their number should be greatly reduced; otherwise therapy must be reevaluated.

4. The number of CSF cells and the glucose and protein levels slowly return to normal and may still be abnormal at 48 hours. If the clinical course is satisfactory, it may not be necessary to perform a third LP.

5. The duration of treatment is at least 14 days but should be at least 21 days for gram-positive enterococci and 28 days for gram-negative enteric bacilli.

BACTERIAL MENINGITIS IN ADULTS

With treatment, fatality rates of adult bacterial meningitis are usually less than 10%, but severe neurologic sequelae are possible. The two leading causes in the adult are pneumococci *(S. pneumoniae)* and meningococci *(N. meningitidis).*

1. Pneumococcal meningitis is usually preceded by pneumonia; is often associated with alcoholism, debilitation, and old age; and usually occurs sporadically, except in developing countries. Confused elderly patients should be assumed to have meningitis until a clear and adequate diagnosis can be made.

2. Meningococcal meningitis occurs in epidemics (serogroups A or C) in the pediatric age group and may be acquired by susceptible adults.

3. Meningitis caused by gram-negative enteric bacteria is almost always a disease of the hospitalized or nursing home patient and often follows bacteremia from other foci, such as cellulitis or urinary tract infection, or may be seen in patients with head penetrating head trauma.

Treatment:

1. *Initial therapy:* Penicillin G, aqueous, 2 million units IV every 2 hours and chloramphenicol 1 g IV every 6 hours. See Table 14-3 for drug dosage and regimens.

2. Patients are customarily treated through 5 afebrile days but not less than 1 week for meningococci, 10 days for *H. influenzae,* and 14 days for pneumococci.

COMPLICATIONS OF MENINGITIS

1. *Seizures:* Drug therapy for seizures is outlined in Chapter 11. These seizures may be transient and do not require prolonged anticonvulsant (antiepileptic drug) therapy, or they may persist for many years after brain destruction and scar formation. If a patient has a seizure during the acute episode, treat him or her with anticonvulsants for 1 year. After that time, the drug may be withdrawn, according to the guidelines in Chapter 11.
2. *Raised intracranial pressure:* This is usually a transient problem caused by cerebral edema; if necessary, treat with fluid restriction or mannitol, or steroids (see Chapter 12). CSF shunting may be necessary if progressive ventricular enlargement occurs.
3. *Subdural effusions:* These are especially common after *H. influenzae* meningitis in children; suspect subdural effusions with persistent fever and focal seizures. The effusions are usually treated by repeated subdural taps, but they occasionally require neurosurgical intervention.
4. *Subdural empyema:* This is similar to a subdural effusion except that the fluid contains live organisms (pus) and is consequently much more dangerous. Immediate surgical drainage and reassessment of antibiotic therapy are indicated.
5. *Infarction:* Venous infarcts may be caused by cortical thrombophlebitis, venous sinus thrombosis, or both. Cortical thrombophlebitis usually appears early with seizures that are difficult to control. Sagittal sinus thrombosis will manifest as raised intracranial pressure and stroke, predominantly with lower-extremity findings. Arterial infarcts secondary to an inflammatory arteritis accompanying bacterial infection may not be evident until the recovery phase from the acute toxic illness, particularly in pneumococcal meningitis.
6. *Prolonged fever:* A prolonged fever may be a result of a local infection at the IV site, subdural effusion, inappropriate or inadequate antibiotic therapy, drug fever, or the presence of an unsuspected second organism.
7. *Syndrome of inappropriate antidiuretic hormone (SIADH) secretion:* This syndrome is a frequent occurrence during the early phases of meningitis. Diagnosis is made by finding low serum osmolality and high urine osmolality. This is usually prevented by fluid restriction.
8. *Communicating hydrocephalus:* The infection may interfere with proper reabsorption of CSF, but more commonly, hydrocephalus is a late complication. The symptoms include deterioration of mental and behavioral function and bilateral corticospinal tract signs, especially increased reflexes in the lower extremities. The diagnosis is suggested by ventricular enlargement on a CT scan or MRI. If the condition does not spontaneously resolve, CSF shunting by a neurosurgeon may be necessary.

9. *Obstructive hydrocephalus:* This is suggested by an abnormal increase in head circumference and widening of sutures in infants or young children. In older children and adults, there will be progressive mental deterioration and ataxia, and the CT scan or MRI will show ventricular enlargement. Shunting by a neurosurgeon is often required. Acute obstruction results in coma and death if the pressure is not relieved promptly.

Prognosis: The prognosis of bacterial meningitis depends on the following:

1. The nature of the infectious agent and the severity of the initial process (convulsions and coma)
2. The age of the patient
3. The duration of symptoms before treatment
4. Appropriate and early antibiotic therapy

BRAIN ABSCESS

1. A brain abscess resembles that of any other mass lesion, such as a tumor. Fever and leukocytosis may be minimal or absent, and thus do not rule out the diagnosis.
2. Abscesses are very irritating to brain tissue and cause edema, increased intracranial pressure, and seizures.
3. Predisposing factors include acute and chronic sinusitis and otitis, cyanotic congenital heart disease, penetrating head wounds, and chronic pulmonary infection.
4. A CSF culture is usually negative; a cell count is normal or slightly elevated, and the protein level is slightly elevated.
5. All types of organisms cause abscesses; if neurosurgical intervention is undertaken, both aerobic and anaerobic cultures must be performed.
6. A CT scan or MRI usually shows a "doughnut sign"–an area of low density with a rim of higher density (capsule) and marked surrounding cerebral edema.
7. If a CT scan or MRI demonstrates an abscess, an LP should be avoided because of the risk of brain herniation.
8. Sinus and mastoid radiographs should be performed to look for a source of infection in all cases.

Treatment:

1. Antibiotics against anaerobic *Streptococcus* and *Bacteroides* infections are given IV. Recommended drugs are metronidazole 500 to 750 mg/day in 3 or 4 doses and crystalline penicillin G, 100,000 to 400,000 units in 4 to 6 doses daily IV (up to 24 million units daily IV) if the organism is unknown.
2. Treatment of the cerebral edema usually requires dexamethasone 2 to 6 mg every 4 to 6 hours.
3. Neurosurgical drainage of the abscess with instillation of antibiotics locally is required, unless therapy is instituted very early at a "cerebritis" stage.
4. The duration of therapy remains empirical; however, a minimum of 4 to 6 weeks is generally accepted as sufficient in most patients.

TUBERCULOUS MENINGITIS

The incidence of tuberculous meningitis is on the rise in the United States. It should be suspected particularly in recent immigrants, in socially disadvantaged populations, in immunosuppressed patients, or in those with AIDS.

1. The diagnosis is elusive because of the following factors:
   a. The onset is usually gradual without meningeal signs. Symptoms are nonspecific—apathy, anorexia, malaise, and low-grade fever. Later, there may be drowsiness, seizures, cranial nerve palsies, and other focal (particularly brainstem) signs, and papilledema. The illness develops over weeks, not days.
   b. Tuberculous meningitis is seen in association with a disseminated disease in young patients. In adults, the disease (secondary reactivation) usually manifests as a CNS disease without dissemination.
   c. Only one third of patients have evidence of active pulmonary disease, whereas one third have a negative purified protein derivative (PPD) test.
   d. Stains for acid-fast bacilli in CSF sediment are frequently negative, and cultures take 4 to 6 weeks to become positive.
2. Strongly suspect the diagnosis under the following conditions:
   a. In a patient with a history of exposure to TB.
   b. In any case in which there is evidence of active TB, especially in young adults and children.
   c. In any patient with meningitis in whom the intermediate PPD is positive (especially if there is a recent conversion). CSF findings usually consist of increased lymphocytes with or without neutrophils, a decreased glucose level, and a marked increase in the protein level.

Note: Tuberculoma does not present as a meningitis, but as a mass lesion.

3. For the reasons mentioned before, virtually all CSF with increased cells, even if the glucose level is normal, should be stained and cultured for acid-fast bacilli. Cultures and stains have a higher probability of being positive if the CSF is allowed to stand and the resulting proteinaceous precipitate is examined.

Treatment:

1. Once the diagnosis has been made on clinical grounds and adequate cultures have been obtained, treatment must be started immediately; a delay of weeks until the culture is positive may lead to irreversible brain damage.
2. Treat the meningitis routinely with triple therapy:
   a. Isoniazid (INH) 15 mg/kg/day by mouth to a maximum of 300 mg/day, for 1 year
   b. Rifampin 600 mg/day by mouth, or 10 mg/kg/day, for 1 year
   c. Ethambutol hydrochloride 25 mg/kg/day by mouth initially, which should be decreased to 15 mg/kg/day as soon as possible after the treatment course is established, then maintained for 1 year

Note: Pyridoxine 10 to 20 mg/day should be given with isoniazid to prevent polyneuropathy.

3. Second-choice drugs that may be substituted for one or more of the above follow:
   a. Pyrazinamide 20 to 40 mg/kg/day for a total of 3 g/day by mouth
   b. Streptomycin 1 g/day intramuscularly (IM)

Caution:

1. Antibiotic recommendations change from time to time, and consultation with an expert in infectious disease is recommended. Treatment must be monitored with repeated CSF examinations. The antibiotics listed here have a serious potential for toxicity with prolonged use; for example, ethambutol has been associated with optic neuropathy, and streptomycin may cause vestibular damage.
2. Slow acetylators (American Indians, Eskimos, Middle Easterners) do not tolerate high doses of isoniazid, and the addition of rifampin exacerbates this problem. A maximum dose of isoniazid 300 mg, combined with rifampin 600 mg, should be used.

MENINGITIS CAUSED BY FUNGAL DISEASE

1. The diagnosis is often elusive.
2. The onset is often gradual.
3. Systemic symptoms may be mild initially.
4. A CSF examination may show nonspecific findings of normal or low glucose, increased cell, and increased protein levels. These findings evoke a large differential diagnosis: herpes simplex encephalitis, tuberculous meningitis, leptospiral meningitis, secondary neurosyphilis, partially treated pyogenic meningitis, sarcoidosis, cerebral abscess, or subdural empyema.
5. In suspicious cases, obtain CSF for cryptococcal antigen as well as cultures of blood and CSF for *Cryptococcus* organisms.
6. The index of suspicion should be especially high in *immunocompromised* or *debilitated* patients. Patients with Hodgkin's disease or AIDS are particularly susceptible.
7. Common organisms are *Cryptococcus neoformans* (low-grade fever, cough, mental disturbance, eye abnormalities) and *Coccidioides immitis* (prolonged respiratory symptoms, subacute meningitis). However, in autopsy series (especially in medical centers with large numbers of immunocompromised patients), the most frequently identified fungal cause of a CNS infection is *Candida albicans*.

Treatment:
1. Amphotericin B 0.6 mg/kg/day IV, in conjunction with flucytosine 150 mg/kg/day, are life saving in most fungal infections. Because of their potential toxicity, these drugs should be administered by a clinician experienced in their use.
2. The course of treatment is determined by a clinical response and a CNS response documented by repeated CSF evaluation.

3. Occasionally intraventricular administration of amphotericin B is necessary to control the infection.

NEUROSYPHILIS

1. The clinical signs of symptomatic neurosyphilis are protean (stroke, dementia, a CNS mass lesion, meningitis, hydrocephalus); for this reason, CSF testing for syphilis must be done on every patient undergoing an LP; the diagnosis is most often made in this serendipitous manner.
2. The serologic tests for syphilis follow:
   VDRL, RPR, and automated reagin test (ART)—nontreponemal tests
   FTA-ABS test
   Microhemagglutination–*Treponema pallidum* (MHA-TP) test
   Treponema pallidum immobilization (TPI) test
   a. Nontreponemal cardiolipin antibody tests (VDRL, RPR) are the tests of choice on CSF.
   b. Treponemal tests confirm the diagnosis on serum samples; however, the tests are of low sensitivity and specificity on CSF.
   c. A decrease in serum nontreponemal titers documents adequate therapy.
3. Patients with a positive serum test for syphilis should have an LP to rule out asymptomatic neurosyphilis.

Treatment:
1. Neurosyphilis is a treatable disease; the progression may be stopped in all cases, and most patients will show improvement.
2. The following are several acceptable choices of antibiotic therapy:
   a. Aqueous penicillin G 2 to 4 million units IV every 4 hours for 10 days, followed by penicillin G benzathine 2.4 million units IM weekly, for 3 doses.
   b. Amoxicillin 3 g/day by mouth plus probenecid 1 g/day for 10 days, or aqueous procaine penicillin G IM 2.4 million units/day plus probenecid 500 mg at bedtime for 10 days, followed by penicillin G benzathine 2.4 million units IM weekly for 3 doses.
   c. For patients allergic to penicillin, tetracycline 500 mg by mouth at bedtime for 30 days can be substituted.
3. Patients with neurosyphilis must be followed with periodic serologic testing and repeat CSF examinations for 3 years.

ASEPTIC MENINGOENCEPHALITIS

1. Aseptic meningoencephalitis is the diagnosis given to a patient who shows evidence of inflammation of the meninges and brain tissue but shows no evidence of bacteria, fungi, spirochetes, or parasites. The CSF examination shows a slight increase in the number of cells, usually lymphocytes, with normal glucose levels and a slight elevation of protein.

Caution: Although laboratory tests do not find the organism, this is not conclusive evidence that organisms are indeed not present.

2. Aseptic meningitis is most commonly caused by viruses. The differential diagnosis, however, is wide and includes the following:
   a. Parameningeal infections.
   b. Carcinomatous or lymphomatous meningitis. CSF cytologic tests and flow cytometry will identify these.
   c. Rarer conditions include Behçet's disease, Vogt-Koyanagi syndrome, Mollaret's meningitis (some evidence suggest this may be caused by repeated reactivation of herpes simplex meningitis), and Lyme disease.
3. In cases in which the CSF examination shows an increased cell count, normal glucose level, and moderately increased protein level, the following laboratory tests should be performed:
   a. An acute serum should be drawn and frozen; 3 weeks later a second serum should be drawn, and both should be sent to a laboratory where serum responses to specific infectious processes can be detected. The ability to make a diagnosis of a specific agent is of value for epidemiologic purposes (such as elimination of an arthropod vector), as well as for care of the patient. If no rise in antibody titer is found, there should be a higher index of suspicion that the aseptic meningitis was caused by something other than a viral infection. Laboratories require that the physician specify which titers are to be checked; this should be done on the basis of a clinical picture of meningitis or encephalitis, the season of the year, geographic location, and assorted factors (Table 14-4).
   b. CSF tests for syphilis should be performed in all cases.
   c. Serum tests for Epstein-Barr virus (EBV), herpes simplex, and cytomegalovirus should be performed.
   d. Viral cultures of the CSF, pharynx, and stool are helpful in selected cases.
4. A presumptive diagnosis may be made during epidemics (arboviruses) or when there is a concurrent recognizable illness (such as mumps, measles, or infectious mononucleosis).

Treatment:
1. Supportive therapy, maintenance of fluid and nutrition (see Chapter 12)
2. Control of cerebral edema (see Chapter 13)
3. Control of seizures (see Chapter 11)

VIRAL DISEASES OF PARTICULAR IMPORTANCE
Acute Encephalitis
Herpes simplex **encephalitis.** Herpes simplex encephalitis is the most common sporadic viral encephalitis. It affects primarily the temporal lobes (a focal encephalitis), although brainstem encephalitides do occur.
1. A classic sign of the disease is early personality and behavioral changes (often with memory deficits), followed by lateralizing and localizing neurologic signs, such as hemiparesis or a visual field defect with increased intracranial pressure. Occasionally the patient may have an aseptic viral meningitis without focal findings.

TABLE 14-4
Common Viruses

Virus	Associated factors	Season	Prominent meningitic symptoms	Prominent encephalitic symptoms
ENTEROVIRUSES				
Poliovirus types 1,2,3	Appear in epidemics of gastrointestinal illness	Summer, early fall	X	
Coxsackie virus A9, B1-5				
Echovirus types 3, 4, 6, 9, 11, 18, 30				
ARBOVIRUSES				
Eastern equine	Atlantic Gulf Coast (mosquito vector)			
Western equine	Western United States (mosquito vector)			
Venezuelan equine	Florida, southwest (mosquito vector)			
St. Louis	All United States urban areas (mosquito vector)	Summer, early fall		X
Powassan	Northern United States (tick vector)			
California	All United States, primarily children (mosquito vector)			
Herpesvirus				
Herpes simplex type 1	Adult (mimics temporal lobe tumor)	Sporadic, winter		X
Herpes simplex type 2	Neonatal			
Varicella-zoster	Shingles, chickenpox	Winter, spring		
Epstein-Barr	Associated with infectious mononucleosis			
Cytomegalovirus	Infants, immunosuppressed adults			

Continued

TABLE 14-4
Common Viruses—cont'd

Virus	Associated factors	Season	Prominent meningitic symptoms	Prominent encephalitic symptoms
Myxovirus and Paramyxovirus				
Influenza	Rare	Winter		
Parainfluenza	Croup/bronchitis in young children	Winter		
Mumps	Parotitis; common cause of aseptic meningitis	Spring	X	
Measles (rubeola)	Encephalomyelitis 1-14 days after rash	Peak in April		X
Adenoviruses	Primarily in neonates			X
Arenavirus (lymphocytic choriomeningitis)	Contact with excreta of house mouse	Winter	X	X
Rabies virus	Animal bites			X

2. A CT scan or an MR image of the brain may be normal early in the course. After 48 hours, abnormalities are often apparent in the temporal lobe(s).
3. Early in the course of the illness, an electrocardiogram (EEG) may show characteristic periodic focal spikes from the temporal area with focal slowing or periodic lateralizing epileptiform discharges (PLEDs).
4. There is a reduction in mortality and neurologic sequelae if the diagnosis is established early and treatment with specific antiviral agents is started, particularly if therapy is initiated before coma ensues.

Treatment:
1. The efficacy of acyclovir (acycloguanosine) is established. Acyclovir 10 to 20 mg/kg IV every 8 hours should be administered for 10 days; the stabilization or improvement of clinical symptoms should be evident within 48 hours of beginning therapy. Renal function tests should be monitored.
2. Steroids (dexamethasone 10 mg IV initially, followed by 4 mg IV every 6 hours) may be used to reduce cerebral edema.
3. For herpes simplex encephalitis, cultures of CSF, throat swabs, and stools are of no use in revealing the organism but should be performed to rule out other pathogens.
4. A CSF herpes simplex polymerase chain reaction (PCR) is sensitive and specific for the diagnosis.
5. Since herpes infection is ubiquitous in the population and infections outside the nervous system are so common, acute and convalescent titers are usually not helpful unless immunoglobulin M (IgM) titers are elevated.

   Summer encephalitides. The following diseases occur in epidemics and are usually secondary to arboviruses:
1. Equine encephalitis should be suspected anywhere in the United States when the horse population first becomes affected; with eastern equine encephalitis, 80% of cases will have neurologic sequelae, whereas western equine encephalitis is milder, with 5% to 10% of cases having neurologic sequelae.
2. St. Louis encephalitis occurs primarily in the far western United States.
3. Venezuelan encephalitis occurs primarily in the southwestern United States.
4. California encephalitis (a tick-borne disease) occurs primarily in the midwestern United States.

Acute and convalescent viral titers need to be obtained, but treatment is symptomatic and supportive.

   Poliomyelitis. Poliomyelitis is now a rare disease in developed countries with compulsory immunization programs. It appears with a febrile illness followed by asymmetric weakness, often involving only one limb (except for bulbar polio) associated with a loss of deep tendon reflexes (see Chapter 15).

   Rabies. Rabies is a disease with the following characteristics:
1. Rabies appears as a brainstem encephalitis.

2. The disease is transmitted by animal bites, domestic or wild; particularly worrisome are unprovoked attacks by wild animals or bites from bats.
3. The most dangerous cases are multiple bites or bites around the face.

Note: In the case of an animal bite, the animal should be impounded and observed. Vaccination should be instituted with a rabies vaccine produced in cultured human diploid cells. Passive immunization with human antirabies antiserum may be used adjunctively. In all suspected cases consult local or state health authorities and an infectious disease specialist.

Chronic Encephalitis

Acquired immunodeficiency syndrome

1. The human immunodeficiency virus (HIV) that is responsible for AIDS resides chronically in the CNS long before clinical signs of systemic AIDS appear, but appropriate serologic tests can confirm the diagnosis within 6 weeks of the onset of infection. However, it can be years after the initial infection before the patient develops AIDS.
2. The neurologic complications of AIDS are a wide spectrum of disorders, from encephalitis and myelitis to neuritis and myositis. Neurologic signs and symptoms in a patient with AIDS may be a result of one or more of the following:
   a. Opportunistic infections in an immunocompromised host: for example, toxoplasmosis, progressive multifocal leukoencephalopathy (PML), cryptococcal and coccidioidal meningitis, cytomegalovirus encephalitis, disseminated *Mycobacterium avium intracellulare*
   b. Unusual primary or metastatic malignancies: for example, primary CNS lymphoma (reticulum cell sarcoma) or metastatic Kaposi's sarcoma
   c. The direct effect of the AIDS virus itself, which seems to have a propensity for causing damage to the deep cerebral white matter (This is called *AIDS-dementia complex [ADC]* and manifests as a dementing illness.)
3. Every patient with unusual or unexplained neurologic signs or symptoms should have a serologic evaluation for the AIDS virus.
4. CSF studies, together with MRI, will often identify an opportunistic infection of the CNS.

Treatment: A treatment specific for any documented opportunistic infection should be administered. Specific antiretroviral agents are used to treat HIV infection.

Progressive multifocal leukoencephalopathy

1. PML is a rare condition, occurring in immunocompromised or debilitated patients, presenting as sequential multifocal neurologic signs.
2. A CT scan or MRI shows multiple white matter lesions.
3. The disease is caused by a papavavirus.

Treatment: There is no effective treatment.

Creutzfeldt-Jakob disease (CJD); subacute spongiform encephalopathy; prion disease.

CJD is a rapidly progressive dementia associated with either myoclonus or extrapyramidal movement disorder caused by an infectious proteionparticle now termed a *prion*, derived by abnormal polymerization of a normal brain protein ("PrP"). No treatment is available (see Chapter 6).

Caution: The nervous system tissue of patients is highly infective, even after a sample is fixed in formalin (although a solution of 15% phenol in formalin or brief immersion of formalin-fixed tissue in formic acid solution does appear to inactivate the agent). Fluids and tissues of demented patients should therefore be handled with care, unless the cause of dementia is certain. Tissue from these patients should never be used for transplantation.

Subacute sclerosing panencephalitis
1. SSPE is a slowly progressive dementing and degenerative disease occurring primarily in children (caused by reactivation of a latent form of an altered measles virus), years after clinical measles. Its incidence has decreased since a widespread compulsory measles immunization in North America, but it is still prevalent in underdeveloped countries.
2. The four clinical stages of SSPE are identified as follows:
   Stage I–Personality, behavioral, and cognitive changes, often with apraxia and agnosia
   Stage II–The onset of characteristic slow myoclonus that is periodic, often involving the trunk and axial structures
   Stage III–The progression of focal neurologic signs
   Stage IV–A neurovegetative state followed by death
3. A characteristic EEG change of periodic complexes (usually generalized) in a relatively normal background occurs in late stage I or early stage II.
4. Markedly elevated measles antibody titers are identifiable in the CSF.
Treatment: No curative treatment is available. Reports suggest that isoprinosine (Inosiplex) or intrathecal interferon arrests the disease for a while in some cases.

Progressive rubella encephalitis.
Progressive rubella encephalitis occurs in children with congenital rubella (see Chapter 16) after 8 to 19 years and is characterized by progressive dementia, seizures, ataxia, and spasticity. CSF tests show increased lymphocytosis, mildly increased protein, and markedly increased gamma globulin. Serum and CSF show markedly increased rubella antibody titers.
Treatment: There is no effective treatment.

Postinfectious Encephalopathies
There are a number of uncommon acute toxic encephalopathies and acute and subacute hemorrhagic and nonhemorrhagic leukoencephalopathies that are best managed at a specialized center. However, prompt recognition and initial management of Reye's syndrome are imperative before referral.

Reye-Johnson syndrome
1. Reye-Johnson syndrome appears with vomiting, then a rapid decrease in consciousness in children with preceding viral infections (usually influenza B).

2. Differential clinical staging criteria have been proposed, but generally, if the patient reaches the state of coma, the point of irreversibility may have been passed.
3. A massive cerebral edema may be evident as papilledema or on CT scan or MRI of the brain. An LP and measurement of CSF pressure *should not* be done without preparation for medical (by mannitol) or surgical decompression. Management usually requires an ICU with the ability to do continuous intracranial pressure monitoring.
4. Treatment of the syndrome is aimed primarily at decreasing intracranial pressure, supporting vital functions, and preventing complications of a comatose patient (see Chapter 13).
5. There is a probable role of aspirin or salicylates in causing this disease, with recent data indicating a strong association. Therefore the present recommendation is that no salicylates be given to children with fever. Some evidence also suggests that the risk may be similar in adults.

Herpes Zoster

1. The varicella (chickenpox) virus resides asymptomatically in the dorsal root ganglia and for unknown reasons may occasionally migrate along sensory roots, causing pain and later, herpes zoster (shingles), a vesicular skin eruption in root distribution.
2. Pain may precede the eruption of skin vesicles by several days, making a diagnosis obscure until the eruption occurs.
3. Patients should be evaluated for underlying immune deficiency, especially lymphomas, HIV infection, or diabetes mellitus.
4. Acyclovir is a useful treatment, decreasing pain and new vesicle formation. The dosage is acyclovir 15 mg/kg IV in three divided doses daily for 5 to 10 days. In otherwise healthy patients, prednisone 60 to 80 mg daily by mouth for 2 to 3 weeks may reduce the risk of postherpetic neuralgia.
5. Complications follow:
   a. Postherpetic neuralgia occurs in about 15% of patients with shingles. Treatment is symptomatic: carbamazepine 200 mg 3 or 4 times daily after meals or gabapentin (Neurontin) 400 to 1200 mg daily. Topical preparations containing capsaicin (the active ingredient in hot peppers) may also alleviate this condition.
   b. Ophthalmic zoster carries the danger of corneal scarring. Treatment is with local steroids and antibiotics; patients should be referred to an experienced ophthalmologist for care.
   c. Geniculate zoster will present with a peripheral facial palsy. Management is the same as with Bell's palsy (see Chapter 15).

BIBLIOGRAPHY

Bell WE, McCormick WF: *Neurologic infections in children,* ed 2, Philadelphia, 1981, WB Saunders.
Bell WE, McGuinness GA: Current therapy of acute bacterial meningitis in children. II. *Pediatr Neurol* 1:201-209, 1985.
Booss J, Thornton GF, editors: Infectious diseases of the central nervous system, *Neurol Clin* 4:1-325, 1986.

Corey L, Spear PE: Infections with herpes simplex viruses, *N Engl J Med* 314:749-757, 1986.

Hirsh MS, Schooley RT: Treatment of herpesvirus infections, *N Engl J Med* 309:963-969, 1986.

Hook WH, Marra CM: Acquired syphilis in adults, *N Engl J Med* 326:1060-1067, 1992.

Johnson GM, Scurletis D, Carole NB: A study of 16 fatal cases of encephalitis-like disease in North Carolina children, *NC Med J* 29:464-473, 1963.

Johnson RT: *Viral infections of the nervous system,* New York, 1982, Raven Press.

McArthur J: Neurologic manifestations of AIDS, *Medicine* 66:407-437, 1987.

Navia BA, Jordan BD, Price RW: The AIDS dementia complex: clinical features, *Ann Neurol* 19:517-524, 1986.

Smith AL: Neurologic sequelae of meningitis, *N Engl J Med* 319:1010-1013, 1988.

Steele AC: Lyme disease, *N Engl J Med* 321:586-596, 1989.

Whitley RJ: Viral encephalitis, *N Engl J Med* 323:242-250, 1990.

15

Focal and Diffuse
Weakness of
Peripheral Origin

Although generalized weakness may be caused by a variety of medical problems (such as anemia or cardiac failure) or by psychiatric disturbances, in this chapter weakness is assumed to be a result of disease of the peripheral nervous system (PNS) (muscle or nerve) or the central nervous system (CNS). Sometimes it is difficult to differentiate PNS disease from CNS disease. The following guidelines may be helpful:

1. Hyperactive muscle stretch reflexes and extensor plantar responses (Babinski's reflex) are associated with CNS disorders.
2. Hypoactive muscle stretch reflexes generally indicate a weakness of PNS origin, except in the acute phase of CNS disease or in a long-standing, extremely severe CNS disease.
3. The involvement of an arm and a leg on the same side suggests CNS disease.
4. Changes in muscle bulk (such as atrophy or hypertrophy) suggest PNS disease.
5. Trophic changes in the skin and hair, especially if associated with changes in muscle bulk, suggest PNS disease.

Once the clinician has determined that the weakness is of PNS origin, Tables 15-1 and 15-2 may be helpful for determining whether the problem primarily involves the muscle or the nerve.

DIFFUSE WEAKNESS OF PERIPHERAL ORIGIN
Polyneuropathy
Diabetic neuropathy. The following three types of neuropathies are associated with diabetes, and a patient may have one or any combination of all three neuropathies:

1. Diabetic peripheral neuropathy

▶   a. The usual signs are paresthesias, hyperesthesias, pain in the feet, and painless foot trauma; suspect neuropathy when either an

TABLE 15-1
Differentiation of Nerve and Muscle Disease on Clinical Examination*

Sign	Nerve	Exceptions	Muscle	Exceptions
Reflexes	Absent early	In anterior horn cell disease, reflexes preserved	Usually present	In end-stage muscle disease and in polymyositis, reflexes are diminished or absent.
Distribution of weakness	Distal	Weakness occurs occasionally in anterior horn cell disease and lead poisoning; weakness is proximal.	Proximal	Myotonic dystrophy has distal weakness.
Sensory disturbance	Usually present	In anterior horn cell disease, sensory disturbances are absent; motor symptoms appear first in some neuropathies.	Absent	In inflammatory myopathy, nerve terminal branches can be involved; pain may be misinterpreted as sensory disturbances.
Autonomic disturbance	Often present	Autonomic disturbances are absent in anterior horn cell disease.	Absent	In inflammatory myopathy, nerve terminal branches can be involved.
Atrophy	Early	Atrophy is absent in early anterior horn cell disease.	Late	Common in muscular dystrophy or the congenital myopathies.
Hypertrophy	Rare	Hypertrophy is absent in plexiform neurofibroma.	Common in Duchenne's dystrophy	—
Cramps	With initiation of exercise	—	After exercise	—

*Characteristic findings are (1) myotonia, which are found in myotonic dystrophy, myotonia congenita, and periodic paralysis, and (2) fasciculations, which indicate anterior horn cell disease but may be benign in situations such as excess caffeine intake.

TABLE 15-2
Laboratory Features That May Be Helpful in Corroborating Clinical Differentiation of Nerve or Muscle Involvement

Test	Nerve	Exceptions	Muscle	Exceptions
Creatine phosphokinase (CPK)	Normal	Elevated factitiously after injections and trauma; elevated 2-3 times normal in anterior horn cell disease	Markedly elevated 8-200 times normal	End-stage muscle disease, rare cases of inflammatory muscle disease, and "congenital" myopathies
Needle electromyogram (EMG)	Fibrillations and fasciculations (large-amplitude units)	Possibly normal less than 3 wk from onset; in severe disease electrical activity not detectable	Small motor units	Fibrillations, which may occur in inflammatory disease
Nerve conduction velocity	Usually a decrease	Usually normal in anterior horn cell disease and selective axonal disorders	Normal	—
Muscle biopsy	Small atrophic fibers and grouping of fiber types	Normal less than 3 wk from onset or sampling error	Necrotic muscle fibers and abnormal fiber architecture, which are common	Sampling error

exaggerated withdrawal response to plantar stimulation or summation (e.g., recurrent pinpricks suddenly become painful) is present (see Chapter 1).
   b. Some degree of peripheral neuropathy is evident in almost all diabetic patients.
   c. Significant peripheral neuropathy is usually associated with absent ankle reflexes.
   d. Severe diabetic peripheral neuropathy (pseudotabes) may be characterized by recurrent spontaneous pain (described as "deep in the bones"), a loss of pain sensation in the joints, sensory ataxia, and the development of perforating ulcers.

Note: It is sometimes necessary to differentiate peripheral polyneuropathy (a symmetric involvement of all peripheral nerves, usually resulting from a metabolic disturbance and affecting the distal portions of extremities more than the proximal) from mononeuritis multiplex (an involvement of multiple individual nerves, often asymmetric and proximal and usually the result of vasculitis). Both types of peripheral neuropathy may occur in diabetic patients. The "stocking" component of the symmetric peripheral neuropathy is always clinically more evident before the "glove" component.

2. Diabetic autonomic peripheral neuropathy
   a. The patient with diabetic autonomic peripheral neuropathy commonly complains of excessive sweating or a loss of sweating in a portion of the body and symptoms resulting from postural hypotension.
   b. Other symptoms may include impotence, atonic bladder, palpitations, and abnormalities of gastrointestinal motility.
   c. Individuals with diabetic autonomic peripheral neuropathy are susceptible to heat stroke.

3. Diabetic lumbosacral radiculoplexoneuropathy
   a. Previously known as *diabetic amyotrophy,* diabetic lumbosacral radiculoplexoneuropathy is characterized by weakness and atrophy of the quadriceps muscles; nocturnal pain in the groin, thigh, back, and perineum; and the presence of fasciculations.
   b. Sensory loss is minimal for patients with this polyneuropathy; the knee reflex may be absent whereas the ankle reflex is present.
   c. This neuropathy is important to diagnose because an improvement is often noted with better blood glucose control.

Treatment:
1. Pain should not be treated with narcotics. Gabapentin (Neurontin) 100 to 400 mg by mouth 3 times a day, carbamazepine 200 mg by mouth 2 times a day and topiramate (Topamax) 25 mg by mouth 2 times a day offer good pain control.
2. The value of glycemic control in all forms of diabetic neuropathy is generally accepted. Neuropathic pain reduces quickly and clinical signs improve with euglycemia.
3. The value of immunotherapy is unclear.

Polyneuropathies associated with deficiency states and metabolic disorders. Polyneuropathies associated with deficiency states and metabolic disorders are extremely common and, in most instances, closely resemble the diabetic polyneuropathies, although there are some individual characteristics in each.

Vitamin B$_{12}$ deficiency

1. The clinical presentation of a vitamin B$_{12}$ deficiency (pernicious anemia, subacute combined degeneration, combined systems disease) is variable because the patient may have only one or more of the following disturbances:
   a. Peripheral neuropathy: the patient may experience a moderate to severe involvement of sensation and, in later stages, distal muscle atrophy and weakness.
   b. Spinal cord involvement: the patient may have posterior-column symptoms, such as markedly diminished or absent vibratory and position sensation (particularly in the lower extremities), as well as sensory ataxia; on examination, the patient will fall from a standing position with the eyes closed (a positive Romberg's test). Spasticity from corticospinal tract involvement with paraparesis or quadriparesis (tetraparesis) occurs; on clinical examination, bilateral extensor plantar responses (a Babinski's reflex) will usually be present. This is called *subacute combined degeneration of the cord.*
   c. Dementia: in the patient, dementia may be clinically indistinguishable from other forms of dementia (see Chapter 6).
   d. Neuropsychiatric disorder: the patient may have prominent behavioral and personality changes, particularly depression.
   e. Optic nerve atrophy: the patient may experience impaired vision.

Remember: It may be difficult to demonstrate spasticity or posterior-column disturbance with severe peripheral neuropathy, and demonstrating sensory disturbance may be difficult with significant dementia.

2. A diagnosis is best established by finding high levels of serum methylmalonic acid. Low serum vitamin B$_{12}$ levels are helpful in establishing a diagnosis but may not be abnormal even with tissue deficiency. A Schilling test is rarely necessary in modern practice.
3. Anemia or disturbances of blood cell morphologic structures may be absent and should not be used as criteria for excluding this diagnosis.

Treatment: Treatment should be started only *after* the diagnosis is *definitely established*. We suggest replacement with vitamin B$_{12}$ 1000 µg intramuscularly *(IM)* daily for 5 days, followed by 1000 µg IM every 2 weeks for life. The literature does not support the requirements of vitamin B$_{12}$ in a deficient state, and these patients may require a higher maintenance dose for life.

Caution: The administration of folic acid may mask the hematologic abnormalities of vitamin B$_{12}$ deficiency and can worsen the neurologic symptoms.

Folic acid deficiency

1. Folic acid deficiency is often indistinguishable from vitamin B_{12} deficiency, except that dementia is usually the most prominent neurologic symptom.
2. A diagnosis is established by low serum folate levels.

Treatment: Before folic acid is administered, vitamin B_{12} deficiency must be definitely excluded. Folic acid 5 mg should be administered daily.

Thiamine deficiency–alcoholic polyneuropathy

Thiamine deficiency is most common in alcoholic patients (see Chapter 8) with absent ankle reflexes, paresthesias, and minimal motor weakness.

Other metabolic causes of peripheral polyneuropathy

1. Chronic renal failure is associated with peripheral polyneuropathy.
2. The remote effect of carcinoma, particularly bronchogenic carcinoma, can cause polyneuropathy. (Serum antibody assays are available to support this cause of peripheral polyneuropathy.)
3. Drug-induced peripheral polyneuropathy can occur with many agents, including vincristine, cisplatin, nitrofurantoin, dapsone, isoniazid (INH), and disulfiram.
4. Heavy metal poisoning, such as arsenic, lead, mercury, and thallium, are the most common metal poisonings associated with peripheral neuropathy. Specific features of these polyneuropathies are summarized in Table 15-3.

Genetic metabolic causes

1. Metachromic leukodystrophy, Krabbe's leukodystrophy

Guillain-Barré syndrome. Guillain-Barré syndrome (Landry-Guillain-Barré-Strohl syndrome, acute inflammatory polyradiculoneuropathy, "French polio," ascending polyradiculoneuropathy) is a polyneuropathy with the following characteristics:

▶ 1. The syndrome causes an acute symmetric progressive weakness that is usually greater distally than proximally and is usually worse in the legs than the arms; usually the weakness has an ascending paralysis that affects motor nerves more than sensory nerves.
2. The reflexes are absent early in the disease.
3. The facial nerves may be involved.

Caveat: Bilateral facial weakness of rapid onset accompanied by a motor polyneuropathy is most often caused by Guillain-Barré syndrome.

4. Sensory loss is variable but usually mild; when present, position and vibration senses are more affected than the pinprick sensation. Patients, however, often have some sensory symptoms at the onset.
5. The onset is subacute 80% of patients peak within 2 weeks. More than half of the patients have a history of an antecedent "flulike" illness that has resolved by the time of the onset of polyradiculoneuropathy; 10% of patients have had surgery 1 to 4 weeks before the onset; a postimmunization occurrence has been reported.

TABLE 15-3
Principal Metal Toxins

	Arsenic	Lead	Mercury	Thallium
Clinical tip-off	Red hands and burning feet with hyperhidrosis	Peripheral neuropathy that may appear to be a single nerve involvement (such as a wristdrop or footdrop)	Severe spontaneous arm and leg pain	Alopecia
Exposure	Homicide attempts; insecticides; medicinal arsenic; Paris green; accidental contamination; Fowler's solution (potassium arsenite)	Industrial ingestion; tetraethyl gasoline; lead paint; burning lead batteries; eating from pewter or dishware with a glaze containing lead; melting lead for purposes of molding	Ingestion of methyl mercury (Minamata disease), especially from fish in polluted areas; industrial exposure; antifungal treatment of grain	Homicide; insecticide; rodent poison
Clinical syndrome	"Stocking-glove," mainly sensory neuropathy; severe pain and paresthesias, especially of feet; "burning feet and hands," red hands with hyperhidrosis and subsequent motor neuropathy involving distal muscles of hands and feet	Primarily a motor neuropathy that frequently may appear as though single nerves are involved, such as the radial nerve (wristdrop), the median nerve (thenar atrophy), or the peroneal nerve (footdrop); painful joints; cerebral edema in children	Dementia with primary motor neuropathy; occasional sensory stocking-glove neuropathy; acrodynia (pink disease) in infants and young children	Distal sensorimotor neuropathy of stocking-glove type with alopecia
Diagnosis	24-hour urine analysis; hair analysis; blood arsenic level	Blood lead level; 24-hr urine analysis	24-hr urine analysis	24-hr urine analysis
Treatment	Penicillamine 250 mg 4 times a day (may also use BAL or EDTA)	Penicillamine 250 mg 4 times a day (may also use BAL or EDTA)	Penicillamine 250 mg 4 times a day (may also use BAL or EDTA)	Diphenylthio-carbazone or sodium dicarbamate

BAL, Dimercaprol; *EDTA,* ethylenediaminetetraacetic acid.

6. Autonomic function may also occur, but manifestations are variable and include bladder disturbance, fluctuating blood pressure with postural hypotension, anal sphincter weakness, gastrointestinal motility disturbances (including dysphagia), and sluggishly reactive pupils; abnormalities of cardiac rhythm may occur; a loss of sweating in lower extremities may result in increased sweating in the upper extremities.

7. After the first few days of symptom onset, the CSF protein is elevated and only a few lymphocytes are present, usually less than 10 cells/μl (so-called albuminocytologic dissociation). Peak levels of CSF protein (may be greater than 2000 mg/dl) occur between 4 to 6 weeks after the onset of illness and may continue to rise as clinical improvement occurs.

8. A maximum deficit occurs between 3 days and 4 weeks; a spontaneous recovery occurs from 6 weeks to 6 months.

9. Routine nerve conduction velocities are normal in up to 10% of patients; tests of F-wave latency and the H-reflex are usually abnormal.

10. Neurologic complications of arsenic poisoning or of acquired immunodeficiency syndrome (AIDS) may closely mimic Guillain-Barré syndrome and should be excluded by appropriate tests.

11. The first sign of chronic inflammatory demyelinating polyneuropathy may mimic Guillain-Barré syndrome. However, such patients have multiple relapsing episodes at varying intervals and of varying duration, often without complete recovery between exacerbations.

Treatment:

1. The availability of an intensive care nursing unit is vital for managing the acute life-threatening complications of Guillain-Barré syndrome (see also Chapter 20).

2. Respiratory function must be closely monitored initially with frequent (at least hourly) bedside measurements of forced vital capacity (FVC) and negative inspiratory force (NIF), which is a direct pulmonary reflection of muscular strength. Respiratory function must be closely monitored even in patients with no apparent respiratory involvement, since rapid progression of weakness over several hours may lead to respiratory failure. If the FVC falls below 25 ml/kg or the NIF falls below 25 cm, mechanical ventilation should be instituted. The frequency of monitoring of respiratory function may be reduced as the patient shows signs of clinical improvement.

Caution: The use of paralyzing agents (such as succinylcholine) to facilitate endotracheal intubation may lead to dangerous hyperkalemia.

3. Ventilatory assistance must be provided at the first sign of dyspnea or decreased blood oxygen saturation. Dysphagia can result in aspiration; enteral tube feeding may be necessary. Paroxysmal hypertension, cardiac arrhythmias, and abnormal thermoregulation can occur and must be individually treated. Intercurrent infections must be treated vigorously. Prophylaxis against deep venous thrombosis should be started.

4. Plasma exchange or intravenous immunoglobulin (IVIg) therapy should be started as soon as the diagnosis is made. Therapeutic benefits include rapid improvement, a shorter period of ventilator support, and better outcome at 6 months. Overall, 70% of treated patients will be ambulatory at 3 months, but only 45% will be ambulatory if ventilatory support is required. Poor prognostic features are a low-amplitude compound muscle action potential (CMAP) amplitude on nerve conduction studies, old age, and respiratory failure requiring mechanical ventilation.

5. Treatment of the precipitating illness may be necessary; about 5% of cases have a preceding mycoplasmal infection requiring antibiotic therapy. Also, the syndrome of inappropriate antidiuretic hormone (SIADH) may occur in some patients and should be treated with careful fluid restriction.

6. Nursing care and physical therapy are necessary adjuncts. Frequent turning of the patient is important to avoid pressure sores. Pressure on peripheral nerves (especially the ulnar nerve at the elbow and the peroneal nerve at the fibular head) can destroy the still-intact nerve axons, as well as the delicate regenerating myelin, resulting in permanent nerve palsies; this should be avoided by appropriate patient positioning and cushioning. A passive range of motion is important to prevent contractures. Early mobilization of the extremities is necessary to avoid the development of thrombophlebitis with subsequent pulmonary embolization; low-dosage anticoagulation therapy may also be useful in preventing this complication.

7. Corticosteroids have no benefit in treating Guillain-Barré syndrome. In chronic relapsing polyneuropathy however, there is a definite benefit with corticosteroid therapy.

Diseases of the Anterior Horn Cell

Amyotrophic lateral sclerosis

▶ 1. Amyotrophic lateral sclerosis (ALS) is characterized by gradually progressive muscle weakness associated with muscle atrophy and fasciculations. The initial weakness may be proximal and resemble a muscle disease. The onset is usually asymmetric, and bulbar musculature may be affected first. Signs of upper motor neuron disease (hyperactive reflexes and extensor plantar responses) may be present initially.

Caveat: The simultaneous occurrence of upper and lower motor neuron paralysis in the same muscle (spastic hyperreflexia along with fasciculations and atrophy) suggests ALS.

2. ALS has no significant sensory abnormalities.

3. Occasionally, minor elevations of serum creatine phosphokinase (CPK) levels up to 3 times more than normal and the elevation of the CSF protein level to 70 to 80 mg/dl may be noted.

4. The diagnosis of ALS is usually established based on clinical and electrodiagnostic criteria.

5. Since the disease is fatal within several years in 80% of patients, ALS must be very carefully differentiated from the following potentially treatable conditions:
    a. Diseases of the cervical spinal cord (see Chapter 18), such as syringomyelia, spondylitic myelopathy, and tumors (fasciculations only in the upper extremities and upper motor neuron signs in the lower extremities)
    b. Diabetic amyotrophy (improvement with blood glucose control)
    c. Benign fasciculations (often seen in patients with excessive caffeine intake)

Treatment:

1. The intellect in ALS is preserved; careful counseling of the patient and family concerning the poor prognosis are mandatory.
2. If dysphagia is present, a feeding gastrostomy may make the patient more comfortable and improve his or her quality of life.
3. The use of ventilatory assistance in these totally paralyzed patients (eventually even eye movements become paralyzed) will lead to suffering a prolonged and agonizing death.
4. Further information on services available to patients with ALS can be obtained from the Muscular Dystrophy Association, 3300 E. Sunrise Dr., Tucson, AZ 85718; (800)572-1717; website: www.mdausa.org, or from the ALS Association, 27001 Agoura Road, Suite 150, Calabasas Hills, CA 91364; (818)340-7500; website: www.alsa.org.

Inherited anterior horn cell disease (spinal muscular atrophies [SMAs])

1. In infancy, the atrophy afflicts patients as *Werdnig-Hoffmann disease.* There are two forms of the disease—type I and type II spinal muscular atrophy.
   ▶ a. Werdnig-Hoffmann disease is characterized by a "floppy" baby (Fig. 15-1) with progressive weakness and feeding difficulties.
    b. Paradoxical breathing resulting from intercostal muscle weakness, is a cardinal sign of the disease.
    c. In the infant, fasciculations of the tongue are best seen at its lateral edges. Polyminimyoclonus of fingers—rapid abduction-adduction movements—are caused by fasciculations of intrinsic hand muscles.
    d. Death usually occurs in the first 2 years of life resulting from respiratory insufficiency in Type I spinal muscular atrophy. A patient with Type II atrophy has a slower course and a longer survival.
    e. This disorder is caused by an autosomal recessive gene located on chromosome 5.
2. In childhood or adolescence, the atrophy is termed *Kugelberg-Welander disease.* The disease is a Type II spinal muscular atrophy.
   ▶ a. The disease is characterized by a progressive, proximal weakness sometimes associated with pseudohypertrophy of the calves.
    b. In the patient, fasciculations may be visible in the extremities and tongue or seen on an electromyogram (EMG). Upper motor neuron signs are absent.
    c. This disorder may result from an autosomal recessive or autosomal dominant gene.

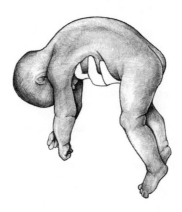

FIG. 15-1 A 1-year-old "floppy baby" with infantile spinal muscular atrophy (Werdnig-Hoffmann disease). Note that there is a marked lack of muscle tone.

3. A diagnosis is made on the basis of the clinical presentation, evidence of denervation on the findings of EMG studies, and characteristic pathologic conditions indicated by histochemically stained muscle biopsies. Currently, the gene can be tested for directly.

Treatment:

1. There is no specific treatment, but physical and occupational therapy should be directed toward maintaining limb function and preventing deformity and respiratory infections.
2. Genetic counseling is necessary.
3. Emotional support for the family should be provided.
4. Further information on services available to patients can be obtained from the Muscular Dystrophy Association.

Charcot-Marie-Tooth disease

▶ 1. Charcot-Marie-Tooth disease is also known as *peroneal muscular atrophy syndrome, dominantly-inherited hypertrophic polyneuropathy, or hereditary motor and sensory neuropathy.*
2. This disorder represents a group of hereditary neuropathies with different modes of inheritance and pathologic features.
3. The neuropathies are characterized by a slowly progressive foot deformity (pes cavus and hammertoes) and atrophy of the lower legs resulting in "stork legs" or "inverted champagne bottle legs" (Fig. 15-2). The most common early sign is a bilateral footdrop.
4. A diagnosis is suggested by appropriate clinical findings, family history, and abnormal nerve conduction studies.
5. The clinical signs of this disorder and the mode of inheritance varies from family to family, but the symptoms of affected individuals within a single family tend to be similar.

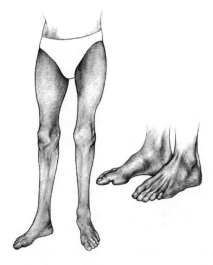

FIG. 15-2 Patients with the peroneal muscular atrophy syndrome (Charcot-Marie-Tooth disease) have a "stork legs" appearance caused by atrophy of the lower leg and distal one third of thigh musculature. Hammertoes and pes cavus may also be early signs of this disorder.

6. In some families, other neurologic signs may include sensory loss, enlarged nerves, and cerebellar ataxia.

Treatment: There is no specific treatment for this disorder, although disability is usually mild and compatible with a long life for the patient. Genetic counseling is necessary. The prevention of injuries to limbs that have reduced sensibility is imperative. Supportive physical and occupational therapy can often be provided through the Muscular Dystrophy Association.

Poliomyelitis

▶ 1. Poliomyelitis is an acute viral infection of the anterior horn cells. The weakness is often preceded by gastroenteritis and heralded by back and radicular pain.

2. The disease is usually asymmetric with flaccid weakness.

3. There may be paralysis of the bulbar muscles.

4. Aseptic meningitis occurs in the early stage of the disease.

5. A diagnosis is confirmed by acute and convalescent serologic titers and stool cultures.

▶ 6. Many years after the acute paralysis with varying degrees of subsequent recovery, a patient occasionally may experience an apparent progressive weakness, sometimes accompanied by pain. This might be a result of the premature loss of anterior horn cells (postpolio syndrome) that presumably have been overtaxed in having to maintain massive motor units.

Treatment:
1. There is no specific treatment for poliomyelitis.
2. Monitor respiratory function early in the disease.
3. Use bracing and prosthesis for weak limb(s).
4. The disease is now rare in North America because of prevention with appropriate vaccination. Vaccinate individuals who have been in contact with the patient, if not previously done.
5. There is no known treatment for postpolio syndrome.

Diseases of the Neuromuscular Junction

Myasthenia gravis

▶ 1. Myasthenia gravis is an acquired autoimmune disease of the neuromuscular junction.
2. Patients usually have ocular symptoms, such as double vision and droopy eyelids.
3. The symptoms may remain localized to the eyes (ocular myasthenia gravis) or may involve muscles of the extremities and the trunk (generalized myasthenia gravis).
4. Weakness is characteristically fatigable, and patients often complain of experiencing weakness at the end of the day.
5. A clinical examination should include an assessment of fatigability. Ask the patient to maintain a sustained upward gaze for at least 3 minutes without interruption and observe him or her for ptosis (Fig. 15-3). Have the patient perform repetitive muscle contractions

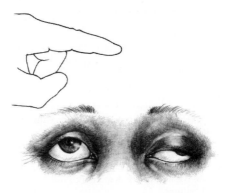

FIG. 15-3 In myasthenia gravis, fatigable weakness is evident on the examination of eye movements. There is usually ptosis, which becomes more evident as the patient attempts to sustain an upward gaze.

related to the complaint and observe him or her for evidence of developing weakness. For example, if the patient complains of weakness while climbing stairs, repetitive deep knee bends will become progressively more difficult to perform. If the patient complains of weakness in the hands, repetitive squeezing of a manometer cuff will show a progressive decrease in power. If the patient complains of difficulty in swallowing, repeated sips from a large glass of water will be normal at first but will subsequently result in choking.

6. The involvement of respiratory and pharyngeal muscles may occur with variable severity in the disease and can lead to fatal respiratory failure or aspiration.

7. Myasthenia gravis is an autoimmune disorder associated with the presence of acetylcholine receptor antibodies. Approximately 40% are associated with thymic pathologic conditions. Approximately 85% of those are thymic hyperplasia and 15% are arethymomas.

8. The following diagnostic tests can help diagnose the disorder:
   a. Acetylcholine receptor antibody testing (The antibodies are elevated in greater than 90% of patients with generalized myasthenia gravis.)
   b. Electrodiagnostic studies, including repetitive motor nerve stimulation showing a characteristic decrementing pattern and single-fiber EMG
   c. A Tensilon test in which edrophonium (Tensilon) chloride is injected into the patient with an observation of the clinical improvement in motor power
   d. A chest computed tomographic (CT) scan or magnetic resonance imaging (MRI) to look for thymic enlargement

9. In certain circumstances, a myasthenic crisis (an acute or subacute onset of respiratory failure) may be induced by drugs or an infection. This is a neurologic emergency (see Chapter 20). Some of the drugs that can produce a myasthenic crisis are curare, succinylcholine, aminoglycosides, dihydrostreptomycin, kanamycin, polymyxin, lincomycin, tetracycline, oxytetracycline, gentamicin, and quinine (tonic water).

10. During the neonatal period, 20% of infants born to myasthenic mothers have transient feeding difficulties, a weak cry, breathing difficulties, floppiness, and other myasthenic symptoms (transient neonatal myasthenia), and they require only supportive treatment. Persisting myasthenia after the neonatal period is caused by several congenital myasthenia syndromes resulting from inborn errors and not an autoimmune dysfunction. Repetitive nerve stimulation, before and after an edrophonium or neostigmine injection, makes the diagnosis. An intercostal muscle biopsy with special stains is needed to determine the presynaptic or postsynaptic defects and to classify the congenital myasthenic syndrome.

Treatment:
1. Acetylcholinesterase inhibitors: these inhibitors (such as pyridostigmine) are used for symptomatic therapy.

2. Plasma exchange: plasma exchange is indicated with significant bulbar involvement or a myasthenic crisis when patients are in respiratory failure (see Chapter 20).
3. Immunosuppression: steroids are useful for long-term immunosuppression in myasthenia gravis. Clinical worsening is expected to occur 7 to 10 days after starting steroids. This is predictable, and patients should be monitored closely during this period. Hospitalization may be necessary. Other immunosuppressive agents, including cyclosporine, axathioprine, and mycophenolate mofetil (CellCept), are used as steroid-sparing agents.
4. Thymectomy: the role of thymectomy in myasthenia gravis remains unclear. It is of little debate that thymectomy should be performed in patients with radiologic evidence of thymic enlargement.

Caution: Myasthenia gravis is a rare neurologic disorder. Myasthenic patients are fragile and should be followed regularly by a neurologist.

Lambert-Eaton (myasthenic) syndrome

1. The Lambert-Eaton syndrome resembles myasthenia gravis with complaints of tiredness and weakness, but ocular involvement is rare, unlike in myasthenia gravis. Patients often complain of a dry mouth and constipation.
2. The patient's strength may improve temporarily after voluntary muscle contraction, but prolonged effort results in fatigue.
3. The patient's muscle tendon reflexes are depressed but may improve after exercise.
4. The response to edrophonium is usually equivocal, and the diagnosis is established by characteristic findings with repetitive motor nerve stimulation.
5. Some 50% to 60% of cases are associated with an occult malignancy (particularly small cell carcinoma of the lung).
6. Antibodies against the voltage-gated calcium channel (VGCC) are identified in affected patients. Rarely, patients also have antiacetylcholine receptor antibodies and may have the signs and symptoms of both myasthenia gravis and the Lambert-Eaton syndrome.
7. The diagnosis may be made using the following studies:
   a. Electrodiagnostic studies, including repetitive nerve stimulation and single-fiber EMG
   b. Antibody testing for VGCC antibodies

Treatment:

1. Search for an occult malignancy, particularly small cell carcinoma of the lung.
2. Plasmapheresis and prednisone are beneficial in treating these patients.
3. A symptomatic improvement of strength and exercise tolerance may be achieved with pyridostigmine or 3,4-diaminopyridine 40 to 200 mg/day. Potential side effects include seizures and a confusional state.

Botulism

1. Botulism presents as a subacute paralysis of extraocular muscles with subsequent involvement of pharyngeal muscles.
2. Patients commonly complain of blurred vision and constipation in addition to generalized motor weakness.
3. A respiratory compromise secondary to skeletal muscle weakness occurs 24 to 48 hours after the onset.
4. Botulism is caused by the ingestion of toxin produced by *Clostridium botulinum*, which may be found in improperly canned acidic foods, such as green beans or salsa. The cause is rarely secondary to wound botulism.
5. A diagnosis can be confirmed by characteristic findings on repetitive nerve stimulation.

Treatment:

1. Polyvalent botulinum antitoxin should be administered, and the stomach and intestinal contents should be removed.
2. Respiratory failure is a major concern and should be monitored and treated in a manner similar to the respiratory problems of Guillian-Barré syndrome.

Diseases of the Muscle

Myotonic dystrophy

▶ 1. Myotonic dystrophy (Steinert's disease) is an autosomal dominant dystrophy characterized by complaints of a muscular stiffness (caused by myotonia) that is relieved after repetitive activity. It is associated with slowly progressive distal weakness, especially in the upper extremities.
2. Myotonia is a delayed relaxation of muscles, clinically recognized by the following studies:
   a. Have the patient make a tightly clenched fist for 30 seconds and observe his or her difficulty in opening the hand.
   b. Percussion of the thenar eminence with a reflex hammer will cause the patient's thumb to oppose the little finger and remain so for several seconds.
   c. Percussion of the patient's gastrocnemius produces a transient hard lump in the gastrocnemius.
   d. The findings of an EMG show a characteristic pattern with "dive-bomber" sounds.
3. Facial features are often distinctive in the patient with this disorder (Fig. 15-4); other characteristics include pronounced frontal balding, ptosis, cataracts, cardiac conduction defects, glucose intolerance, disturbed gastrointestinal motility, sleep problems (daytime somnolence), and psychologic disturbances (depression).
4. It is a systemic disorder associated with mild mental subnormality and diabetes mellitus resulting from an excessive number of triple repeats in the gene. The patient's family history reveals the phenomenon of anticipation—the appearance of symptoms earlier and earlier in succeeding generations.

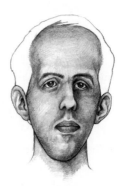

FIG. 15-4 Patients with myotonic dystrophy have the characteristic facial features of frontal baldness, depression of the temporal region (caused by atrophy and the loss of bulk of the temporalis muscle), and a long, thin face with a pointed chin.

5. Myotonic dystrophy may first appear in a floppy baby with respiratory distress and difficulty in feeding, usually in myotonic infants born to myotonic mothers. Mothers may have been minimally involved and previously undiagnosed.

6. Some other diseases with myotonia include myotonia congenita and hyperkalemic periodic paralysis.

Treatment:

1. Most patients do not require treatment of the myotonia, but for a few patients with incapacitating myotonia, phenytoin 100 to 400 mg/day is the preferred drug for relieving symptoms. Quinidine, procainamide, and imipramine can also be used.

2. Genetic counseling should be provided.

3. Cardiac evaluations are mandatory, and a pacemaker insertion may be necessary to prevent fatal cardiac arrhythmias.

4. Depressive psychologic (and other personality) disturbances may be improved by imipramine hydrochloride 50 to 150 mg at bedtime.

5. Pregnant women with myotonic dystrophy should be warned that there may be difficulty with the delivery and that the infant may have respiratory and feeding difficulties (a neonatal presentation of myotonic dystrophy).

Dystrophinopathies

Duchenne's muscular dystrophy

▶ 1. Duchenne's muscular dystrophy (DMD) is an x-linked muscular dystrophy. It is a hereditary disorder that affects only boys and is first manifested around 3 years of age by difficulty in running and climbing stairs.

2. On clinical examination, the following signs are seen:

   a. The calves are larger than normal and have a rubbery feel on palpation.

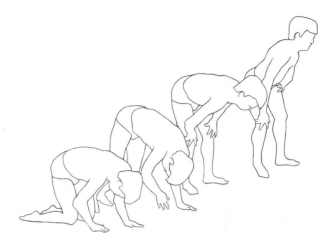

FIG. 15-5 In Duchenne's muscular dystrophy, the patient will get up from the floor with Gowers' maneuver. The boy will "walk up" his body with his hands as he arises.

  b. When the patient attempts to go from a lying to a standing position, he will try to climb up on his legs (Gowers' maneuver) (Fig. 15-5).
3. The serum CPK level is extremely high (8 to 200 times greater than normal).
4. The diagnosis is confirmed by an extremely high serum CPK level, by characteristic pathologic findings in histochemically stained muscle biopsies, and by biochemical analysis of muscle specimens revealing absence of the membrane protein *dystrophin* manufactured by a gene on the short arm of the X chromosome. DNA studies can reveal the exact gene mutation (most often a deletion) in the patient or in female carrier relatives.
5. An associated intellectual impairment is common in patients with the disorder.
6. A slowly progressive variant form of the disease with an onset in late childhood or adolescence is termed *Becker's muscular dystrophy.*
Treatment: Patients should be referred to the local clinics directed by the Muscular Dystrophy Association, which provides diagnostic facilities, genetic counseling, physical therapy, appliances such as braces and wheelchairs, and social services.
Inherited muscle diseases not associated with a dystrophic abnormality
Inherited muscle diseases that aren't associated with a dystrophic abnormality include: congenital muscular dystrophy, severe congenital autosomal recessive muscular dystrophy (SCARMD), and limb-girdle muscular dystrophy.

Polymyositis and dermatomyositis

1. The patient with polymyositis or dermatomyositis has subacute onset of proximal weakness. (A common complaint is difficulty in climbing stairs.)
2. Neurologic examination findings show evidence of proximal weakness demonstrated by difficulty performing deep knee bends or rising from a chair without support (Fig. 15-6).
3. The patient may have skin lesions, including malar flush, reddening at the base of the fingernails, a scaly rash over the extensor surface of the joints, and subcutaneous calcifications.
4. Characteristic pathologic findings are seen in histochemically stained muscle biopsies.
5. Approximately 10% to 20% of adults with dermatomyositis have an occult malignancy.
6. The serum CPK level is usually elevated, often above 1000 ml.

Treatment: Prednisone in a dosage of 1 to 2 mg/kg daily (children) or 100 mg daily (adults) will often result in a remission, but treatment with other additional immunosuppressive drugs may be necessary.

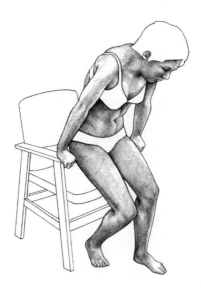

FIG. 15-6 The proximal muscle weakness found in polymyositis results in difficulty rising from a chair. Note that the patient must use her arms to push off the chair to come to a standing position.

Viral myositis

Viral myositis is a direct inflammation of muscle during a systemic viral illness that presents with pain and, less often, weakness and is usually self-limited with good recovery.

Inclusion body myositis

1. Inclusion body myositis (IBM) is the most common type of inflammatory myopathy in adults.
2. The diagnosis is based on the clinical phenotype of the distribution of weakness that is characteristic with a predominant distal weakness coupled with pathologic features on a muscle biopsy.
3. There is no effective treatment for IBM yet. Some reports showed response to IVIg therapy.

Muscle weakness associated with systemic disease

1. The patient with the type II muscle fiber atrophy has proximal weakness of subacute or chronic onset.
2. The disorder is associated with disuse ("disuse atrophy") or with various chronic disorders, such as cachexia, hypercorticism ("steroid myopathy"), hyperparathyroidism, cancer ("carcinomatous myopathy"), or hyperthyroidism ("thyroid myopathy").
3. Nerve conduction studies and serum CPK levels are usually normal. The EMG examination shows the presence of myopathic motor unit potentials.

Treatment:

1. Weakness is generally reversible if the underlying cause can be corrected.
2. This potentially treatable cause of muscle weakness must be carefully differentiated from the untreatable causes of proximal muscle weakness.

Malignant hyperthermia

1. Malignant hyperthermia is characterized by a sudden onset of marked hyperthermia (a body temperature of 42° C or 107° F and higher) during general anesthesia with halogenated anesthetics (halothane, enflurane) or succinylcholine. Other symptoms include extreme muscular rigidity, hyperkalemia, tachycardia, tachypnea, severe metabolic and respiratory acidosis, and myoglobinuria.
2. It is frequently familial and is occasionally associated with neuromuscular diseases, including central core disease and myotonia congenita. Several different gene defects related to skeletal muscle ion channels have been identified as causes of malignant hyperthermia.
3. Susceptible patients often have elevated serum CPK levels in preoperative blood studies.

Treatment:

1. Death occurs in more than 60% of patients in whom treatment is delayed. Immediate IV administration of dantrolene in a dosage of 1 to 10 mg/kg will usually abort an episode. Follow with oral dantrolene 1 to 2 mg/kg 4 times a day for 1 to 3 days to prevent recurrence.
2. Prevention of the disease is most important. If there is a family history of anesthetic-associated deaths, the known precipitating anesthetic

agents should be avoided. If surgery in a known susceptible individual is indicated, preoperative treatment with dantrolene 1 to 2 mg/kg every 6 hours for 1 or 2 days before surgery with a last dose of 2 mg/kg 3 hours before surgery may prevent development of the syndrome.

FOCAL WEAKNESS OF PERIPHERAL ORIGIN

Nerve Lesions

Localized weakness is frequently a result of injury of the peripheral nerve, plexus, nerve root, or nerve cell body (Fig. 15-7). In most cases, there is both a motor and a sensory disturbance. The specific site of the nerve injury is recognized by the pattern of muscle weakness and by the distribution of the cutaneous sensory disturbance. Sometimes it is difficult to determine the exact muscle involvement by clinical examination, and in

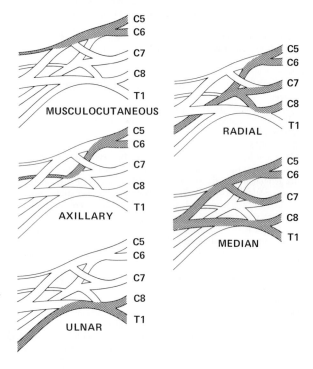

FIG. 15-7 A diagram of the relationship among cervical nerve roots, brachial plexus, and peripheral nerves.

such circumstances, the findings of an EMG may determine the specific muscles involved. Since most clinicians do not often evaluate patients with peripheral nerve lesions, help is available from a thin, inexpensive paperback book from the Medical Research Council that can be carried in a physician's bag: *Aids to the examination of the peripheral nervous system* (Her Majesty's Stationery Office, England).

Although specific causes of focal peripheral nerve weakness are not discussed in this chapter, root lesions are most commonly caused by a herniated intervertebral disc, plexus lesions by trauma or infection, or peripheral nerve lesions by trauma, pressure, or vascular occlusion. Multiple individual nerve lesions may occur in a single extremity (as in trauma, vascular injury, or infection) or in multiple extremities (mononeuritis multiplex). The descriptions of common peripheral weakness patterns should be recognized by the clinician.

Root lesions

Common cervical root syndromes involve the C6 and C7 roots and are discussed in Chapter 18. The relationship of the cervical roots, brachial plexus, and peripheral nerves are shown in Fig. 15-7. Common lumbar root syndromes involve the L4, L5, and S1 roots and are discussed in Chapter 17.

Peripheral nerve lesions

Radial nerve (Fig. 15-8)

▶ 1. A radial nerve lesion is characterized by weakness of extension of the wrist and fingers (wristdrop) and only a small area of sensory loss along the dorsum of the base of the thumb (anatomic snuff-box).

2. The lesion is known as *Saturday night palsy* because paralysis commonly occurs from prolonged pressure on the nerve in the upper arm, such as might occur with an intoxicated person in a semistuporous state resting with an arm hanging over a park bench.

Treatment:

1. If the injury is caused by pressure, a spontaneous recovery will usually occur between 2 and 6 months.

2. Until recovery occurs, a cock-up splint for the wrist may make the hand more functional.

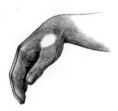

FIG. 15-8 With a radial nerve palsy, there will be a wristdrop (caused by weakness of the radial-innervated wrist extensor muscles) and a small patch of sensory disturbance in the area of the "anatomic snuff-box."

Median nerve

1. Median neuropathy at the wrist (carpal tunnel syndrome). The syndrome has the following characteristics:

▶ a. The patient will complain of pain and paresthesias in the hand, especially of the thumb and index finger. The patient may also complain of pain more proximally in the forearm, upper arm, or shoulder. The pain is frequently worse at night, often awakening the patient; pain relief may be obtained by rubbing or shaking the hand and arm or letting the hand hang over the side of the bed.

   b. Although the patient may complain of a reduced sensibility in the thumb and index finger, actual sensory loss may be difficult to demonstrate on formal testing.

   c. Weakness and atrophy of the thenar muscles are usually late signs of the syndrome.

   d. Tinel's sign (Fig. 15-9) is obtained by lightly tapping the median nerve at the wrist with such a tap reproducing the symptoms. Hyperextension or hyperflexion of wrist may produce the same effect.

   e. The syndrome may be bilateral but is usually worse in the dominant hand.

   f. Finding prolongation of the distal latency on nerve conduction velocity studies of the median nerve at the wrist, and slowing of the median nerve conduction across the wrist establishes the diagnosis.

   g. The syndrome is associated with rheumatoid arthritis (collagen vascular disease), hypothyroidism, obesity, acromegaly, gout, and multiple myeloma; carpal tunnel syndrome initially appearing during a pregnancy usually resolves after delivery.

Treatment:

1. Treatment of any underlying disease is necessary.

2. Symptomatic relief is usually obtained with a wrist splint, which keeps the wrist in a neutral position and prevents repetitive motion.

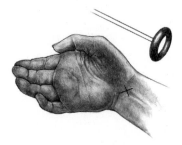

FIG. 15-9 Tinel's sign is a burning-tingling sensation in the fingers, produced by tapping over the median nerve at the site of entrapment under the carpal ligament in the carpal tunnel syndrome.

3. Most patients with the carpal tunnel syndrome do not necessarily require surgery, although sectioning of the carpal ligament will relieve pressure on the nerve in severe cases.

Ulnar nerve

▶ 1. Characteristic clinical features of ulnar nerve lesions include the following:
   a. In a slight or early injury:
      1) A weakness of finger extension (especially the ring and little fingers)
      2) A weakness of little finger abduction
      3) A slight weakness of wrist flexion
   b. In a severe or long-standing injury:
      1) Atrophy of the hypothenar eminence
      2) Atrophy of the intrinsic hand muscles with hollowing between the metacarpal bones (especially evident in the space between the thumb and index finger; Fig. 15-10)
      3) A clawhand or "beer stein holder's hand" deformity
   c. A sensory loss of the little finger and medial half of the ring finger
2. The most common location of an injury is at the condylar (ulnar) groove at the elbow; the most common modes of injury are pressure and arthritis. A previous fracture or a shallow condylar groove predisposes to injury; *tardy ulnar palsy* refers to recurrent injuries to the ulnar nerve at the elbow, resulting in a slowly progressive loss of ulnar nerve function (frequently involving the dominant hand).

Treatment:

1. Padding the patient's elbow and educating him or her to avoid ulnar nerve injury at the elbow may result in the return of ulnar nerve function.
2. Anterior surgical transposition of the nerve may be necessary to avoid repeated injury.

Caveat: The radial, ulnar, and median nerves all supply the muscles of the thumb. Extension is served by the radial nerve, adduction is served by the ulnar nerve, and opposition is served by the median nerve (Fig. 15-11).

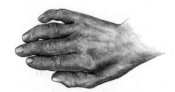

FIG. 15-10 Lesions of the ulnar nerve produce atrophy of the interossei of the hand, which is evident as a "guttering" between the carpal bones.

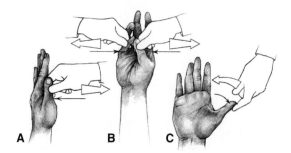

FIG. 15-11 Functional integrity of the radial, median, and ulnar nerves can be tested by examining the strength of the thumb. **A,** Adduction—ulnar-innervated muscles. **B,** Opposition—median-innervated muscles. **C,** Extension—radial-innervated muscles.

Idiopathic facial palsy (Bell's palsy)

▶ 1. A facial palsy is characterized by an acute or a subacute onset of complete or partial unilateral paralysis of the facial muscles, including the forehead (Fig. 15-12). This paralysis may be associated with a previous nonspecific viral illness and is not associated with any other neurologic abnormalities.
  2. The patient may complain of hypersensitivity to noise on the same side resulting from paralysis of the stapedius muscle.
  3. If the injury to the facial nerve is proximal to the chorda tympani, loss of taste on the anterior two thirds of the tongue on the same side as the paralysis can be demonstrated by careful examination; however, patients rarely complain of any change in taste.
  4. The patient may complain of difficulty chewing because of an accumulation of food in the paralyzed cheek (resulting from buccinator muscle paralysis); there is no true dysphagia.

Caution: Bell's palsy is an idiopathic disorder with a good prognosis for spontaneous recovery. However, it must be differentiated from other causes of facial paralysis, including the following:

1. If there is decreased hearing or a decreased corneal reflex, suspect a cerebellopontine angle tumor, such as an acoustic neuroma (schwannoma) or meningioma.
2. If there are vesicles in the external auditory canal, suspect the Ramsay Hunt syndrome (infection of the geniculate ganglion with herpes zoster); there may be an underlying lymphoma.
3. Chronic otitis media or mastoiditis may damage the facial nerve.
4. Since the facial nerve passes through the parotid gland, an infection or inflammation (including sarcoidosis) of the parotid can cause facial nerve paralysis.

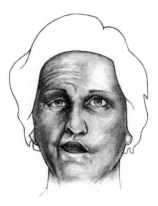

FIG. 15-12 The patient with Bell's palsy (facial nerve palsy) will demonstrate an unwrinkled forehead, widely opened eyes (with weakness of eyelid closure), flattening of the nasolabial fold, and a droop of the corner of the mouth.

5. Peripheral facial palsy may be an early neurologic sign of Lyme disease. Look for the characteristic erythema migrans at the site of the tick bite, and obtain appropriate Lyme titers.

Treatment:

1. Spontaneous recovery usually occurs.
2. Corticosteroids have not been shown to be beneficial, although it is a common practice to administer prednisone 80 mg every day for 5 days if the patient is seen within 3 days of the onset or if pain in or behind the ear is prominent.
3. The eye is vulnerable because lid closure is impaired, and the cornea must be protected with ophthalmic ointments, patches, or goggles.

Peroneal nerve

1. The patient with a peroneal nerve lesion has a footdrop ("slapping foot"). The lesion causes weakness of extension of the foot and toes and weakness of eversion (turning out) of the foot. In long-standing or severe lesions, there is wasting of the anterolateral compartment of the lower leg (Fig. 15-13).
2. Sensory loss may sometimes be demonstrated over the lateral and anterior portions of the lower leg and dorsum of the foot.
3. Injury to the common peroneal nerve in the lateral knee (where the nerve courses around the head of the fibula) often results from the following situations:
   a. Sitting with the legs crossed
   b. Pressure during sleep, coma, or anesthesia
   c. Pressure by casts, garters, boots, or braces
   d. Trauma or laceration to the area of the fibular head (as in climbing over a barbed wire fence)

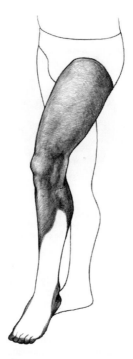

FIG. 15-13 In long-standing or severe lesions of the peroneal nerve, there is wasting of the anterolateral compartment of the lower leg.

Caveat: A peroneal nerve injury resembles an L5 root lesion; however, the internal hamstring reflex is diminished in an L5 root lesion but not in a peroneal nerve lesion (see Chapter 17), and the posterior tibial muscle (which inverts a plantar-flexed foot) is weak in an L5 root lesion but not in a peroneal nerve lesion.

Lateral femoral cutaneous nerve

▶ 1. The patient with a lateral femoral cutaneous neuropathy (meralgia paresthetica) has a sensory disturbance on the lateral aspect of the thigh (Fig. 15-14). The abnormal sensation may be a reduced sensibility, a pins-and-needles feeling, or burning discomfort, and may be exacerbated by touching the skin (as from clothing or stockings), or by prolonged standing or walking.
2. Since the lateral femoral cutaneous nerve is a sensory nerve to the skin, weakness is never present.
3. Symptoms are a result of compression of the lateral femoral cutaneous nerve in its passage under the inguinal ligament.

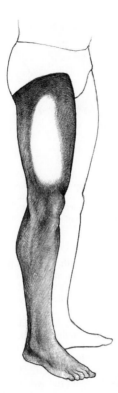

FIG. 15-14 Meralgia paresthetica is an uncomfortable (burning) sensation in the distribution of the lateral femoral cutaneous nerve. Both the hypersensitivity to sensory stimulation and the loss of normal sensibility can usually be demonstrated in this distribution.

    4. This condition commonly occurs in cases of obesity, pregnancy, diabetes, or trauma to the inguinal area or after wearing tight-fitting corsets.

Brachial plexopathy

    Lesions of the brachial plexus are difficult to diagnose but should be suspected when there is more extensive involvement than would be produced by a lesion of a single nerve or root.

Upper trunk of the brachial plexus lesion

▶ 1. The patient with a brachial plexopathy of the upper trunk (Erb-Duchenne palsy) has weakness about the shoulder and the elbow. The arm may dangle at the side with the fingers slightly flexed and

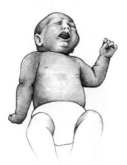

FIG. 15-15 An Erb-Duchenne palsy (a lesion of upper trunk of brachial plexus) will result in an inability to abduct and externally rotate the arm, with weakness of wrist extension leading to the characteristic "porter's tip" posture. Such an injury is not uncommon in infants as a result of traction on the head and neck during delivery.

the palm facing backward (the so-called porter's tip position; Fig. 15-15). This is caused by the inability to abduct and externally rotate the shoulder and to supinate and flex the forearm.

2. Biceps and brachioradialis reflexes are absent in patients with this condition.

3. Sensory loss is minimal with this condition but, if present, may be found over the lateral shoulder, thumb, and index finger.

4. The patient with this condition usually complains of a diffuse discomfort or pain in the shoulder.

5. These lesions are produced by a sudden traction that pulls the shoulder downward or pulls the neck in the direction opposite to the shoulder; this may occur during anesthesia, motorcycle accidents, or "rucksack paralysis" or as a birth injury, usually in large babies with shoulder dystocia during delivery.

Note: An upper trunk plexus injury resembles a C6 root lesion; external rotation and abduction of the shoulder are severely affected in the upper trunk plexus lesion but not in the C6 root lesion. Also, sensation is often intact in the upper trunk plexus lesion, but a sensory disturbance is usually present in the C6 root lesion (see Chapter 18). MRI of the spinal cord and spine may be necessary to rule out cervical spine disease.

Lower trunk of the brachial plexus lesion

▶ 1. The patient with a brachial plexopathy of the lower trunk (Klumpke-Dejerine palsy) has weakness of the forearm flexors and all intrinsic muscles of the hand; in long-standing or severe lesions, there will be atrophy of the intrinsic muscles of the hand, recession of the thumb into the plane of the hand, and extension of the wrist.

2. The triceps reflex is absent in these patients.

3. Often there is no sensory disturbance with this condition but, if present, it may be found along the posteromedial aspect of the forearm and the ulnar side of the hand.
4. The patient will frequently complain of a diffuse pain in the shoulder and axilla.
5. The condition may be associated with Horner's syndrome (ptosis, miosis, and facial anhidrosis on the same side as the injury) caused by damage to preganglionic sympathetic nerve fibers in the T1 root.
6. The lesion results from a sudden upward pull on the shoulder (e.g., a parent jerking upward on the arm of a falling child).

Note: Nerve transplantation operations are possible but controversial because of an incomplete recovery of brachial plexus lesions. The exact timing and indications should be determined with a neurosurgeon experienced in this kind of surgery.

Brachial plexus neuritis
▶ 1. The patient with brachial plexus neuritis (brachial plexitis) has a sudden onset (usually at night) of severe pain in the shoulder or arm, which is exacerbated by arm movement and elbow flexion. This is followed (within 2 weeks of the onset of the pain) by progressive weakness usually involving the shoulder girdle musculature innervated by the upper trunk of the brachial plexus, with lesser diffuse involvement of the musculature innervated by the rest of the plexus.
2. The patient's reflexes will be variably reduced depending on the extent and degree of the involvement.
3. Sensory loss is minimal or not detectable in these patients.
4. The condition may involve both arms but is usually asymmetric with greater involvement in the dominant arm.
5. The CSF is normal in these patients.

Treatment: Spontaneous recovery usually occurs but may take up to 2 years. Contractures may develop unless physical therapy range-of-motion exercises are undertaken until the strength returns.

Other Lesions Causing Focal Weakness
Focal myositis
1. With focal myositis, muscle inflammation may occur secondary to bacterial infection (a *Staphylococcus* or *Streptococcus* abscess), a parasitic infestation (toxoplasmosis, trichinosis, *Toxocara* infection), or granulomatous disease (tuberculosis [TB], histoplasmosis, actinomycosis, sarcoidosis).
2. The patient has swelling, weakness, pain, and tenderness in the affected muscles. This may be confused clinically with peripheral nerve, plexus, or root lesions but may be differentiated by finding an elevated serum CPK level.
3. A definitive diagnosis may be made by muscle biopsy with histochemical staining, bacterial and fungal stains, and cultures.

Treatment: Treatment is of the basic disease process. A fasciotomy may be necessary to prevent ischemic necrosis if associated swelling is marked.

BIBLIOGRAPHY

Beckmann JS: Disease taxonomy: monogenic muscular dystrophy, *Br Med Bull* 55(2):340-357, 1999.

Bedlack RS, Sanders DB: How to handle myasthenic crisis: essential steps in patient care, *Postgrad Med* 107(4):211-214, 2000.

Bril V, Kojic J, Dhanani A: The long-term clinical outcome of myasthenia gravis in patients with thymoma, *Neurology* 51(4):1198-1200, 1998.

Carrieri PB, Marano E, Perretti A, Caruso G: The thymus and myasthenia gravis: immunological and neurophysiological aspects, *Ann Med* 31S:52-56, 1999.

Cook JD, Tyre R, Gascon GG: Motor unit diseases from infancy to adolescence. In: Elzouki A, Harti H, Nazer H, editors: *Clinical textbook of pediatrics,* Philadelphia, 2001, Lippincott, Williams & Wilkins.

Dubowitz V: *Muscle disorders in childhood,* ed 2, London, 1995, WB Saunders.

Emery AE: The muscular dystrophies, *Br Med J* 317(7164):991-995, 1998.

Fletcher DD, Lawn ND, Wolter TD, Wijdicks EF: Long-term outcome in patients with Guillain-Barré syndrome requiring mechanical ventilation, *Neurology* 54(12):2311-2315, 2000.

Heitmiller RF: Myasthenia gravis: clinical features, pathogenesis, evaluation, and medical management, *Semin Thorac Cardiovasc Surg* 11(1):41-46, 1999.

Jaretzki A III, Barohn RJ, Ernstoff RM et al: Myasthenia gravis: recommendations for clinical research standards. Task Force of the Medical Scientific Advisory Board of the Myasthenia Gravis Foundation of America, *Neurology* 55(1):16-23, 2000.

Medical Research Council: *Aids to the examination of the peripheral nervous system,* England, 1976, Her Majesty's Stationery Office.

Melillo EM, Sethi JM, Mohsenin V: Guillain-Barré syndrome: rehabilitation outcome and recent developments, *Yale J Biol Med* 71(5):838-839, 1998.

Ouvrier RA, McLeod JG: *Peripheral neuropathy in childhood: international review of child neurology series,* New York, 1999, Cambridge University Press.

Schapira AH, editor: Griggs RC: *Muscle diseases: blue book of practical neurology,* ed 3, Woburn, Mass, 1999, Butterworth-Heinemann.

Tawil R: Outlook for therapy in the muscular dystrophies, *Semin Neurol* 19(1):81-86, 1999.

Urtizeberea JA: Therapies in muscular dystrophy: current concepts and future prospects, *Eur Neurol* 43(3):127-132, 2000.

Wolfe GI, Barohn RJ: Cryptogenic sensory and sensorimotor polyneuropathies, *Semin Neurol* 18(1):105-111, 1998.

WEBSITES

Muscular Dystrophy Association: www.mdausa.org

Muscular Dystrophy Family Foundation: www.mdff.org

Myositis Association of America: www.myositis.org

Myasthenia Gravis Foundation of America: www.myasthenia.org

Parent Project for Muscular Dystrophy Research: www.parentdmd.org/index.html

Washington University neuromuscular homepage: www.neuro.wustl.edu/neuromuscular

16

The Child Who Is Not Developing or Learning Normally

Children are frequently brought to the physician for an evaluation of neurologic problems. Apart from the focal neurologic symptoms described in other chapters of this book, children may be referred for an evaluation of deviation from the expected normal pattern of development. In this chapter, neurologic problems are categorized according to the age at which the child is most likely to require evaluation and treatment. For many of the disorders, a multidisciplinary approach to evaluation and treatment is required. For the child under 3 years of age, the physician most likely needs to coordinate the services of these various disciplines, usually delivered through community early intervention programs. However, for the child over 3 years of age, school systems (as required by Public Law 94-142, Education for All Handicapped Act of 1975) may coordinate services with the physician acting as a member of the multidisciplinary team. Table 16-1 lists some of the problems.

Every child under 3 years of age who visits a primary care physician should be screened for developmental delays as part of the general physical examination or well-baby visit. This task can be simplified by providing a growth and developmental questionnaire for parents to fill out in the waiting room; by routinely plotting height, weight, and head circumference measurements (see Appendix A); and by training an office assistant or nurse to administer the Denver Developmental Screening Test (see Appendix A). Observations of the child's behavior in the waiting room by a perceptive receptionist or secretary are also helpful. Remember that during the first two years of life, the child's responses are limited and consist mainly of motor responses. After that period, the child's language develops and makes the assessment of intellectual functioning easier. Once the child enters school, abnormalities of attention and learning and various types of behavior disorders may also become evident.

TABLE 16-1
Developmental, Learning, and Behavioral Problems by Age

Age of child (yr)	Assessable responses	Types of abnormalities
Infants and toddlers (birth to 3 yr)	Developmental screening Gross motor Speech Dysmorphic features Neurometabolic urine screening Denver Developmental Screening Test	Cerebral palsies Dysgenetic ("funny-looking kid") syndromes Inborn errors of metabolism Chromosomal disorders Autism Rett syndrome
Preschool years (3-6 yr)	Language Fine motor Adaptive and social development	Hearing loss, visual impairment Mental retardation syndromes Developmental language disorders Autistic spectrum disorders
School age (6-12 yr)	Cognitive development Emotional or social development Moral development Behavioral development Minor neurologic signs ("soft signs") through special neurologic examination	Hyperactivity-attentional disorders Learning disability syndromes Childhood depression Conduct disorders Oppositional-defiant disorders Petit mal epilepsy Tourette's syndrome Obsessive-compulsive disorder
Adolescence (12-18 yr)	Emotional health Neuropsychologic assessments	Attentional disorders Written language disabilities Adolescent adjustment reactions Psychiatric disorders, bipolar disorders Alcohol and drug abuse

One of the most important roles of the physician is to determine whether the child's deviation from normal is the result of slow development, developmental arrest, or developmental deterioration, since this will determine the types of disease processes considered and hence the evaluation undertaken (Fig. 16-1). The rate of acquisition of new

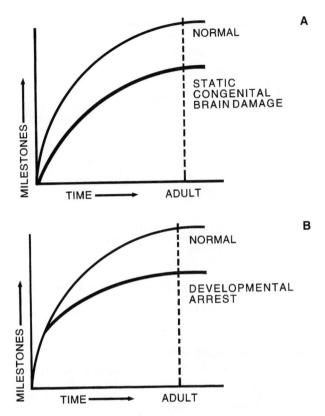

FIG. 16-1 A, In slow development, the child starts slowly and gradually falls further behind his normal peers because the rate of development is also slow. This type of developmental curve is seen in the child with a static congenital encephalopathy or with Down syndrome. **B,** Developmental arrest occurs in the child who has shown normal development from birth but stops acquiring new skills. This type of developmental curve may be found in the child who has been successfully treated for bacterial meningitis or has sustained significant head trauma. (CAUTION: This type of curve may also be seen in the early phases of a degenerative process when the natural acquisition of developmental milestones may balance the deterioration.)
Continued

milestones provides dynamic clues to developmental disabilities. By schematically graphing time against the courses of abnormal development for any given series of developmental milestones, it is possible to show three different schematic graphs. Children with slow development (Fig. 16-1, *A*) require an evaluation by psychosocial and educa-

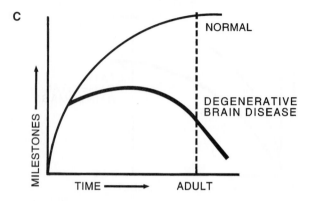

FIG. 16-1 cont'd   C, Deterioration of functioning (the actual loss of previously acquired milestones) implies an ongoing destructive process in the brain. This type of curve may be found in hydrocephalus, untreated galactosemia, or phenylketonuria or in rare central nervous system (CNS) neurometabolic diseases.

tional services and referral to appropriate community resources. The presence of developmental arrest (Fig. 16-1, *B*) or a deterioration of functioning (Fig. 16-1, *C*) will almost always require a referral to a specialized diagnostic center.

INFANTS AND TODDLERS
How to Identify an Infant Who Is Not Developing Normally
Obtain the infant's history to determine whether he or she has any of the risk factors listed in Box 16-1. The infant at risk for later developmental, learning, or behavioral problems is one:
1. Whose prenatal and perinatal history reveals certain risk factors (Box 16-1)
2. Who acquires illnesses that may injure the brain, such as head trauma, meningitis or encephalitis, stroke, brain tumor, and malnutrition
3. Whose rate of acquisition of developmental milestones deviates from the normal expectancy

Note: Risk factors are not only biologic, but more important, are often psychosocial, such as poor maternal-child interaction, inappropriate parenting by primary caregivers, and child abuse or neglect. Other risk factors include poverty, with its attendant cultural deprivation and accompanying emotional and nutritional deprivation. Wealth, with its tendency for overindulgence, can also inhibit emotional and behavioral development. The physician cannot alter the nonbiologic risk factors but can exert great indirect influence by compassionate parent education and sensitive referral to psychologic and social services. Any infant in the high-risk category should receive special attention.

BOX 16-1

Factors That Place an Infant in the High-Risk Category for Future Abnormal Development Necessitating Careful Physician Follow-up

---

1. Maternal diabetes
2. Maternal toxemia
3. Maternal viral infection (rubella, HIV)
4. Maternal alcoholism or drug addiction (cocaine)
5. Teenage mother
6. Mothers over 35 years of age, especially if first pregnancy
7. Fetal distress during delivery
8. Breech delivery
9. Premature delivery
10. Infant small for gestational age (assessed by Dubowitz scale)
11. Neonatal respiratory distress
12. Neonatal seizures
13. Neonatal infection (especially meningitis)
14. Prolonged neonatal jaundice

HIV, Human immunodeficiency virus.

Caveat: The majority of medical causes of mental retardation tend to fall into the following broad categories:

Perinatal hypoxia and ischemia
Infection—prenatal, perinatal or early infantile
Down syndrome and other autosomal chromosome disorders
Fragile X syndrome
Other cerebral dysgenesis (including neuronal migration disorders)
Phenylketonuria and other inborn errors of metabolism
Nonchromosomal dysmorphic syndromes

Obtain a *history* of developmental milestones in the infant, in particular looking for evidence of the following signs:
1. The absence of a social smile after 8 weeks of age
2. Poor head control while sitting on the mother's lap after 4 months of age
3. An inability to sit unsupported after 8 months of age
4. An inability to play games such as peekaboo, bye-bye, and pat-a-cake after 12 months of age
5. An inability to walk independently by 15 months of age
6. A persistent hand preference before 12 months of age
7. A delay in speech and language milestones (Tables 16-2 and 16-3)
8. Peculiar postures or modes of crawling (e.g., lying frog-legged, crawling on one side, kicking of legs symmetrically after 4 months of age)

TABLE 16-2
**Important Speech and Language Milestones
(ages 6-30 mo)**

Receptive language	Age (mo)	Expressive language
Turns to sound of bell	6	Cries, laughs, babbles
Waves "bye-bye" Knows meaning of "no" and "don't touch"	9	Imitates sounds and makes dental sounds during play ("dada")
—	12	1-2 words ("dada," "mama," "bye")
Responds to "come here"	15	Jargon (speechlike babbling during play)
Points to nose, eyes, hair	18	8-10 words (a third are nouns); puts two words together ("more cookies"); repeats requests
Points to a few named objects and obeys simple commands	24	Asks one- to two-word questions ("where kitty?")
Repeats two numbers and can identify by name "what barks" and "what blows"	30	Uses *I, you, me;* names objects, uses three-word simple sentences

TABLE 16-3
Important Speech Milestones (ages 3-6½ yr)

Receptive language	Age (yr)	Expressive language
Responds to prepositions *on* and *under*	3	Masters consonants *b, p, m*
Responds to prepositions *in,* *out, behind, in front of*	4	Speaks in four- to five-word sentences; uses future and past tenses; masters consonants *d, t, g, k*
Can repeat a sentence of seven words	5	Masters consonants *f, s, v;* names *red, yellow,* *blue, green*
—	6½	Masters consonant *th;* uses sentences of six to seven words; says numbers up to thirties

Neurologic/Neurodevelopmental Examination of the Infant

The essential parts of the pediatric neurologic examination include the following:

1. Measure the infant's frontal-to-occipital head circumference (Fig. 16-2) and plot it on an appropriate growth chart (see Appendix A). Values less than the 5th percentile or greater than the 95th percentile are abnormal. Serial measurements are more reliable than single measurements. Growth should be along a percentile line, and deviation is abnormal. Head circumference growth should be correlated with growth in height and weight.

2. Perform transillumination of the infant's head (Fig. 16-3) in the newborn period and before 1 year of age. Use a flashlight with an appropriate rubber adaptor to perform the examination in a light-tight, darkened room after appropriate dark adaptation. A small rim of light on the scalp should surround the rubber adaptor symmetrically in similar positions on each side of the head and in the midline posteriorly at the base of skull. Excessive transillumination suggests an absence of brain tissue, necessitating further evaluation. A Chun gun,* a high-intensity illuminator, can be used in a lighted room. This procedure has generally been neglected with the advent of neurosonography, computed tomographic (CT) scans, and magnetic resonance imaging (MRI).

3. Examine the skin for café au lait spots, vitiliginous spots, hairy patches over the midline, ichthyosis, nevi, and port-wine stains (or other neurocutaneous stigmata). A Wood's lamp (ultraviolet lamp) may be helpful in detecting vitiliginous patches, particularly in light-skinned subjects.

4. Observe the patient for abnormal facial features in the eyes, ears, nose, and chin and question whether the child looks significantly different from the parents.

5. Observe the infant's leg postures, particularly looking for the following signs:
   a. Frog legs (suggests hypotonia; see Fig. 16-4).
   b. Kicking legs symmetrically beyond 4 months of age (suggests spastic diplegia)
   c. Kicking only on one side (suggests spastic hemiplegia involving the less mobile side)

6. Observe the infant's neck response. An asymmetric tonic neck response from 2 to 6 months of age is normal; it is abnormal if the infant is unable to move out of the posture (too obligatory) or if the response persists beyond 6 months of age (Fig. 16-5).

7. Observe the infant for a Moro's (or startle) reflex (Fig. 16-6) in the waking state, which is normally present from birth to 3 months of age. Persistence of the reflex after 3 months is abnormal. Asymmetry in this reflex at any time is abnormal and may suggest hemiparesis, brachial plexus injury, or a spinal cord defect.

---

*This is an illuminator with a pistol grip and trigger, originally designed by Dr. Raymond Chun, former chief of pediatric neurology at the University of Wisconsin.

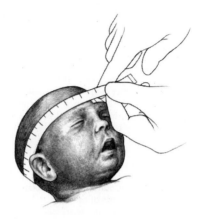

FIG. 16-2 The occipital-frontal circumference (OFC) is measured by using a steel or paper centimeter tape measure, which is placed over the forehead and the occipital protuberance (see also Appendix A).

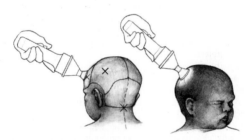

FIG. 16-3 Transillumination of the head. A flashlight with a rubber adaptor is placed over the symmetric frontal and parietal skull areas. The rim of light around the edge of the rubber adaptor is usually no more than a few millimeters and should be symmetric. (The illustrated rim is abnormal.) The flashlight is placed in the midline below the occipital protuberance to inspect posterior fossa transillumination.

8. Observe the infant for excessive opisthotonic posturing, either spontaneously or on being handled. This is an early sign of cerebral palsy, which may be present before obvious diplegia or other major motor deficits.

9. In testing the infant on the pull-to-sit (traction) test, observe the arm resistance as well as head control. By 5 months of age, the infant's head should come up with the body and not lag. The infant should

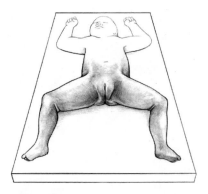

FIG. 16-4 Frog-legged posture, suggesting hypotonia. Extremities are abducted proximally and flexed at the elbows and knees.

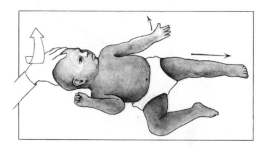

FIG. 16-5 Tonic neck response. With the infant supine, the arm (and leg) extend on the side that the head is turned, whereas the other arm (and leg) flex ("fencing posture").

pull symmetrically against the examiner with both arms (Fig. 16-7). A persistent head lag indicates axial hypotonia. An asymmetrical arm pull suggests a hemiparesis.
10. Test the infant for joint hyperextensibility by extending his or her knee beyond 180 degrees, extending the wrist back on the arm and dorsiflexing the foot on the shin. Abnormalities indicate ligamentous laxity or muscle hypotonia.
11. Lift the infant under the armpits. A hypotonic child will slip through the hands.
12. Observe the infant's postural responses at 6 months of age in a sitting position (Fig. 16-8).

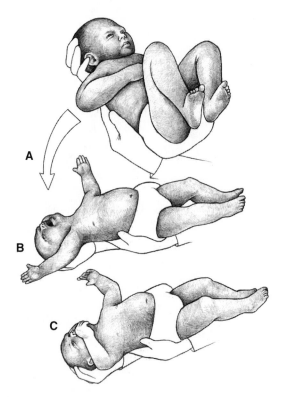

FIG. 16-6 Moro's (startle) reflex is elicited by suddenly extending the baby's head (**A**). The normal response has two phases: first, sudden extension and abduction of the arms and extension of the legs (**B**); and second, slower adduction of the arms (**C**).

    a. When pushed to the side, the infant should extend the arms to catch himself or herself.

    b. When pushed backward, the infant should extend the legs. Asymmetry suggests hemiparesis, and nonextension of the legs suggests a diparesis.

13. Test for the parachute response (Fig. 16-9).
14. Administer the Denver Developmental Screening Test on the initial visit and on the next few subsequent visits, if a developmental delay is suspected. Serial developmental assessments are more predictive of a later outcome than single assessments (see Appendix A).

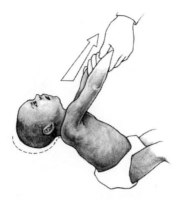

FIG. 16-7 Pull-to-sit (traction) maneuver. This is tested from the newborn period to 6 months of age. The pull of the child's arms and the degree of head lag are observed.

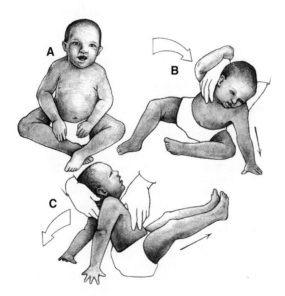

FIG. 16-8 A, Responses to thrust in an infant in the sitting position. **B,** When pushed to the side, the baby extends outward the arm on that side, as if to catch the fall. **C,** At 6 months of age, when the infant is suddenly pushed backward, the legs should kick out symmetrically.

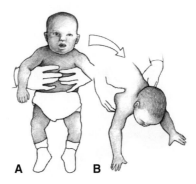

FIG. 16-9 The parachute response appears at 8 months of age. It is elicited by suspending the baby in the upright position **(A)** and then rapidly propelling the head toward the examining table (but stopping short of hitting the table). The arms should thrust out symmetrically, as if to break the fall **(B)**.

Laboratory Studies

1. If there is *developmental delay,* the following screening procedures may be done:
   a. Urine neurometabolic screening. If an inborn error of metabolism is suspected, screen blood for amino acids and urine for organic acids, or, if regionally available, perform tandem mass spectroscopy using a blood spot on filter paper.
   b. Neurosonography. This simple portable procedure (necessitating no radiation exposure or sedation) should be performed in all neonates with an abnormal head circumference or dysmorphic features or in whom intraventricular hemorrhage or hydrocephalus is suspected.
   c. Thyroid testing. Serum thyroid-stimulating hormone (TSH), triiodothyronine (T_3), thyroxine (T_4) and blood lead levels should be tested.
   d. Other laboratory tests. If a congenital intrauterine infection is suspected, TORCH (Toxoplasmosis, Rubella, Cytomegalovirus, Herpes) titers need to be done.*
   e. Genetic screening. If dysmorphic features are prominent, chromosome karyotyping and high-resolution studies are warranted. Evaluation for chromosome breakage syndromes and the fragile X syndrome requires special media and methods, and the cytogenetics laboratory must be alerted. Some chromosomal disorders (Angelman's and Miller-Dieker syndromes) require fluorescent in situ hybridization (FISH) studies.
   f. Skull x-ray tests. Review x-ray tests specifically for abnormal calcification, suture synostosis or splitting, and beaten copper appearance.

---

*A recent recommendation would replace the acronym TORCH with the acronym STARCH (Syphilis, Toxoplasmosis, AIDS, Rubella, Cytomegalic inclusion disease, and Herpes simplex) to emphasize the importance of HIV as a cause of congenital infection.

g. MRI. If developmental anomalies of the brain are suspected, (e.g., lissencephaly, polymicrogyria, or other neuronal migration disorders), MRI of the brain is warranted.

2. If there is *developmental regression*, referral to a center with a pediatric neurologist is indicated (see 3d to 3f in this section).

3. Diseases that have *developmental arrest and then regression* tend to fall into the following few categories:

   a. Previously diagnosed cerebral palsy that turns out to be a misdiagnosis and is really a slowly progressive, rather than static, encephalopathy.

   b. Complications of developmental brain anomalies, such as the development of hydrocephalus.

   c. Resistant seizure syndromes, such as infantile spasms, Lennox-Gastaut syndrome, and infantile myoclonic epilepsy.

   d. Infectious diseases, such as AIDS, subacute sclerosing panencephalitis (SSPE), and rare slow virus infections, including progressive rubella encephalopathy and progressive multifocal leukoencephalopathy.

   e. Neurometabolic diseases, such as certain aminoacidurias, organic acidurias, leukodystrophies, lysosomal storage diseases, peroxisomal diseases, and mitochondrial diseases involving primarily gray or white matter or both.

   f. Rare syndromes of episodic neurologic disturbance, associated with lactic acidosis, hyperammonemia, hypoglycemia (organic acidurias, mitochondrial diseases), or degenerative disorders of unknown cause, such as neuronal ceroid lipofuscinosis. Neuroimaging studies of the brain, particularly MRI and MR spectroscopy, can be very helpful diagnostically in suggesting a neurometabolic disease.

IDENTIFIABLE CAUSES OF DEVELOPMENTAL DELAY

Neonatal Hypothyroidism

Neonatal hypothyroidism includes the following characteristics:

1. Profound mental retardation will develop if treatment is delayed beyond the neonatal period. If treatment is instituted in patients under 3 months of age, 80% of infants may be normal; if treatment is delayed beyond 3 months of age, less than 30% of infants will be normal.

2. The patient may be a lethargic, floppy infant with poor sucking.

3. Prolonged neonatal jaundice is often present.

4. The presence of the triad of a large tongue, abdominal distention, and constipation is rare and is usually found only in severe cretinism.

5. The diagnosis is confirmed by a heel-stick blood sample analysis for T_4; this is done as a routine neonatal screening in most states.

Treatment: Immediate oral T_4 supplementation, desiccated thyroid 15 mg at bedtime. The patient should be monitored closely with thyroid studies.

Phenylketonuria

Phenylketonuria (PKU) includes the following characteristics:

1. The patient is usually a normal-appearing neonate who fails to gain weight and has feeding difficulties in the first weeks of life.

2. Seizures, poor growth, and profound mental retardation will develop if the condition is untreated.
3. There is an autosomal recessive pattern of inheritance.
4. The diagnosis is confirmed by a heel-stick blood sample (drawn after milk feeding) analyzed for the phenylalanine level (this screening procedure is done by law in all states) or by a positive urine ferric chloride test.

Treatment: A diet low in phenylalanine (e.g., formula such as Lofenalac) is necessary. Genetic counseling should be provided to the family.

Galactosemia

Galactosemia includes the following characteristics:

1. The patient is a normal-appearing infant who develops vomiting, diarrhea, and seizures of variable severity after several days or weeks of milk feeding, including breast feeding.
2. Prolonged neonatal jaundice is often present.
3. Blood glucose levels are in the hypoglycemic range only if assayed immediately after a milk feeding.
4. There is an autosomal recessive mode of inheritance.
5. Cataracts, hepatosplenomegaly, seizures, and profound mental retardation will develop if the condition is untreated.
6. The diagnosis is confirmed after a feeding by finding low blood glucose and positive urine glucose (Clinitest tablets) but negative urine glucose (glucose oxidase urine dipsticks); quantitative galactose levels can also be obtained.

Treatment: A galactose-free diet is necessary. Genetic counseling should be provided to the family.

Down Syndrome

1. The clinical diagnosis of Down syndrome is made by the following criteria:
   a. Oblique palpebral fissures
   b. Epicanthal folds
   c. Brushfield's spots (light speckling) of the iris
   d. A flat nasal bridge
   e. Clinodactyly of the fifth fingers and bilateral transverse palmar creases
   f. Wide spacing between the first and second toes
   g. Hypotonia
2. Down syndrome is more frequent in pregnancies of women over 40 years of age.
3. There is a high incidence of associated problems, such as congenital heart disease, tracheoesophageal fistula, duodenal atresia, megacolon, and lymphoreticular malignancies.
4. The diagnosis is confirmed by chromosomal studies; 95% of cases have trisomy 21, and the remainder have translocations or mosaicism.
5. Hip radiographs show a characteristic change in the acetabulum.
6. Progressive upper cervical spine abnormalities may result in spinal cord compression symptoms in late childhood or early adolescence.
7. Progressive personality changes and intellectual deterioration begin in the late twenties or early thirties, and by 40 years of age all patients have histopathologic Alzheimer's disease.

Treatment:
1. Although no specific medical treatment is available, there is evidence that early intensive developmental stimulation programs and early special education programs, as well as psychosocial support, result in achievement of higher functioning than what might have been predicted in the past. The degree of psychomotor retardation varies from mild to moderate and allows placement into trainable or educable special education classes. Employment as adults in sheltered situations is possible, and independence in self-care is the rule.
2. The recurrence risk after trisomy 21 is 1% to 2%. Referral to a pediatric clinical geneticist is recommended.
3. Support groups for families are available.
4. Patient and physician information materials can be obtained from the National Down Syndrome Society, 666 Broadway, New York, NY 10012; (800) 221-4602 or the National Down Syndrome Congress, 7000 Peachtree-Dunwoody Road, NE, Lake Ridge 400 Office Park, Building #5, Suite 100, Atlanta, GA 30328; (800) 232-NDSC; website: www.ndsccenter.org.

Fragile X Syndrome
Fragile X syndrome includes the following characteristics:
1. It is associated with moderate-to-severe mental retardation.
2. Dysmorphic features include large ears, a prominent jaw and forehead, a broad nose, a high-pitched voice, and macroorchidism.
3. It is often associated with seizures.
4. The disease is an X-linked disorder affecting primarily males, but females are carriers and may be mildly affected.
5. Chromosome studies show excessive breaks when cultured in special media.

Note: Because special culture media are required to demonstrate the chromosomal abnormality, it is imperative to alert the laboratory if this diagnosis is considered. However, DNA testing for the expansion of the number of triplet repeats in the fragile X region is a more sensitive and specific test.

Treatment:
1. No specific medical treatment is available, but seizures should be treated symptomatically (see Chapter 11); genetic counseling of the family is necessary.
2. Patient and physician information materials can be obtained from the FRAXA Research Foundation, PO Box 935, West Newbury, MA 01985; (978) 462-1866; website: www.fraxa.org.

Congenital Intrauterine Infection
1. Depending on the type and duration of the prenatal infection, the child may vary from a small-for-dates, premature, severely microcephalic infant with hepatosplenomegaly, purpura, and severe jaundice, to a normal-appearing child who does well in infancy but develops poorly in late childhood.

2. The most common agents are in the TORCH groups, but other agents include the hepatitis B virus, enterovirus, and increasingly, HIV.
3. The diagnosis is confirmed by determination during the neonatal period of elevated (preferably from umbilical cord blood) serum immunoglobulin M (IgM) (and disease-specific IgM). The agents can sometimes be cultured from the patient's stool, urine, or throat. Serologic tests are available through state health laboratories.
4. Skull radiographs or CT scans of the brain reveal punctate periventricular calcifications in cytomegalovirus infection and larger, scattered calcifications of toxoplasmosis.
5. The degree of neurologic impairment varies with the severity of the infection, as follows:
   a. Seizures and severe retardation are more common with herpes simplex, toxoplasmosis, and cytomegalovirus infection.
   b. Visual disturbances are more common with toxoplasmosis and rubella (cataracts), and hearing loss alone is common with cytomegalovirus infection.
   c. Hearing impairment together with autism is more common with rubella. A progressive rubella encephalitis continuing after the neonatal period and through the first year is now recognized.
   d. Cytomegalovirus is the most common infectious cause of mental retardation and is also the most underdiagnosed.
   e. Developmental delay, a "failure to thrive," and recurrent infections can be associated with HIV-related central nervous system (CNS) involvement, as either progressive or static encephalopathy. Neonatal HIV infection is transmitted by less than 40% of infected mothers either in utero or at delivery. Confirmation of the infection is difficult because of the presence of maternal antibodies in the infant up to 6 months of age. Prevention of maternal-infant transmission is imperative. An infectious disease specialist needs to be consulted if there is suspicion of HIV infection, AIDS-related complex (ARC), or AIDS.

Treatment:
1. In congenital syphilis, procaine penicillin G 50,000 units/kg intramuscularly (IM) in 1 daily dose for 14 days must be administered.
2. Toxoplasmosis is treated in the infant younger than 1 year of age with pyrimethamine 1 mg/kg/day orally (with leucovorin calcium 5 mg twice weekly) and sulfadiazine 50 mg/kg/day orally in divided doses for 21 days. If there is evidence of active disease, additional corticosteroid (prednisone) 1 to 2 mg/kg/day may be necessary. Complicated cases requiring additional or other courses of treatment should be referred to an infectious disease center. Chorioretinitis should be managed by an ophthalmologist.
3. Since the child with any congenital infection is potentially contagious, contact with other infants and with pregnant women should be avoided. (Excretion of high titers of virus may continue for several months in congenital cytomegalovirus and rubella infections.)
4. General supportive care is available only for rubella and cytomegalovirus, whereas acyclovir is available for herpes simplex encephalitis (usually secondary to type 1 or genital herpes).

5. Currently zidovudine (azidothymidine [AZT] or Retrovir) and the protease inhibitors are available for the treatment of AIDS, but the mother should be counseled about the risk of having another infected child.

Static Congenital Encephalopathy with Predominant Motor Involvement

1. Static encephalopathies (cerebral palsies) are defined as a group of disorders where there is a major *motor* deficit secondary to a brain lesion acquired at or around the time of birth. Hypoxia and ischemia, infection, hemorrhage, and brain anomalies account for the majority of static encephalopathies.
2. The infant with static encephalopathy has a delay in achieving motor milestones, whereas social and behavior development may be normal. The infant often has normal or above-normal intelligence, but 40% have varying degrees of mental retardation.
3. Neonatal intensive care units have been a major reason for the survival of very low–birth weight (<1500 gm) and extremely–low birth weight (<1000 gm) babies, but they probably increase the risk of long-term neurologic and developmental disabilities, including cerebral palsies.
4. Some specific patterns of motor involvement can be recognized. Children may display combinations of the following patterns (mixed forms) and may show variation over time (note that the mixed forms have a worse prognosis):
   a. Hemiplegia or hemiparesis (the involvement of arm and leg on the same side; undergrowth and abnormal posturing of that side).
   b. Diplegia or diparesis (both legs are involved with minimal to absent involvement of the upper extremities), the most common form. Usually there is delayed standing, early walking on tiptoes, and walking with scissoring or the knees crossing, and in the first years of life, hypotonia and decreased reflexes, but later with increased tone and hyperreflexia.

Note: The term *paraplegia* refers to acquired leg paralysis secondary to a spinal cord injury usually at the thoracolumbar level.

   c. Tetraplegia or tetraparesis (the involvement of both legs and arms; very poor head control and trunk control on sitting), which is better described as a bilateral hemiplegia, since the lesions responsible are usually bilateral hemispheric.

Note: The term *quadriplegia* usually refers to paralysis of the arms and legs secondary to a cervical spinal cord injury.

   d. Ataxic/atonic (hypotonia in infancy, then marked unsteadiness and incoordination when the upright posture is attempted).
   e. Choreoathetosis (an abnormal choreoathetoid posturing of the arms and legs), the least common pattern of motor involvement. The infant usually has hypotonia, which then evolves into rigidity and choreoathetoid movements.

5. The patient's speech may be abnormal in tone, rate, rhythm, and pronunciation resulting from impairment of the motor aspects of articulation, whereas basic language expression and reception are normal. The most severe motor speech disorders, sometimes to the point of anarthria, are seen in the choreoathetoid syndromes. Occasionally the speech disorder is disproportionately severe relative to the involvement of the extremities and compared to the preservation of intellect.

6. Epilepsy occurs in one third or fewer of cases, primarily in those with spastic cerebral palsies (hemiplegic, diplegic, or tetraplegic). When some combination of a major motor defect, mental retardation, and epilepsy occurs, with or without deafness or blindness, the term *multiply handicapped* is often applied. Such distinctions are important because they determine the appropriate intervention programs.

7. The observation of postures—early excessive opisthotonos, obligatory spontaneous asymmetric tonic neck postures, and the persistence of developmental reflexes that should have been inhibited—is important in the neurologic examination. The persistence of the asymmetric tonic neck reflex after 6 months of age and the absence of a parachute response after 1 year of age augur for a poor prognosis for walking.

8. Many diagnoses of "cerebral palsy" attributed to birth asphyxia are now known to be a result of the following prenatal causes:
   a. Preexisting brain malformations that may predispose the newborn to neonatal problems, including asphyxia.
   b. Placental abnormalities with consequent fetal ischemia or embolization, resulting in brain injury.

Note: A pathologic study of the placenta should be performed in any infant with neonatal difficulties to identify causative placental abnormalities.

   Caveat: "Minimal cerebral palsy" occurs in a number of children, and presents as clumsiness, "visual-perceptual" difficulties, or sometimes attentional-hyperactivity disorder. The diagnosis is made on finding minimal but definite neurologic signs, such as shortened Achilles tendons with hyperactive lower extremity reflexes and a Babinski's reflex, or mild but definite signs of congenital hemiparesis. Usually the children have no functional handicap from the motor deficits.

Treatment:
1. Physical and occupational therapy and developmental stimulation programs must be established *early,* preferably in the first year of life, to permit maximal socialization and education of the child and minimize the development of fixed joint deformities.

2. The child with "pure" spastic diplegia or hemiplegia responds best to treatment.

3. Many forms of neurodevelopmental therapies, which are usually administered along with routine physical-occupational therapy, are available.

4. The medical and surgical treatment of spasticity or dystonia ranges from oral antispastic drugs (diazepam, baclofen [Lioresal]), botulinus

toxin injections, baclofen infusion pumps, dorsal rhizotomies, tendon-lengthening and tendon-release operations to "functional neurosurgery." Follow-up care needs to be monitored and coordinated, particularly since multiple disciplines, especially orthopedics and physical-occupational therapy, but also neurology and neurosurgery, are involved. Regional crippled children's service clinics are available. If the family can identify with one central primary physician or agency as the care coordinator, compliance of therapeutic regimens by the family is better ensured.

5. Information for physicians and patients may be obtained from Cerebral Palsy Associations of New York State, 330 West 34th Street, 13th floor, New York, NY 10001; (212) 947-5770; website: www.cerebralpalsynys.org.

Caution: In patients with cerebral palsies in whom there is a change in motor or mental functioning for the worse or in whom there is a family history of cerebral palsy or early deaths from neurologic conditions, suspect hereditary neurometabolic disease or familial brain dysgeneses, and refer to a pediatric neurologist.

PRESCHOOL YEARS (Ages 3 to 6)
Identifying the Child Who Is Not Developing Normally
During the preschool years, a child develops language and behavioral patterns that indicate temperament or personality. A delay in speech and language is the most important disorder to assess during this period. Speech or language delay is the most consistent predictor of later learning disabilities, particularly in reading and writing. Motor disabilities are less commonly noted for the first time during this period.

Parents may bring their child to the physician with a primary complaint of delayed speech or language. However, the astute physician must be able to recognize delayed or aberrant speech and language during the following visits:

1. During routine physical examinations
2. During follow-up examinations of children who were identified earlier as high risk
3. During an examination for another complaint such as a cold

In the child's preschool years, physicians should become aware of the following risk factors that warn of academic or behavioral difficulties when he or she begins first grade:

1. The presence of attention-deficit hyperactivity disorder (ADHD). ADHD can be suspected by reports from nursery school or kindergarten teachers that a child is more "immature" than expected for his or her age. Parents will report discipline problems and problems in playing with peers.
2. Delayed speech and language. If a language disorder (developmental dysphasia or acquired aphasia) is present, there is a high risk for a specific learning disability involving a delayed acquisition of reading and writing skills (dyslexia and dysgraphia). Speech disturbances (develop-

mental articulation disorders or stuttering) alone do not presage learning disabilities. A developmental language disorder is a specific delay in acquiring comprehension and the production of speech and language when hearing and cognition are normal.

The Landau-Kleffner syndrome is an acquired language disorder associated with seizures and electroencephalographic (EEG) epileptiform abnormalities that has a subacute onset but a chronic course. Milder forms of the autistic spectrum disorders (pervasive developmental disorders) may appear either with a language delay or language regression.

3. Poor academic skills. A lack of achievement of academic readiness skills at the end of kindergarten (e.g., counting, reading and writing the alphabet, naming colors) are predictive of readiness for the first grade.
4. Lack of drawing abilities. Poor drawing abilities for age, clumsiness, or incoordination do not necessarily presage academic learning disabilities, although they may lead to difficulties in handwriting and in art classes.

The physician has many therapeutic services available to patients at this age. Private or public community agencies, Headstart programs, preschool handicapped programs, and formal speech therapy are available in most communities even before the formal kindergarten period. Various nursery schools that provide more than babysitting by incorporating child-development approaches are becoming more widely available. The special services of special education departments of the public school systems are mandated to provide educational services for preschool children, beginning at 3 years of age, under the Education for All Handicapped Act, depending on state law.

IDENTIFIABLE DISORDERS
Hearing Loss

1. A deviation from the normal rate of development of sound reception and expression (Tables 16-2 and 16-3) suggests a possible hearing impairment.
2. There may be a delay in the development of speech and an abnormal tone or quality of speech sounds. For example, with mild hearing loss, words with high-frequency sounds will be misunderstood by the child, and the high-frequency sounds in words will be omitted from the child's speech. ("Stop" will be heard and spoken as "top.")
3. The most common and frequently neglected cause of hearing loss is middle ear disease.
4. The child with hearing loss may display autistic features.
5. The child will be fascinated by loud sounds (especially vibrating bass sounds) and the parents may complain that the child turns the volume of the radio or television too loud.
6. The child with hearing loss may develop lip-reading skills and gestures and pantomime to communicate.
7. A diagnosis necessitates detailed audiometric testing by an audiologist experienced with young children. Recording of brainstem auditory-evoked potentials may be necessary in younger children.

Caution: An apparent normal response to a bell in office testing is an inadequate assessment of the child with possible hearing loss. Screening audiograms in the school usually will not detect the child with anything less than profound hearing loss.

Treatment: Thorough otologic and audiologic assessment is usually necessary. Amplification devices or cochlear transplants may be helpful in some children. Modification of the classroom environment or special schooling for the deaf may be necessary.

Mental Subnormality

1. In the child with normal hearing (after thorough audiologic testing) who has a delay in speech or language, the most common cause is a global deficit in intellectual-cognitive skills (i.e., mental subnormality or retardation).
2. The most important gross language milestone is a *two- to three-word sentence (must be a subject-verb sentence) between 24 and 30 months of age.*
3. Testing by a psychologist experienced in assessing children must be done to discriminate the presence of the intellectual-cognitive deficit. Tests such as the Bayley Scales of Infant Development (BSID), the Stanford-Binet Form L-M, the Wechsler Preschool and Primary Scale of Intelligence (WPPSI), and the Kaufman Assessment Battery for Children (K-ABC) are useful. Extreme caution must be exercised in predicting the child's future performance potential based on test numbers alone.
4. Mental retardation is documented not only by intellectual-cognitive testing, but also by social-behavioral testing. Significant deficits in both areas must be present for the diagnosis to be accurately applied.
5. Mental retardation is actually only a description of a symptom complex (intellectual-cognitive and social-behavioral deficit that occurs before 18 years of age) and may be the result of multiple causes.
6. The following conditions may mimic mental retardation (pseudomental retardation):
   a. The most common condition is a developmental language disorder (developmental dysphasia). This condition will cause test results showing a low Wechsler full-scale IQ score, with the verbal scale IQ score usually 15 to 20 points below the Performance Scale IQ score.
   b. Multiple specific disabilities but a normal intellectual potential, as indicated by normal adaptive behavior, age-appropriate play and social functioning, and average or better IQ subtest scores on subtests indicative of a cognitive ability (Wechsler Similarities and Information subtests).
   c. A borderline intellectual potential that is complicated by specific developmental disabilities, attention disorders, emotional disorders, or sensory impairments.
   d. Other conditions include deafness or severe hearing impairment (presenting as speech and language delay), behavioral disorders (including childhood depression), ADHD, bilingualism (and ethnic-cultural differences), and pharmacologically induced cognitive dysfunction.

7. Etiologic screening: Look for treatable causes. More and more genetic diseases are being treated by dietary restrictions, cofactor supplementation, detoxification, bone marrow transplantation (storage diseases), enzyme transfusions, and possibly (in the near future) gene transplantation. Known genetic causes require genetic counseling of the parents and siblings of child-bearing age; referral to a pediatric geneticist is helpful. If any screening tests are positive, refer the patient to an appropriate specialist in neurologic studies, genetics, or metabolism for further in-depth diagnostic assessment.

Infantile Autism

Infantile autism includes the following characteristics:
1. The onset is before 18 months of age.
2. There is an abnormal interpersonal relationship. (The child does not relate to people as "people" but as "objects.") The child avoids eye contact and tactile contact; the child may, for example, use the mother's hand as a "tool" to grasp a doorknob. He or she does not cuddle as an infant.
3. The child displays bizarre mannerisms (motor stereotypies). The repetitive movements resemble tics, such as flapping the arms at the sides, rocking, and other self-stimulating maneuvers (whirling and spinning).
4. The child uses toys inappropriately in a stereotyped manner; for example, trucks are lined up (never rolled), whereas buildings are rolled.
5. The child has aberrant language development.
   a. The child has variable acquisition rates; for example, the child exhibits markedly delayed verbal comprehension and production, but in later childhood there is "cocktail party chatter."
   b. The child acquires reading skills before spoken language skills.
   c. The child uses pronoun inversion (substitutes "I" for "you").
   d. The child exhibits echolalia and perseveration in his or her language.
6. On formal intellectual testing, the child's scores are in the "retarded" range, but the child appears to be functioning at a much higher level.
7. The child may have splinter skills. These are precociously developed but isolated abilities, such as calendar skills (e.g., being able to tell what day of the week it was on September 25, 1896).
8. The child has a compulsive need for a sameness in environment and routine.
9. Autistic children who are aggressive, hyperactive, and nonverbal are often misdiagnosed as suffering from severe or profound mental retardation.
10. Similar disorders with milder features (e.g., a less severe language disability) begin in children after 18 months of age. These autistic-like disorders have been termed *pervasive developmental disorders* or *autistic spectrum disorders.* Patients may experience language regression, rather than delay; exhibit a need for rigidity; and relate poorly to peers. A special case is Asperger's syndrome, in which language is actually superior in vocabulary or syntax but elicits a semantic or pragmatic disorder. The learning problem is often characterized as a "nonverbal learning disability" or a "right hemisphere learning problem."

11. Rett syndrome is a neurodevelopmental disorder affecting female patients, presenting as an autistic, ataxic dementia, with possible upper motor neuron signs and acquired microcephaly, and characteristic hand-wringing and respiratory stereotypes. The regression plateaus and improves later in life. A defect in a regulatory gene (MECP2) is responsible for the disorder.

Treatment:

1. Neuropsychopharmacologic management is entirely symptomatic and empirical and probably should be supervised by a child psychiatrist or psychopharmacologist.
   a. Haloperidol may be used if there is much hyperactive aggression, self-mutilation, or marked motor stereotypies (bizarre mannerisms). Starting dosage: 1 mg 2 to 3 times a day. An alternative medication is risperidone, which is less likely to produce sedation or extrapyramidal reactions.
   b. Clonidine and guanfacine may help control aggressive behavior if it is an expression of emotional impulsivity in a child with ADHD.
   c. Amitriptyline hydrochloride may be used if there is much hyperactivity, trouble sleeping at night, or reversal of the diurnal cycle. Starting dosage: 0.25 mg at bedtime.
   d. Carbamazepine may be used if there is much aggressive behavior and the child also has seizures. Starting dosage: 200 mg 2 to 3 times a day.
   e. Lithium carbonate may be used for sustained hyperactive behavior akin to mania although divalproex sodium is thought to be as effective. Starting dosage: 300 mg every day to 3 times a day.
   f. The CNS stimulants, methylphenidate, dextroamphetamine, and pemoline hydrochloride, may also be used for prominent attentional disturbances or hyperactivity. The long-acting sustained-release preparations have the advantage of once-a-day administration.
2. Psychoeducational management is another option. Refer patients younger than 3 years of age to community infant-stimulation programs; children over 3 years of age should be referred to the public school department of special education for preschool handicapped programs and development of an Individual Education Plan (IEP) under the Education for All Handicapped Act. Physician and parent information may be obtained from the Autism Services Center, PO Box 507, Huntington, WV 25710; (304) 525-8014.

Developmental Hyperactivity

1. The parents of a child with ADHD describe the child as "always on the go" from birth. (The child may even have been more active in utero.) The Conners parent and teacher questionnaires are highly supportive in diagnosing the disorder.
2. The child may never crawl but walks early and runs rather than walks. There are often sleep difficulties in infancy; the child is unable to keep to a sleep schedule, and gives up naps early.
3. The child characteristically is impulsive, distractible, immature, and clumsy, with a short attention span, and has difficulty following directions, often racing from task to task without completing any one task. There is often a history of accident-proneness in the toddler and preschool years.

4. Frequently parents, other caretakers, and peers have difficulty tolerating the child. Behavioral problems may develop.
5. There is an apparent "paradoxical reaction" to certain drugs. Barbiturates (a sedative in normal individuals) markedly increase the child's hyperactivity, whereas stimulants such as amphetamines, methylphenidate, and pemoline reduce the hyperactivity and increase the attention to tasks.
6. Boys are more frequently affected than girls in the hyperactive presentation; girls are more often affected than boys in the inattentive presentation (attention deficit disorder without the hyperactivity).
7. Subtle neurologic signs on special extended neurologic examinations may be demonstrated. Children with ADHD do not perform well with competing stimulus tests or continuous performance tasks.
8. The initial presentation of Tourette's syndrome to the primary care physician can be with hyperactivity and attentional problems, before tics develop. Although obsessive-compulsive traits may be present when tics occur, obsessive-compulsive disorder, if it develops at all, does so in late childhood or adolescence. Motor compulsions must be differentiated from complex motor tics.

Treatment:

1. The physician's immediate task is to educate the parents about both the nature of the condition and the appropriate management of the attentional, behavioral, and academic problems. Parents should be referred to the appropriate literature on dealing with the hyperactive child. Refer to Children and Adults with Attention Deficit Disorder (CHADD).
2. Pharmacologic management is effective if given in conjunction with a comprehensive program of behavioral modification and environmental adjustment in the school and home, along with appropriate pedagogic intervention, cognitive-attentional training, and training in organizational skills. Modification of the school and home environment is necessary—more structure, fewer distractions, short circumscribed tasks, a checklist for developing self-monitoring abilities, and home chores to develop time-management abilities and responsibilities.
3. Pharmacologic management should, if at all possible, be avoided in preschool children. This type of management uses primarily the CNS stimulant drugs methylphenidate, dextroamphetamine, and pemoline. The dosage is clinically titrated to achieve a therapeutic effect. Hyperactivity may abate with a lower dosage than is necessary to improve attentional or behavioral disturbance. Failure with one drug does not necessarily mean that the other drugs will also fail.
4. Before initiating treatment with the selected medication, the physician must establish a baseline assessment of motor, attentional, and behavioral parameters; a variety of standardized questionnaires and continuous performance tests, now often computer administered and scored, are available. The use of central auditory processing tests by an audiologist experienced with children is also a good method for establishing a baseline for attentional tasks and for follow-up monitoring. These measures will ensure that data from a number of sources, other than the physician's own observation of the child in the examining room (which is often misleading), are available for an accurate view of the child's functioning.

a. Methylphenidate (Ritalin) is the usual first drug of choice. If treatment is unsuccessful, discontinue the drug and treat the patient with dextroamphetamine. Medication should be given in a twice-daily regimen, just before breakfast and lunch, to avoid anorexia and maximize absorption. Medication after 4 PM should be avoided to prevent insomnia. Suggested beginning doses are:

1) Methylphenidate 5 mg can be administered twice a day.
2) Dextroamphetamine 5 mg can be administered twice a day.
3) Pemoline may be used as a single morning dose after breakfast (if successful treatment cannot be achieved with either methylphenidate or dextroamphetamine) starting with a dosage of 18.75 mg every morning for younger children or 37.5 mg for older children. Recent reports of serious liver toxicity should make one proceed with caution.
4) A preparation of dextroamphetamine salts (Adderall) has a longer duration of action than methylphenidate.
5) Dextroamphetamine itself comes in a sustained-release preparation, Dexedrine Spansules.
6) A new sustained-release form of methylphenidate, Concerta, is available.
7) All medication should be clinically titrated for efficacy, duration of action, and adverse drug effect (anorexia or insomnia).

b. Medication should be given daily, although some children who display symptoms only during school need not be given the drug on weekends, on school holidays, or during summer vacation.

c. The child should be carefully followed on a weekly basis with upward adjustment of dosage if necessary to achieve the desired therapeutic effect. After a maintenance regimen has been established, height and weight should be monitored and charted at least monthly to detect a growth failure. A drug-free holiday is necessary if growth failure is documented. The child on a maintenance regimen must be followed regularly to monitor for undesirable side effects. Some 4% of children treated with CNS stimulants develop tics, which do not necessarily evolve into Tourette's syndrome.

SCHOOL-AGE YEARS (Ages 6 to 19)

Entry into school can be a traumatic period where intellectual, motor, and emotional disorders may become more prominent. Disorders such as hyperactivity-attentional syndromes may become more obvious during this period. However, difficulty in school performance may be the first indication of a developmental or learning disability. Some specific behavioral and educational disorders may first become evident at this time. Typically, children with attention deficit disorder (ADD) without hyperactivity emerge in late elementary or early middle school, when academic achievement requires organized effort, which may have been compensated for by high native intelligence in the early elementary school years.

This is a particularly trying time not only for the child but also for the family. It is imperative that all professionals provide the family with accurate, comprehensive, and noncontradictory information. Because of the presence of a disabled child, family interactions may be tumultuous, affecting the psychosocial adjustment of siblings and parents, as well as family unity. A well-coordinated support system for the family may be as beneficial as any intervention prescribed for the child individually.

Childhood Depression

1. Endogenous major depression in a child may first present during school age (see Chapter 9).
2. The child's family history is often strongly positive for depression, mania, nervous breakdown, mental illness, suicide, or alcoholism.
3. The child with depression has a history of recurrent episodes of a change in behavior, including the following examples:
   a. A change in activity level, either hyperactivity (especially fluctuating) or reduced activity
   b. School problems secondary to distractibility or decreased attention span or a new learning disability
   c. Excessive moodiness or irritability
   d. An appetite or sleep disturbance
   e. Medically unexplained headaches, recurrent abdominal pain, or recurrent vomiting
   f. Secondary enuresis (see Chapter 5) without demonstrable urologic or neurologic abnormality
   g. Phobias or excessive fears
   h. A preoccupation with death, suicide attempts, setting fires, or running away
4. Sadness and low self-esteem are encountered in long-standing learning disabilities, underachievement, or school failure but in these situations are not associated with the variety of other symptoms characteristic of depression.

Treatment: Antidepressant pharmacotherapy is usually necessary, along with supportive psychotherapy and family therapy, and is generally best accomplished by referral to child psychiatrists, psychologists, or family therapists.

Educational Dysfunction

Many non-CNS factors can account for a below-expected academic performance, including the following:
1. Sensory deprivation (blindness or deafness)
2. Schools with deficient teaching programs
3. Membership in a minority group with different values from those of the predominant culture
4. Bilingualism
5. Primary emotional or psychiatric disturbances

If non-CNS factors cannot be identified as the cause of poor achievement, then one or more of several kinds of educational dysfunction may account for poor academic performance.

1. *Mild to moderate mental retardation:* The child with mental retardation

has global intellectual, cognitive, adaptive, and social-behavioral deficits. Formal psychologic testing, as well as serial developmental and neurologic assessments over time, is required to make this diagnosis.

Caution: Skepticism must be used in evaluating intelligence test scores that report "characteristic of mental retardation." Psychologic tests produce numerous false-negative and false-positive results. Careful detailed neuropsychologic testing is necessary for a precise characterization of mental retardation.

Treatment: Usually public schools have resource rooms or special classes for the educable or trainable mentally retarded child. An IEP is required for each child, according to the Education for All Handicapped Act.

2. *Borderline intelligence:* On formal psychologic testing, the child with borderline intelligence shows cognitive potential below normal but above that of mental retardation. Although not mentally retarded, the child will perform more slowly than normal because his or her potential is lower than normal.

Treatment: The child will require an IEP, usually incorporating more tutoring at a slower pace than that of the comparable regular classroom. This group is correctly referred to as "slow learners." Information for parents on mental retardation and borderline intelligence can be obtained from The Arc of the United States, 500 E. Border St., Suite 300, Arlington, TX 76010; (800) 433-5255; website: www.thearc.org.

3. *ADHD* (attention deficit disorder with or without hyperactivity): In children with ADHD, developmental hyperactivity in which a short attention span and distractibility, and not necessarily motor hyperactivity, is the presenting feature and the reason for academic underachievement. Girls, more than boys, are apt to have attentional disorders without hyperactivity. This group of disorders is one of the most common problems for which schools refer children to physicians. The referral information usually has terms such as *immaturity, underachievement, learning disability,* and *behavioral problem.* Motor hyperactivity tends to abate with age, but the attentional disorder may persist through high school and even into adulthood. The older the child, the more the physician must look for complicating secondary emotional problems, such as a conduct disorder or oppositional-defiant disorder (ODD).

Treatment: All management previously discussed in the section on developmental hyperactivity applies. In addition, continual and clear communication with school teachers and administrators is necessary for effective monitoring of the child's responses to pharmacologic intervention.

4. *Specific learning disabilities:* Children with specific learning disabilities have normal intellectual potential but greater than expected difficulty in acquiring one or more of the basic academic skills of reading, writing, arithmetic, and spelling. The incidence is about 3% of the school population. Specific reading disabilities (developmental dyslexia), with later spelling and written language disabilities (developmental dysgraphia), are the most common specific learning disabilities. Arithmetic disabilities (developmental dyscalculia) are less common.

a. The classic neurologic examination is almost always normal, but subtle neurologic signs can sometimes be demonstrated. A neurodevelopmental evaluation may reveal aberrant or delayed functioning.

b. Test speech articulation with the repetition of test phrases, such as "la-la", "mi-mi", and "go-go."

c. Rapidly screen the child's spoken language with repetition of sentences of varying length and syntax.

d. Screen arithmetic ability in the early school-age child using the addition and subtraction of single digits and in the older school-age child using the multiplication of two-digit numbers by two-digit numbers (written).

e. Note whether errors in reading, writing, or arithmetic may be caused by attentional problems (e.g., skipping lines, wrong lining up of columns) or by impulsive errors (e.g., writing down the first thing to come to mind, frequent erasing). These are clues to an attentional disorder that may be presenting as a learning disability.

f. Ascertain if there is a family history of reading or other learning disabilities or of attentional-activity disorders.

g. Screen for visual-motor problems as the child completes performing the draw-a-person test, drawing a clock, or copying geometric figures.

h. The common specific learning disability syndromes are developmental dyslexia (see Habib in bibliography), developmental dyscalculia (see Shalev), developmental clumsiness or apraxia (see Flory), developmental dysgraphia, and developmental dysphasia (see Leung, Waterstone).

i. Although psychometric testing may be helpful in elucidating these disorders, many psychologic tests produce false-positive and false-negative results. Detailed neuropsychologic evaluation is often necessary to characterize more precisely strengths and weaknesses in a clinically diagnosed learning disability.

j. Learning disability syndromes may occur alone or in combination, and also may be co-morbid with ADHD.

k. Many neurobiologic correlates of learning disabilities are now known and may suggest techniques in the future for a supplementary diagnosis.

l. Physician and parent information is available from the Association for Children and Adults with Learning Disabilities, 4900 Girard Road, Pittsburgh, PA 15227; (412) 881-2253; website: acldonline. org, or the International Dyslexia Association, 8600 LaSalle Road, Chester Building, Suite 382, Baltimore, MD 21286; (410) 296-0232; website: www.interdys.org.

BIBLIOGRAPHY

Aman MG, Collier-Cresppin A, Lindsay RL: Pharmacotherapy of disorders in mental retardation, *Eur Child Adolesc Psychiatry* 9(Suppl 1):98-107, 2000.

Amato M, Donati F: Update on perinatal hypoxic insult: mechanism, diagnosis and interventions, *Eur J Paediatr Neurol* 4(5):203-209, 2000.

Barkley RA: Genetics of childhood disorders. XVII. ADHD, part 1: the executive function, *J Am Acad Child Adolesc Psychiatry* 39(8):1064-1068, 2000.

Bobarth, B: *Motor development in the different types of cerebral palsy,* Woburn, Mass, 1999, Butterworth-Heinemann.

Buitelaar JK, Willemsen-Swinkels SH: Medication treatment in subjects with autistic spectrum disorders, *Eur Child Adolesc Psychiatry* 9(Suppl 1):185-197, 2000.

Clinical Practice Guideline: diagnosis and evaluation of the child with attention-deficit hyperactivity disorder, American Academy of Pediatrics, *Pediatrics* 105(5):1158-1170, 2000.

Daily DK, Ardinger HH, Holmes GE: Identification and evaluation of mental retardation, *Am Fam Physician* 61(4):1059-1067, 1070, 2000.

Denckla MB: Neurological examination for subtle signs (PANESS), *Psychopharmacol Bull* 21:273-300, 1985.

Feldman R, Eidelman AI: Intervention programs for premature infants: how and do they affect development? *Clin Perinatol* 25(3):613-626, 1998.

Filipek PA, Accardo PJ, Baranek GT et al: The screening and diagnosis of autistic spectrum disorders, *J Autism Dev Disord* 29(6):439-484, 1999.

Flory S: Identifying, assessing and helping dyspraxic children, *Dyslexia* 6(3):205-208, 2000.

Gascon G, Johnson R, Burd L: Central auditory processing and attention deficit disorders, *J Child Neurol* 1(1):27-33, 1986.

Gascon GG, Mikati M: Pediatric neurology. In Elzouki AY, Harfi H, Nazer H: *Textbook of clinical pediatrics,* Philadelphia, 2001, Lippincott, Williams & Wilkins.

Gascon GG, Ozand PT: Aminoacidopathies and organic acidopathies, mitochondrial enzyme defects, and other metabolic errors. In Goetz CG: *Textbook of clinical neurology,* ed 2, Philadelphia, 2002, WB Saunders (in press).

Giedd JN: Bipolar disorder and attention-deficit/hyperactivity disorder in children and adults, *J Clin Psychiatry* 61(Suppl 9):31-34, 2000.

Goldstein S, Reynolds CR, editors: *Handbook of neurodevelopmental and genetic disorders in children,* New York, 1999, Guilford Publications.

Habib M: The neurological basis of developmental dyslexia: an overview and working hypothesis, *Brain* 123(12):2373-2379, 2000.

Hechtman L: Assessment and diagnosis of attention-deficit/hyperactivity disorder, *Child Adolesc Psychiatr Clin N Am* 9(3):481-498, 2000.

Hoffman JB, DuPaul GJ: Psychoeducational interventions for children and adolescents with attention-deficit/hyperactivity disorder, *Child Adolesc Psychiatr Clin N Am* 9(3):647-661, 2000.

Howlin P: *Children with autism and Asperger syndrome: a guide for practitioners and carers,* New York, 1999, John Wiley & Sons.

Jensen PS: ADHD: current concepts on etiology, pathophysiology, and neurobiology, *Child Adolesc Psychiatr Clin N Am* 9(3):557-572, 2000.

Leung AK, Kao CP: Evaluation and management of the child with speech delay, *Am Family Physician* 59(11):3121-3128, 3135, 1999.

Levine MD, Carey WB, Crocker AC: *Developmental-behavioral pediatrics,* ed 3, Philadelphia, 1999, WB Saunders.

Madrid AL, State MW, King BH: Pharmacologic management of psychiatric and behavioral symptoms in mental retardation, *Child Adolesc Psychiatr Clin N Am* 9(1):225-243, 2000.

Msall ME, Tremont MR: Functional outcomes in self-care, mobility, communication and learning in extremely low-birth weight infants, *Clin Perinatol* 27(2):381-401, 2000.

Naidu S: Rett syndrome: natural history and underlying disease mechanisms, *Eur Child Adolesc Psychiatry* 6(Suppl 1):14-17, 1997.

Nelson KB, Willoughby RE: Infection, inflammation and the risk of cerebral palsy, *Curr Opin Neurol* 13(2):133-139, 2000.

Nyhan WL, Ozand PT: *Atlas of metabolic diseases,* Philadelphia, 1999, Lippincott-Raven.

Paine R, Oppe T: *Neurological examination of children, vol 20/21, Clinics in Developmental Medicine,* Philadelphia, 1966, JB Lippincott.

Petersen MC, Kube DA, Palmer FB: Classification of developmental delays, *Semin Pediatr Neurol* 5(1):2-14, 1998.

Ramin SM, Gilstrap LC: Other factors/conditions associated with cerebral palsy, *Semin Perinatol* 24(3):196-199, 2000.

Rosenthal M, Griffith ER, Kreutzer JS, Pentland B, editors: *Rehabilitation of the adult and child with traumatic brain injury,* ed 3, Philadelphia, 1999, FA Davis.

Schaefer GB, Bodensteiner JB: Radiological findings in developmental delay, *Semin Pediatr Neurol* 5(1):33-38, 1998.

Shalev RS, Auerbach J, Manor O, Gross-Tsur V: Developmental dyscalculia: prevalence and prognosis, *Eur Child Adolesc Psychiatry* 9(Suppl 2):1158-1164, 2000.

Spencer T, Biederman J, Wilens T: Pharmacotherapy of attention deficit hyperactivity disorder, *Child Adolesc Psychiatr Clin N Am* 9(1):77-97, 2000.

Swaimann KF, Ashwal S: *Pediatric neurology: principles and practice,* St Louis, 1999, Mosby.

Touwen BC: *The examination of the child with minor nervous dysfunction,* ed 2, Philadelphia, 1981, JB Lippincott.

Waterstone T: The child with slow language development, *Practitioner* 244(1612): 636-641, 2000.

Weinberg WA, Harper CR, Brumback RA: Attention, behavior, and learning problems in children: protocols for diagnosis and treatment, Hamilton, Ontario, Canada, 2001, BC Decker.

WEBSITES

American cerebral palsy information center: cerebralpalsy.org

American Medical Association (AMA): health insight: www.ama-assn.org/ama/pub/category/3457.html

American Speech-Language-Hearing Association: www.asha.org

Apraxia: www.apraxia-kids.org

Autism Society of America (ASA): www.autism-society.org

Children and Adults with Attention Deficit Disorder (CHADD): www.chadd.org

Down Syndrome WWW page: www.nas.com/downsyn

Dyscalculia International Consortium: www.shianet.org/~reneenew/DIC.html

Dysgraphia: diagnosis and interventions strategies for disorders of written language: www.udel.edu/bkirby/asperger/dysgraphia_mjkay.html

Family village: a global community of disability-related resources: www.familyvillage.wisc.edu/index.htmlx

International Rett Syndrome Association: www.rettsyndrome.org

Kidshealth.org: kidshealth.org/index2.html

National Organization for Rare Disorders: www.rarediseases.org

Neurogenetics: brain.mgh.harvard.edu:100/ngenethp.htm

NINDS: learning disabilities information: www.ninds.nih.gov/health_and_medical/disorders/learningdisabilities_doc.htm

Online Mendelian Inheritance in Man (OMIM) database: www.ncbi.nlm.nih.gov/Omim

Quackwatch: www.quackwatch.com

Society for the Autistically Handicapped: www.autismuk.com

Support-group.com: www.support-group.com

The Arc of the United States: www.thearc.org

Tourette Syndrome Association: tsa-usa.org

United Cerebral Palsy (UCP): www.ucp.org

17

Low Back Pain

L ow back pain with or without leg pain is one of the most common complaints seen in medical practice. It is estimated that up to 80% of the American population will suffer at least a temporary disability from low back pain. Low back pain is only a *symptom* that can result from several conditions, and hence the term should not automatically be equated with a herniated lumbar disc. Each patient must be evaluated with a detailed history, an adequate physical examination, and relevant investigations so that a correct diagnosis is reached and an appropriate treatment initiated. The causes of low back pain include the following:

1. Trauma:
   a. Acute lumbosacral sprain
   b. Fracture of the lumbar vertebrae
2. Tumors:
   a. Metastases to the spine (Common sources are prostate, breast, and kidneys.)
   b. Tumors compressing the cauda equina
3. Metabolic: Osteoporosis (particularly in postmenopausal women), myeloma, and hyperparathyroidism
4. Degenerative processes involving the intervertebral disc or the joints between the articular processes of adjacent vertebrae (A posterolateral herniation of the nucleus pulposus usually compresses a nerve root.)
5. Other structural lesions of the spine:
   a. Spinal stenosis
   b. Spondylolisthesis
6. Infections of the disc space or vertebrae
7. Inflammatory disorders involving:
   a. Vertebrae (e.g., ankylosing spondylitis)
   b. Meninges (e.g., arachnoiditis)
8. Vascular:
   a. An abdominal aortic aneurysm eroding the vertebrae
   b. Occlusive vascular disease causing radicular or plexus ischemia
9. Direct involvement of the lumbosacral plexus or sciatic nerve (e.g., trauma, tumors, injections into or close to the sciatic nerve)
10. Psychogenic: Especially when litigation is involved

HISTORY

It is of utmost importance that the patient's history be derived *without using leading questions*. Patients with pain problems are often overly susceptible to suggestion. Leading questions may only provide misinformation to the initial examiner and allow the patient to develop a symptom complex that will mislead subsequent examiners. For example, do not ask whether specific activities aggravate the pain; ask whether there are any known factors that aggravate the pain. Do not ask whether the pain goes into the leg; ask whether the pain extends into any other part of the body from the lower back. The answers to such questions may help to differentiate organic from functional problems. With experience, the examiner should (in approximately 15 minutes) be able to take a history regarding the back pain problem that will provide the following information:

1. The chronologic sequence of the events involved in the pain problem leading up to the time of the examination: "Tell me the whole story of your problem from the very beginning."
2. An exact description of the type of pain, its location, extent, and radiation, if any: "Tell me exactly what this pain is like."
3. The factors that precipitate the pain and activities that exacerbate or relieve the pain: "Does anything affect this pain?"
4. A description of any back injury (and whether there is litigation related to that injury): "Have you ever injured your back?"
5. Associated motor or sensory complaints (nature and extent): "Have you noticed any weakness or loss of feeling?"
6. An interference with bowel, bladder, or sexual function: "Do your bowels and bladder work all right? Have you had any problems with your sexual function?"
7. A detailed description of previous therapy for the pain and what effect it may have had: "Have you ever had any treatment for your back? If so, describe it." (Be alert to drug-seeking behavior.)

Hypothesis Formation

From the patient's history, a hypothesis as to the possible source of the pain should be formulated.

1. If the pain is localized to the low back without radiation to the leg, it is unlikely that there is nerve root involvement. Osteoporosis, spinal metastasis, degenerative disc disease, and disc space infections can all present with low back pain alone.
2. If the pain radiates to the lower extremity, consider the following sources:
   a. Root pain:
      1) Worse with factors that increase intraspinal pressure (e.g., coughing and sneezing)
      2) Distribution usually in the L4, L5, or S1 dermatome
   b. Neurogenic claudication:
      1) Related to exertion—especially with iliofemoral occlusive vascular disease
      2) Lumbar spinal canal stenosis: pain worse with exertion

Caveat: Stenosis commonly produces numbness and weakness; vascular disease does not.

    c. Posterior longitudinal ligament involvement (most often a bulging disc that does not stretch a nerve root):
       1) Pain seldom radiates below the knee
       2) Pain is vague and not associated with paresthesia
    d. Hip joint disease and pelvic pathology may also cause lower extremity pain

3. Back pain in the elderly population (over 60 years of age) often presents differently than in the younger adult (under 60 years of age) population, including the following signs:
    a. Back pain is often present at rest.
    b. Spinal claudication is more common and can occur without severe spinal stenosis.
    c. Reflex changes are often evident, but reflexes may be normal if the vertebral column is primarily involved.
    d. Bladder dysfunction is often occult and may only be evident with cystometrogram.
    e. Reduced mobility can obscure significant vascular disease.

Physical Examination

1. Examination of *gait* is an important part of the physical examination of patients with back pain. The physician must pay particular attention to the following signs:
    a. Whether the patient is walking with a list of the spine; this is highly indicative of an organic back problem (Fig. 17-1).
    b. Whether the patient can support his or her weight on the toes and heels; this can indicate motor weakness in muscles below the knee.
    c. Whether the patient can hop on one foot or the other; this can indicate weakness of the quadriceps or gluteus muscles.
2. Examination of the *back* should be carried out with the patient in the upright standing position. Note the following conditions:
    a. Muscle spasm (noted by prominence of paraspinal muscles on one side or flattening of the lumbar lordosis; Fig. 17-2).
    b. List or curvature of the spine. The patient often leans away from the site of his or her pain and the scoliosis becomes more prominent as the patient tries to bend forward.
    c. Any palpable mass or tenderness along the vertebral column (including percussion of the flanks while looking for kidney disease and percussion over the spinous processes with a tendon hammer; Fig. 17-3).
    d. Range of motion in flexion, extension, and sideways bending. Often the patient will keep the spine rigid and do the flexion at the hip.
    e. Dimples, birth marks, abnormal patches of hair (clues to congenital malformation or tumors).
3. The straight leg raising test is the *key to identifying nerve root irritation*. With the patient lying flat on his or her back, passively raise the

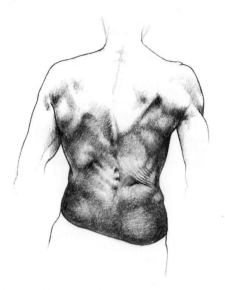

FIG. 17-1 A patient with an organic back pain problem frequently walks with forward flexion of the trunk and with one iliac crest higher than the other. A lateral curve of the spine is often present.

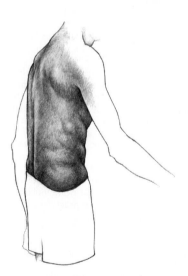

FIG. 17-2 A patient with an organic back problem will often have the lower lumbar curve obliterated. Unilateral paravertebral muscle spasm on one side elevates the iliac crest. This is most commonly seen with a root lesion.

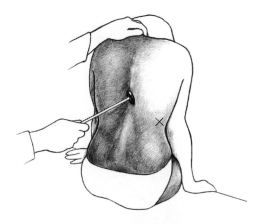

FIG. 17-3 Percussion of the spinous processes will often cause more discomfort over the involved vertebrae. Be certain also to percuss the costovertebral angle in search of renal disease.

extended leg until pain occurs (Fig. 17-4). Normally an 80-degree movement can be made with little discomfort; if the pain is only in the back of the thigh, it is likely to be caused by hamstring tightness and not nerve root tension, irritation, or compression. If the pain radiates to the back as well as to the leg, it often indicates nerve root involvement. When in doubt, use one or more of the following maneuvers to confirm a positive straight leg raising test:

a. The straight leg is lowered until the pain just disappears, then attempt to suddenly dorsiflex the ankle; genuine root pain will be reproduced by this maneuver.

b. Have the patient sit up on the bed with the legs extended at the knee or repeat the test with the patient in the sitting position with his or her legs dangling over the edge of the table (Fig. 17-5). When the leg is extended at the knee, the patient should complain of pain and lean backward to produce the same angle as for the straight leg raising test in the lying position. If the patient experiences no pain in the sitting position, a previous positive straight leg raising test in the lying position probably suggests a nonorganic basis.

c. The patient may be asked to kneel on a chair; in this position the hamstrings are relaxed and the tension on the sciatic nerve is reduced; reluctance to bend forward while in this position suggests a false-positive straight leg raising test.

While the straight leg raising test is performed, hip joint mobility should also be evaluated. This is done by passive rotation of the leg at the hip (Fig. 17-6). A patient with pathologic spinal changes will have no pain or restriction on rotary movements of the hip, but the patient

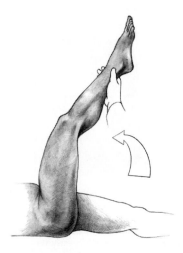

FIG. 17-4 Straight leg raising test. With disc disease, raising the affected leg will often cause pain in the distribution of the affected root. This pain is centered in the buttocks at the sciatic notch and radiates down the leg. Pain at the knee from tight hamstring muscles does not constitute a positive straight leg raising test.

with hip disease (who may appear to have a back pain problem) will show a marked aggravation of the pain when the hip is rotated internally or externally.

Caveat: Disease at the L5 to S1 intervertebral disc space may appear as hip pain.

4. Concentrate on the following aspects of the neurologic examination that may be helpful in confirming nerve root compression:
   a. Unilaterally absent or diminished patellar (L4), internal hamstring (L5), or Achilles (S1) tendon reflexes localize an involved nerve root with reasonable accuracy. Be aware of the patient who may show hyperactive reflexes in the presence of acute back pain caused by tensing the lower-extremity muscles; in such a patient the plantar response will remain flexor.
   b. Absent cremasteric reflexes suggest an upper lumbar root or conus medullaris lesion (Fig. 17-7).
   c. Unequal superficial abdominal reflexes may suggest a thoracic lesion from the T9 to the T12 level (Fig. 17-8).
   d. A dermatomal sensory loss, if typical, is useful in localizing the root involved.

Caution: Never make a diagnosis on the basis of sensory loss alone.

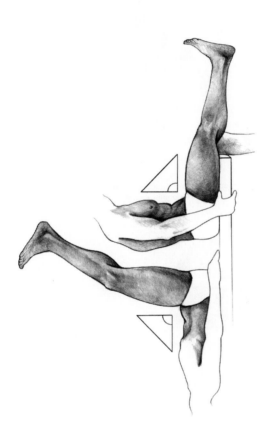

FIG. 17-5 If the examiner suspects the straight leg raising test to be unreliable in the supine position, the examiner can surreptitiously raise the leg while the patient is in the sitting position. If the lesion is organic, radiating pain should be experienced in both positions.

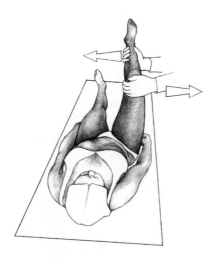

FIG. 17-6 Hip rotation. With the hip and knee flexed, inward rotation of the lower leg will cause pain if there is hip joint disease.

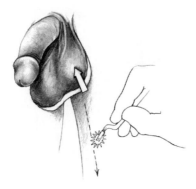

FIG. 17-7 Cremasteric reflex. A light stroke downward on the inner surface of the thigh produces an upward movement of the testicle.

    e. Motor weakness demonstrated by specific muscle testing may confirm a motor root lesion. Muscle testing may also demonstrate involvement of multiple roots.

    f. Bilateral simultaneous muscle testing is a valuable method of detecting hysterical weakness. The patient is unable to coordinate hysterical "giving way" between both extremities (Fig. 17-9).

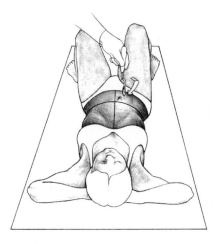

FIG. 17-8 Abdominal reflex. A light stroke toward the umbilicus will normally cause a muscle contraction with movement of the umbilicus toward the stimulus. The pinwheel is a more effective and reliable stimulus than a sharp stick.

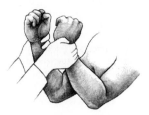

FIG. 17-9 Test comparable muscle strength simultaneously if there is suspicion of a nonorganic process. It is very difficult to give way with one muscle while maintaining strength in another.

5. The physical examination should also include abdominal palpation, palpation of the lower extremity pulsations, and listening for a bruit over the aorta, the iliac arteries, and the femoral arteries.

6. A rectal examination is quite important in evaluating patients with persistent back pain or back and leg pain to detect pelvic pathologic changes and sphincter involvement. The anal reflex, which is often lost in conus medullaris and cauda equina lesions, should also be tested (Fig. 17-10).

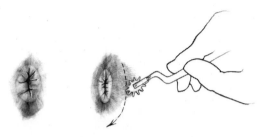

FIG. 17-10 A light stroke with a pinwheel in the perianal area normally causes the anus to pucker.

Clinical Investigations

The patient's history and physical findings should narrow the differential diagnosis. The investigations are chosen on the basis of the most likely diagnoses.

1. Magnetic resonance imaging (MRI) is the procedure of choice except in cases of trauma; computed tomography (CT) is better in identifying fractures but does not show the spinal cord. Order contrast MRI if there have been previous low back surgical procedures or if metastases are suspected.

2. Radionuclide bone scans are particularly useful when metastatic disease is suspected as a cause of low back pain. The scans are also often positive in inflammatory diseases of the spine and in fractures.

3. Damage to a nerve root can be assessed by electromyography (EMG) and nerve conduction studies; a CT scan myelography and MRI show only the anatomic structures. In experienced hands EMG provides accurate localization of the root involved. EMG studies are most useful in identifying peripheral neuropathies that may confuse the picture of root involvement and certainly is not indicated in every case of low back pain.

4. When metabolic bone disease or metastases are suspected, erythrocyte sedimentation rate (ESR) and calcium, phosphate, and alkaline and acid phosphatase assays may be done. When disc space infections or inflammatory disease is suspected, ESR, antinuclear antibodies, and rheumatoid factor assays need to be done. When myeloma is suspected, x-ray studies of other parts of the skeleton, studies of the urine for Bence Jones protein, serum protein electrophoresis, and a bone marrow examination are necessary.

PROTRUDED INTERVERTEBRAL DISC

▶ 1. *The most important diagnostic feature* of a protruded intervertebral disc is the onset of low back pain followed by radiation down one lower extremity.

Caution: All such pain is not caused by disc prolapse; any condition that afflicts the nerve root can have similar symptoms.

2. The initial attack may be provoked by an identifiable precipitating event (e.g., lifting a weight or twisting). Extremely severe trauma may cause a disc to rupture, but by far the most common scenario is repeated minor trauma over many years, plus a genetic susceptibility.

3. The area of pain is usually well localized, and the extension can be traced with a finger. There is a feeling of associated tingling in the distal extension of the pain.

4. During subsequent episodes, which may again be precipitated by physical activity, the pain is often less severe and may disappear within a few days; less severe attacks are usually precipitated by movement and may be relieved by changing the posture or by resting.

5. The pain is improved by flexion of the thigh and knees; in individual patients the pain may be worse at night or during the day. Activity relieves pain in some patients but more commonly aggravates symptoms. The patient will often move about gingerly for fear of aggravating the pain.

6. The patient may complain of extremity weakness, numbness, and paresthesias in localized areas of the leg or foot. Infrequently, there may be interference of the bowel, bladder, or sexual function; these symptoms are more common in midline disc herniation involving the sacral nerve roots of both sides.

7. The physical examination reveals one or more of the following signs:
   a. The patient often stands in a listed position and tends to walk with the affected leg slightly flexed at the knee and thigh. There may be difficulty standing in an upright position with the leg fully extended.
   b. There may be difficulty supporting weight on the toes or heels. Walking on the heels often acutely aggravates the pain.
   c. Hopping is often difficult to perform, but if performed, a tendency for the knee to buckle suggests quadricep weakness and the possibility of an L3 or L4 root lesion.
   d. An examination of the back shows paravertebral muscle spasm with a limitation of bending forward or backward. Bending forward is more often limited in a ruptured disc at the L5 to S1 interspace; bending backward is often limited in a ruptured disc at the L3 to L4 or L4 to L5 interspaces. Frequently scoliosis with a convexity toward the symptomatic side may be seen.
   e. Percussion over the spine may produce radiation of the pain into the affected leg.
   f. The straight leg raising test is positive on the symptomatic side. Occasionally there is a positive crossed straight leg raising test with pain extending into the leg opposite the one being raised. (This is suggestive of an extruded fragment.)
   g. The patient will flex the knees and thighs and roll with the legs flexed in the process of turning over or getting out of bed.

BOX 17-1
Symptoms of Lumbosacral Root Lesions

S1 ROOT LESION (Fig. 17-11)

1. Diminished or absent Achilles tendon reflex (ankle reflex)
2. Sensory deficit in the lateral aspect of the heel and the lateral aspect of the sole of the affected foot
3. Difficulty standing on tiptoe on the affected extremity (suggests calf weakness)

L5 ROOT LESION (Fig. 17-12)

1. Trouble supporting weight on heel or presence of foot drop (The patient may complain that his or her toes get caught on the carpet.)

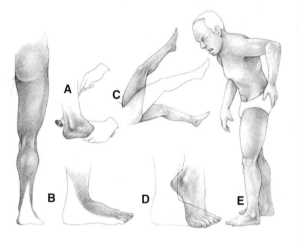

FIG. 17-11 Summary of an S1 root lesion. **A,** Diminished Achilles reflex. **B,** Sensory disturbance over the lateral aspect of the heel and toe. **C,** Positive straight leg raising. **D,** Difficulty standing on tiptoe. **E,** Pain worse bending forward.

    h. More than 90% of ruptured lumbar discs with nerve root compression affect either L5 or S1 roots, producing the neurologic alterations described in Box 17-1.

Caution: Sensory deficits must be interpreted very carefully, taking into account an intuitive assessment of patient reliability and the examiner's experience.

BOX 17-1
Symptoms of Lumbosacral Root Lesions—cont'd

2. Sensory deficits over the anterolateral aspect of the affected leg below the knee and extending to the dorsum of the foot and the big toe
3. Diminished or absent internal hamstring tendon reflex

L4 ROOT LESION
1. Diminished or absent patellar tendon reflex
2. Weakness in the quadricep muscle of the affected leg
3. Sensory deficit extending from the knee down the medial aspect of the lower portion of the affected leg as well as the medial malleolus

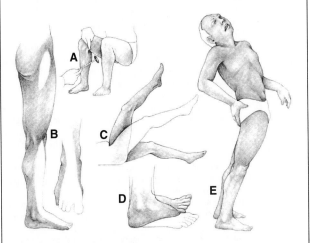

FIG. 17-12 Summary of an L5 root lesion. **A,** Diminished internal hamstring reflex. **B,** Sensory disturbance over dorsum of foot and great toe. **C,** Positive straight leg raising. **D,** Foot drop. **E,** Pain worse bending backward.

8. Investigations
   a. The routine laboratory and plain spine radiographs in protruded lumbar intervertebral discs seldom show diagnostic abnormalities. MRI is the procedure of choice.
9. Management
   a. In acute disc prolapse, at least 6 weeks of conservative treatment should be tried unless there is evidence of spinal cord

compression such as hyperactive reflexes in the legs or Babinski's sign; this constitutes emergency neurosurgical treatment. Conservative management includes the following suggestions:

1) Strict bed rest for a few days (except for bathroom privileges); the bed should be firm (a firm mattress or bed board) and flat. The fetal position with a pillow placed between the thighs is comfortable for most patients.

2) Antiinflammatory agents and mild analgesics and antidepressant medications are helpful during the period of bed rest: Gabapentin (Neurontin) 400 mg by mouth 3 times a day, indomethacin (Indocin) 25 mg 3 times a day, and amytriptyline 25 to 50 mg at bedtime is a suggested regimen. Heating pads delivering both heat and massage are now available. Transcutaneous electrical nerve stimulation (TENS) is useful in patients either with acute low back pain or with low back pain and radicular pain.

3) After recovery from the acute attack, a concerted program of back exercises for at least 6 weeks is recommended.

4) A lumbar roll (a hand towel rolled into a 4-inch roll and secured by rubber bands) in situations where prolonged sitting is necessary (such as in an automobile) helps prevent recurrences.

b. A patient's failure to respond to conservative treatment may result from noncompliance with strict bed rest, an incorrect diagnosis, persistent or worsening nerve root compression, an unstable spine, secondary gain, litigation, or other psychosocial factors. A comprehensive evaluation is needed at this stage to determine the reason for nonimprovement. In some metropolitan areas, a referral to rehabilitation facilities specializing only in low back problems may be useful.

c. Surgical intervention should be considered with the greatest skepticism; extruded disc fragments, spinal cord compression, and progressive objective neurologic deficit are some of the reasons for early surgery. Surgery is successful more often in older patients.

SPRAIN OR FRACTURE

▶ 1. Paravertebral muscle spasm is one of the most common causes of acute low back pain. *The most important clue to the diagnosis* is pain specifically related to an injury that reaches a crescendo (quickly or over a period of days) and gradually tapers to a plateau that may persist for weeks to months.

2. The pain is described as a diffuse backache with associated stiffness, spasm, and limitation of motion. Stiffness may extend up to the neck and down to the pelvis and legs.

3. Extension of the pain is vague unless a fracture has produced nerve root compression. In the facet syndrome (caused by tearing

of the capsule of the facet joint), the pain may extend to the buttock and posterior thigh of the involved side.

4. The pain is relieved somewhat by reclining, changing position, analgesics, and heat. Massage or manipulation often gives temporary relief but may be dangerous in an unsuspected fracture. There is no relationship of the pain to the time of day.

5. Temporary ileus or difficulty in initiating urination may occur in the acute phase of pain.

6. Damage or compression of the spinal cord or nerve root by a fracture may produce deficits in motor, sensory, bowel, bladder, and sexual function.

7. On examination
   a. The gait *should not* be tested during the acute phase until plain x-ray examination has excluded the presence of an unstable vertebral fracture.
   b. Initially there may be palpable swelling or hematoma. Palpation of the back usually reveals an area of focal tenderness over the spinous processes in the region of the injury. Reversal of the spinal curve may be palpable at the level of the compression fracture.
   c. Because a common site of fracture is the T12 vertebra, examination of sensation in the perianal area is mandatory to exclude injury to the conus medullaris without simultaneous nerve root injury. There may be loss of bowel and bladder function, sexual dysfunction in the male patient, and loss of anal reflex or a patulous anal sphincter.
   d. In all patients, careful documentation of reflex, motor, and sensory function is important in the acute phase so that a comparison can be made with follow-up examinations.

8. In the case of low back sprain, spine x-ray film findings reveal few changes other than obliteration of normal spinal curvature resulting from paravertebral muscle spasm.

9. In the case of spinal fracture, spine x-ray studies are the diagnostic tool for identifying the lesion.

Caution: Unsatisfactory x-ray films or films taken too low or too high in the spine result in many fractures being missed.

10. Management
    a. A back sprain is treated like a lumbar disc herniation, both in the acute and chronic phases.
    b. A spinal fracture requires absolute bed rest on a flat, firm surface (bed board) and consideration of surgical treatment by decompression laminectomy or surgical stabilization.

STRUCTURAL BONY LESIONS

1. The conditions that may lead to low back pain caused by structural bony abnormalities include osteoporosis, an old fracture,

and congenital bony abnormalities, such as partially sacralized lumbar vertebrae, unilateral pedicle defect, spondylolisthesis, facet asymmetry, and spinal stenosis.

2. Most of these conditions appear with chronic low back pain of long duration; the patient may trace the onset to injury.

3. The major feature is chronic, nagging, and centrally located back pain without radiation to the lower extremities; the notable exceptions are spondylolisthesis and spinal stenosis where radicular pain spreading to the lower extremities may occur.

4. The pain is precipitated or aggravated by lifting, standing, or prolonged forward bending and is aggravated by work and sexual, physical, and recreational activity. The pain is often relieved by sitting or lying down; it is seldom troubling at night.

▶ 5. *An important diagnostic clue* is that the pain is least troublesome on rising from bed, but increases with activity during the day.

6. There are no complaints of motor, sensory, bladder, bowel, or sexual dysfunction, except in cases of spinal stenosis or spondylolisthesis with nerve root involvement.

7. The results of a physical examination show a normal gait with the ability to walk on the heels and toes, a negative straight leg raising test, and normal reflexes, muscle strength, and sensory perception. The abnormality is easily identified by x-ray films. A CT scan and MRI are of immense help in locating and characterizing the defect.

8. An acute back pain resulting from structural bony abnormality should be treated like an acute herniated disc. Excessive weight in

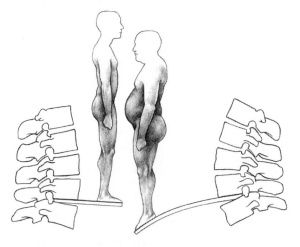

FIG. 17-13 A potbelly increases stress on the lumbar spine. The length of the springboard is proportional to the distance between the navel and the spine.

the abdominal area (potbelly) should be eliminated by a weight-reduction program (Fig. 17-13).

LUMBAR STENOSIS

1. Although also a structural abnormality, lumbar stenosis is mentioned separately, since the clinical presentation is somewhat typical. There is narrowing of the nerve root foramina and spinal canal, resulting in compression of the lumbosacral nerve roots. A congenitally narrow canal with acquired factors, such as hypertrophy of vertebral bone and interspinal ligamentous tissue, as well as displacement of the intervertebral discs, may result in lumbar stenosis.

▶ 2. *The most important diagnostic clue* is the occurrence of symptoms suggestive of *bilateral lumbosacral radiculopathy,* either acutely after minor trauma or insidiously.

3. Typical features of the abnormality include claudication (the pain usually involves the lower extremities, is provoked by exertion, and relieved by sitting), postural aggravation of symptoms (exacerbation of radiating leg pain, paresthesia, and numbness or weakness when standing erect or bending backward; the patient may complain of sudden onset of severe pain in the legs on reaching for objects overhead, which is quickly relieved by bending forward). A typical patient will be one with bilateral sciatica who enters the examining room hunched over and walking with a short cane.

4. The diagnosis is confirmed by findings of MRI or a CT scan of the lumbar spine. The treatment is surgical and consists of wide laminectomy with bilateral foraminotomy.

INFLAMMATORY DISEASE AFFECTING THE SPINE

1. Ankylosing spondylitis is an inflammatory disease that may cause persistent low back pain. This condition is estimated to occur in about 1% of the population. Characteristic features include the following:
   a. An onset between 20 and 40 years of age, often in men.
   b. An insidious onset of chronic low back pain without sciatica.
   c. A feeling of stiffness and pain aggravated by maintaining one position for a long time and improved by mild activity.
   d. The absence of motor or sensory abnormalities; the straight leg raising test is negative.
   e. Possible discomfort on hip rotation with a general reduction in movements of the lumbar spine in all directions.
   f. Confirmation of the diagnosis by the findings of a CT scan or MRI (the involvement of sacroiliac joints, and calcification of anterior and posterior spinal ligaments) and an elevated ESR.
2. Rheumatoid arthritis may lead to persistent low back pain. The most useful diagnostic features include the involvement of other joints and laboratory data supporting the diagnosis.
3. Infections may cause back pain.
   a. Both acute and chronic infection of the spine may present with back pain.

  b. A disc space infection, which may occur after surgery or as a complication of a systemic infection, presents with severe back pain, local spinal tenderness, and paraspinal spasm. MRI, a bone scan, and blood studies are often diagnostic.

  c. Involvement of the spine may also occur in conditions such as tuberculosis, brucellosis, and typhoid. Spinal tuberculosis may present with pain and spinal deformity (gibbus) in the lower thoracic area; a cold abscess may form and compress the spinal cord and produce an acute or subacute onset of paraplegia. The radiologic appearance is characteristic, showing rarefaction and often collapse of the adjacent vertebrae with paraspinal mass.

INTRASPINAL OR SPINAL NEOPLASM

1. Intraspinal or spinal neoplasms occur with metastatic prostatic or breast carcinoma and primary tumors, such as meningioma, neurofibroma, or ependymoma.

▶ 2. *The most important diagnostic clue* is a *steady, relentless progression* of symptoms (as opposed to static or intermittent pain noted with most other causes).

3. With a progressive increase in the severity and constancy of the pain the patient may describe radicular extension of the pain (often with motor and sensory deficits).

4. The pain is aggravated by activity and unrelieved by any therapeutic measures; there is slight improvement on reclining with the knees flexed. Prolonged lying down aggravates the pain and may wake the patient at night. With arousal and ambulation pain may lessen; The pain may be increased by Valsalva's maneuver (but does not necessarily differentiate this cause of pain from other causes of back pain).

5. Progression of the lesion often results in impairment of bowel and bladder control and sexual dysfunction in the male patient.

6. The results of the examination show evidence of a spinal lesion manifested by the following:
   a. Muscle spasm
   b. Area of focal tenderness
   c. Reflex alterations
   d. Sensory deficits
   e. Motor group weakness
   (Examination of the breast or prostate may lead to diagnosis of the underlying metastatic neoplasm in a high percentage of cases.)

7. Primary intraspinal neoplasms have no characteristic laboratory abnormalities.

8. Metastatic spinal neoplasms may exhibit laboratory findings of malignancy such as anemia, an elevated ESR, elevated prostate specific antigen (PSA), and elevation of the alkaline phosphatase and acid phosphatase levels.

9. Results of MRI with contrast may show widening of the spinal canal, erosion of the pedicles, or scalloping of the vertebral bod-

ies. Metastatic neoplasms may show erosion of elements of the vertebral body or osteoblastic changes.

10. Results of a bone scan may show evidence of metastatic lesions when the plain films are negative. Pain usually precedes radiographic changes by several weeks.

Treatment:

1. An early diagnosis may obviate the need for neurosurgical treatment and avoid serious neurologic sequelae in cases of metastatic lesions.

2. A late diagnosis usually necessitates urgent neurosurgical decompression.

3. In almost all cases of malignant neoplasms, chemotherapy or radiotherapy is necessary. Short-term corticosteroid therapy is useful when there is cord compression.

4. Early surgical treatment of benign intraspinal tumors such as neurofibroma and meningioma leads to excellent results.

RETROPERITONEAL LESIONS

▶ 1. *The most important diagnostic clue* of retroperitoneal lesions is the pain, which is described as deep and burning and radiates from the abdomen through to the back. When the nerve plexus is involved, there is usually acute neuralgic pain or burning paresthesia that may radiate from the abdomen to the back, groin, or the lower extremities.

2. The pain may be related to the ingestion of food and may be aggravated by lying flat, emptying the bladder, or moving the bowels; pain may occur related to menstrual flow.

3. The patient's level of activity has little or no effect on the pain.

4. Examination:

   a. The back examination and neurologic examination are normal, unless the lumbosacral plexus has been affected.

   b. Percussion of the costovertebral angle may produce pain. (This maneuver does not produce pain in other causes of back pain.)

   c. Hyperextension of the leg at the thigh may produce pain if there is psoas muscle irritation.

   d. Rectal examination findings may reveal a presacral or pelvic mass.

   e. Evidence of lumbosacral plexus involvement may be present.

5. Laboratory studies may show evidence suggesting inflammatory or neoplastic disease.

6. Routine spinal radiographs are seldom helpful; a CT scan with contrast of the abdomen is often useful in identifying the lesion.

7. Special studies, such as a gastrointestinal (GI) series or intravenous pyelography (IVP), may be of value in the diagnosis.

8. EMG studies may be useful in determining the extent and severity of lumbosacral plexus involvement.

9. Treatment must be directed toward the primary disease process.

PSYCHOGENIC PAIN

▶ 1. *The most important diagnostic clue* of psychogenic pain is that the patient is inconsistent with regard to the chronologic history, description of pain, factors affecting the pain, and the relationship of the pain to the time of day; if the pain is injury related, the circumstances of the injury are usually presented in explicit detail in contrast to the vague description of the nature of the pain problem.

2. The patient's history may be misleading if the patient has had previous exposure to leading questions by other examiners.

3. Sometimes the patient may purposely mislead the examiner.

4. Examination:
   a. The patient exhibits overreaction to the examiner's physical contact.
   b. The patient reacts to palpation in a manner disproportionate to the lack of objective findings in the examination.
   c. The patient frequently exhibits an oscillatory giveaway weakness on muscle testing and exhibits vague, indefinite, and unphysiologic sensory alterations.
   d. The appearance and attitudes of the patient may vary from inappropriate cheerfulness to indifference and apathy, inappropriate distress, and hostility.
   e. Simultaneous muscle testing (Fig. 17-9) or an inappropriate straight leg raising test (Fig. 17-5) may give clues to an underlying disorder.

5. Do not be misled by nonspecific laboratory and radiographic findings.

Treatment: Appropriate management of the underlying emotional problem is often indicated without denying the distress the patient is experiencing from the problem.

BIBLIOGRAPHY

Argoff CA, Wheeler AH: Spinal and radicular pain disorders, *Neurol Clin* 16(4):833-850, 1998.

Blumer D: Psychiatric and psychological aspects of chronic pain, *Clin Neurosurg* 25:276-283, 1978.

Bratton RL: Assessment and management of acute low back pain, *Am Fam Physician* 60(8):2299-2308, 1999.

Condon RH: *Modalities in the treatment of acute and chronic low back pain.* In Finneson BE, editor: *Low back pain,* Philadelphia, 1981, JB Lippincott.

Donelson RG: Identifying appropriate exercises for your low back pain patient, *J Musculoskeletal Med* 8(12):14-29, 1991.

Frymoyer JW: Back pain and sciatica, *N Engl J Med* 318(5):291-300, 1988.

Hall S, Bartleson JD, Onofrio BM et al: Lumbar spinal stenosis: clinical features, diagnostic procedures, and results of surgical treatment in 68 patients, *Ann Intern Med* 103(2):271-275, 1985.

Hardy RW, Plank NW: *Clinical diagnosis of herniated lumbar disc.* In Hardy RW Jr, editor: *Lumbar disc disease,* New York, 1982, Raven Press.

Kelsey JL, White HH, Pastides H et al: The impact of musculoskeletal disorders on the population of the United States, *J Bone Joint Surg Am* 61(7):959-964, 1979.

Mills K, Page G, Siwek R: *Color atlas of low back pain,* Philadelphia, 1990, FA Davis.

Nakano K: *Neurology of musculoskeletal and rheumatic disorders,* Boston, 1979, Houghton Mifflin.

Patel AT, Ogle AA: Diagnosis and management of acute low back pain, *Am Fam Physician* 61(6):1779-1786, 2000.

Ponte DJ, Jensen GJ, Kent, BE: A preliminary report on the use of the McKenzie protocol versus Williams protocol in the treatment of low back pain, *J Orthop Sports Phys Ther* 6:130-139, 1984.

Shields CB, Williams PE Jr: Low back pain, *Am Fam Physician* 33(3):173-182, 1986.

Wheeler JH, Peterson JA: *Back pain relief,* Champaign, Ill, 1997, Sagamore Publishing.

18

Cervical Spine Disease

The grave implications of quadriparesis from spinal cord involvement, or the severe disability of an arm from nerve root damage, make it imperative that symptoms relating to the neck be thoroughly investigated. Otherwise, management of cervical spine disease usually consists of treating a "pain in the neck." However, this chapter is titled "Cervical Spine Disease" rather than "Neck Pain" because a number of conditions affecting the cervical spine may occur without any symptomatic neck pain. Cervical spine disease may be classified as follows:

1. With neurologic involvement:
   a. Acute spinal cord trauma
   b. Tumor
   c. Disc disease
   d. Spinal canal stenosis
   e. Infection
   f. Cervical spondylosis
2. Without neurologic involvement:
   a. Meningeal irritation
   b. Sprain, strain, or fracture
   c. Degenerative or inflammatory disease
   d. Lesion of the vertebrae
   e. "Tension" or emotional disturbances
   f. Cervical spondylosis

HISTORY

Patients with neck pain should be interviewed with particular attention to neurologic dysfunction. In most respects the same types of questions should be used to assess the patient with cervical spine disease as in the patient with low back pain (see Chapter 17). In addition, the following information may be specifically important in disease of the cervical spine:

1. As in other pain syndromes, information should be gathered through nonleading questions. For example, "What happens when you bend your head forward?" If the patient has shocklike feelings in the legs or arms on flexion or extension of the neck, Lhermitte's sign is present.

2. If the patient volunteers sensory or motor symptoms, obtain specifics as in low back pain.
3. Part of the examination must include careful observation of the patient during the history taking. Such observation often gives clues as to the extent of the disability. Particular attention should be paid to a patient's facial expression during head movements. (A patient who freely moves the head without evidence of pain during the history taking but complains of pain during examination is suspect.) Pay attention to the manner in which the patient changes position. (For example, the neck will be held stiffly during head movements in the patient with painful organic spine disease.)

EXAMINATION

1. Hyperactive tendon reflexes in the lower extremities (patellar and Achilles reflexes) combined with upgoing (extensor) plantar responses (Babinski's reflex) suggests spinal cord involvement.
2. Hyperactive tendon reflexes in the lower extremities and upgoing plantar responses, associated with hypoactive or absent reflexes in the upper extremities (biceps, triceps, or brachioradialis), localizes the lesion to the cervical spinal cord. This could occur with the following:
   a. An extrinsic lesion involving both nerve roots and spinal cord (extramedullary lesions as in meningioma or bony tumors)
   b. A lesion involving the central portion of the spinal cord (intramedullary lesions as in tumor or syringomyelia).
3. The presence of a sensory level indicates spinal cord involvement. This may be best demonstrated by instructing the patient to run his or her fingers up the trunk until the sensation changes (Fig. 18-1). In lesions of the central portion of the spinal cord, there is selective loss of pain and temperature sensations in the arms and trunk with sparing of the sacral region (Fig. 18-2).
4. Hyperactive tendon reflexes in all four extremities and upgoing plantar responses associated with a normal jaw reflex indicate high cervical cord disease.
5. Brown-Séquard syndrome indicates pathologic changes in the lateral half of the spinal cord (weakness, hyperreflexia, Babinski's reflex [extensor plantar response], and loss of position and vibration sensation in the lower extremity on one side, associated with a deficit in pinprick and temperature sensation in the other leg).
6. A diminished deep tendon reflex in one arm associated with a normal reflex in the other arm suggests unilateral nerve root involvement and is usually accompanied by other motor and sensory deficits in the distribution of that nerve root (Table 18-1).
7. Examination of the neck should be carried out with the patient in the sitting position with the hands folded in a relaxed position on the lap.
   a. Palpate the cervical and occipital muscles for spasms or masses.
   b. Palpate the posterior cervical triangle for masses or tenderness (Fig. 18-3).

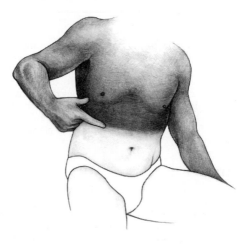

FIG. 18-1 The cooperative patient may be able to outline a sensory change with his own finger more accurately than an examiner with multiple pinpricks.

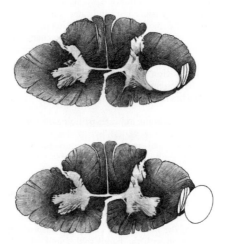

FIG. 18-2 In the spinothalamic tract, the sacral pain fibers are more lateral than cervical pain fibers; destructive lesions in the center of the cord may spare the sacral fibers and sacral sensation. An extrinsic lesion may damage the sacral fibers first and produce a sensory disturbance in the sacral area, as well as a bladder disturbance.

TABLE 18-1
Localizing Findings in Cervical Radiculopathy

Nerve root	Muscle involved	Motor weakness	Sensory loss	Reflex abnormality
C5	Deltoid	Shoulder abduction	Lateral upper arm	Biceps
	Supraspinatus	Shoulder abduction	Lateral upper arm	Biceps
C5, C6	Biceps	Elbow flexion	Thumb and index fingers	Biceps
C6	Extensor carpi radialis	Wrist extension		Brachioradialis
C7	Triceps	Elbow extension	Middle and index fingers	Triceps
	Flexor carpi radialis	Wrist flexion		
C8	Flexor digitorum	Finger flexion	Little and ring fingers	Finger flexor
T1	Interossei	Abduction and adduction of fingers	Medial forearm and medial upper arm	

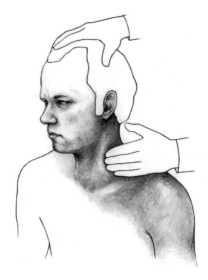

FIG. 18-3 Palpation posterior to the sternocleidomastoid muscle may reveal masses and tenderness of the roots or upper brachial plexus.

    c. Assess the bulk and strength of the sternocleidomastoid muscles.
    d. Palpate and percuss the spinous processes for abnormalities or tenderness.
    e. Determine the passive range of motion in flexion, extension, side bending, and rotation of the neck.
    f. Use the following maneuvers to reproduce radicular pain caused by nerve root compression:
        1) Hyperextend and tilt the patient's neck to the affected side and apply downward pressure over the vertex (Spurling's maneuver, Fig. 18-4); this may cause pain in the affected root. If it does not, strike the head lightly with your fist.
        2) A light blow to the top of the head with the neck in the normal position may also cause pain in the distribution of the affected root.

Caution: Do not perform these tests on patients with suspected cervical spine trauma or instability.

    g. Look for Lhermitte's sign. Flexion of the neck produces shock-like sensations down the back or arms and indicates probable meningeal or dorsal column abnormalities.

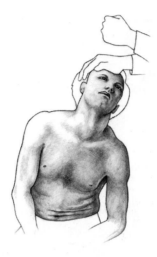

FIG. 18-4 Spurling's maneuver. Extension and tilting of the neck toward the affected arm may reproduce the pain by further compressing a nerve root in its exit from the foramen. Light percussion on the head may accentuate this phenomenon.

8. Horner's syndrome (ptosis, miosis, decreased sweating) may occur in diseases that affect the cervical cord or the T1 root.
9. Examination of sensation over the posterior part of the head can reveal sensory impairment from a lesion involving the second and third cervical roots (Fig. 18-5).
10. Hyperabduction and external rotation of the shoulder will obliterate the pulse in a thoracic outlet syndrome (see chapter 15) or cause severe pain in periarthritis of the shoulder (Fig. 18-6).

ACUTE SPINAL CORD TRAUMA

1. In a patient with acute cervical trauma, evaluation and management must be carried out simultaneously.

Caution: Until a thorough evaluation has been carried out, the neck must be immobilized as completely as possible with sandbags, a wrap-around collar, or head-halter traction, with the head and shoulders supported on a board.

2. Adequate suctioning, administration of oxygen, and the maintenance of a good airway are important if the patient has paralysis.

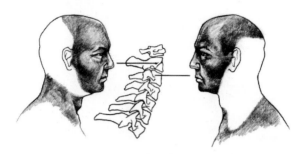

FIG. 18-5 A fracture of the upper cervical vertebrae may result in a sensory loss in the distribution of the C2 or C3 root. Failure to detect this sensory loss in upper cervical spine fractures may lead to dislocation of upper cervical vertebrae and severe quadriparesis or death. REMEMBER: The C1 root innervates the meninges and has no cutaneous representation, and the root of C2 exits above the vertebral body of C2.

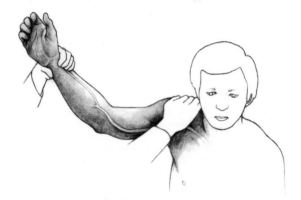

FIG. 18-6 Rotation of the shoulder posteriorly when the arm is held in the illustrated position, may obliterate the radial pulse at the wrist and be a clue to the thoracic outlet syndrome. As the shoulder is rotated posteriorly, the pulse should be obliterated in the affected arm before the normal arm.

Caution: Under no circumstances should the head be hyperextended for the insertion of an endotracheal tube. It is safer to do a tracheotomy if no other means of maintaining a good airway are possible.

3. Circulatory stability must be maintained, since acute cervical cord injury often results in peripheral vasodilation and shock. Volume expanders are usually not necessary; vasopressors are usually indicated (see Chapter 13).

4. An indwelling urinary catheter should be inserted to prevent over-distention of the bladder.

5. The level of spinal cord injury can be best evaluated by using a pin-prick to determine the sensory level, beginning in an anesthetic area and extending upward to the area where sensation is perceived. Do not forget to examine sensation in the arm and hand beginning with the lower dermatome in the axilla (T2) and ending with the higher dermatome over the deltoid (C4).

6. If there is no paralysis or cervical fracture, muscle function should be assessed by testing the ability of the patient to perform antigravity movements in the legs and by testing the strength of the elbow flexion and extension, wrist extension, grip, and finger extension.

7. Deep tendon reflexes should be tested. In the acute phase, these reflexes may be diminished or absent (spinal shock).

8. An accurate history of the details surrounding the injury should be obtained as soon as possible. The history is most reliable immediately after the injury.

9. The patient should be examined carefully for associated injuries, especially fractures of the long bones, rupture of abdominal organs, and injury to the chest or lungs.

Remember: The patient with paralysis and sensory loss may not be able to feel the pain of a broken bone or ruptured viscus below the level of the lesion.

10. Radiographic examination should be performed after the patient's vital functions have been stabilized.

   a. If the patient has paralysis from a cervical spine injury, a single, good lateral radiograph will usually reveal the pathologic changes. Adequate visualization of *all cervical vertebrae and the top of the first thoracic vertebra* requires that the shoulders be depressed by pulling the patient's arms toward the feet while taking the radiograph. If the radiographic findings are normal but a neurologic deficit is present, magnetic resonance imaging (MRI) or a computed tomographic (CT) myelogram is indicated.

   b. If the patient does not have paralysis or neurologic dysfunction, lateral views (as described before) and anterior-posterior (AP) cervical spine radiographs should be obtained. Views of the odontoid (through the mouth) are important to rule out a fracture through the base of the odontoid. If no fracture is demonstrated, oblique views, flexion-extension views, and occasionally, tomograms or a CT scan should be performed to evaluate suspicious areas.

Treatment:

1. For the patient with paralysis or severe spinal fracture, referral to an appropriate specialist is indicated.

Caution: The patient should always be transported with the neck immobilized, preferably in head-halter traction.

2. High-dose methylprednisolone should be started within 8 hours of the injury at a dose of 30 mg/kg intravenous (IV), followed by a continuous infusion of 5.4 mg/kg/hr for 23 hours.
3. The patient having cervical pain with no fractures or neurologic deficit probably has neck strain or sprain. Treat such a patient with the following methods:
   a. Bed rest with the patient lying flat with the neck flexed 30 degrees. Stretch the neck using head-halter traction with no more than 1.5 kg of weight.
   b. Treat the pain with medication on demand and a muscle relaxant around the clock (a combination of diazepam 2 to 5 mg, with aspirin 650 mg 3 times a day, may be effective).
   c. During the ambulatory phase, support the patient's neck with a soft, wraparound cervical collar.
   d. Remove the collar after 1 to 2 weeks and begin an intensive program of physical therapy consisting of heat, massage, and range-of-motion exercises to restore mobility to the cervical spine.

TUMOR

Tumors of the cervical spine can be primary bone or intraspinal tumors, or secondary tumors, such as multiple myeloma, lymphoma, or metastatic carcinoma. (Common primary sources include breast, prostate, lungs, and kidneys.) Spinal cord damage can occur either from compression by metastatic tumor in the epidural space (more commonly) or by direct invasion of spinal cord parenchyma.

▶ 1. *The most important diagnostic clue* of a patient with a tumor is a relentless progression of pain or neurologic deficit (as opposed to static or intermittent pain noted with other causes).
2. Initial symptoms may vary with the location of the tumor.
   a. A bone tumor (involving the vertebrae) usually presents with neck pain that progresses to radicular pain (pain in the arm).
   b. A neoplasm within the spinal canal may present with progressive motor or sensory deficits and radicular pain (pain extending into the arm) or Lhermitte's sign.
3. The examination may show the following:
   a. A stiffly held neck
   b. Palpable masses, commonly in the posterior triangle or over the paraspinal areas
   c. Areas of focal tenderness over the cervical spine
   d. Fasciculations and atrophy of the muscles of the upper extremities with hyperactive tendon reflexes in the lower extremities and Babinski's reflex, which suggests compression of the spinal cord by an extrinsic or intrinsic tumor (Table 18-2)
4. Cervical spine radiographic findings may be negative (with tumors growing in the spinal canal) or may show destruction (as a result of bony or metastatic tumors) or erosion (from pressure effects by intraspinal tumors).
5. MRI with contrast is mandatory in a patient with a suspected spinal tumor.

TABLE 18-2
Differential Diagnosis of Combination of Atrophy of Arm Muscles and Spasticity of Legs

Disorder	Age at onset	Diagnostic features	
		Clinical	Investigative
Spondylitic myelopathy	>50	Progressive spasticity and sensory ataxia with fasciculations restricted to one or two myotomes in the upper extremities	Spondylitic changes often with narrowing of foramina or spinal canal on plain radiographs, CT scan, MRI, or myelography
Amyotrophic lateral sclerosis (ALS)	>40	Generalized fasciculations (including bulbar muscles) with hyperactive tendon reflexes even in atrophic muscles and lack of sensory symptoms or signs	Normal radiographs, CT scan, MRI, or myelography
Cervical syringomyelia	<40	Dissociated sensory loss (absent pain and thermal sensation with intact touch) in the upper extremities and trunk with sacral sparing; fasciculations limited to a few myotomes of upper extremities	Widening of cord on myelogram and CT scan; best seen on MRI
Extramedullary tumor	Any age	Radicular pain and paresthesia, with loss of touch and pain below the level of compression	Typical appearance on myelogram; CT scan and MRI valuable

CT, Computed tomographic; *MRI,* magnetic resonance imaging.

6. A bone scan is often helpful in identifying abnormalities, especially when multiple metastatic lesions are suspected.

7. Primary neoplasms of the cervical spine have no characteristic laboratory abnormalities, but secondary neoplasms may exhibit laboratory findings of malignancy, such as anemia, an elevated erythrocyte sedimentation rate (ESR), elevation of serum alkaline or acid phosphatase levels, and monoclonal gammopathy.

Treatment:

1. Acute or subacute signs of spinal cord compression constitute a neurologic emergency. Immediate referral to an appropriate specialist is necessary if the diagnosis is suspected. A cerebrospinal fluid (CSF) sample should be obtained if contrast material is injected into the subarachnoid space.

Caution: If bone erosion is present, support the neck in a collar (preferably a Philadelphia hard collar).

2. Immediate management of spinal cord compression from metastatic lesion consists of dexamethasone 100 mg IV immediately, followed by 24 mg 4 times a day for 3 days, and then 20 mg for 3 days.

PROTRUDED CERVICAL DISC

▶ 1. *The most important diagnostic clue* that a patient has a protruded cervical disc is the patient frequently awakens with pain in the neck, followed within hours or days by the development of pain radiating in the distribution of the affected nerve root. (This is in contrast to a tumor in which there is a longer duration of cervical pain before radicular involvement.)

2. A protruded cervical disc may appear with a history of trauma.

3. The pain is usually aggravated when the patient assumes an upright position and is often relieved when the patient lies supine with the arm abducted at the shoulder.

4. Valsalva's maneuver often exacerbates the pain.

5. An examination may reveal the following:
   a. A limitation of the range of neck motion.
   b. A positive Spurling's maneuver.
   c. Neurologic deficits in the distribution of the affected nerve root. Approximately 80% of all ruptured cervical discs compress either the C6 or the C7 nerve root. The salient features are given in Table 18-1 and in Figs. 18-7 and 18-8.

FIG. 18-7 A C6 root lesion. The sensory disturbance is primarily over the thumb and the lateral aspect of the index finger (**A**); this sensory disturbance is most easily appreciated on the palmar surface of the hand. Decreased biceps and brachioradialis reflexes (**B**) and weak flexion of the elbow (**C**) and weak extension of the wrist (**D**) may also be present.

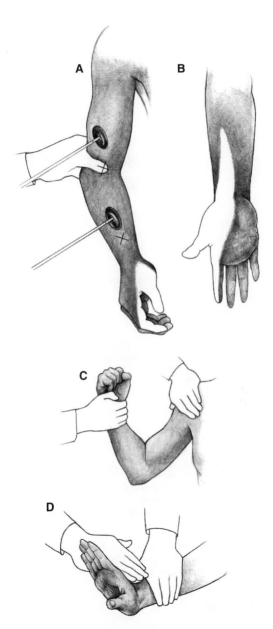

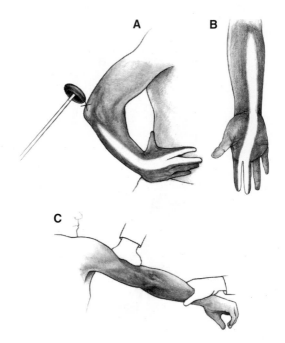

FIG. 18-8 A C7 root lesion. The sensory disturbance occurs in the index and middle fingers (**A**), and this is also most easily appreciated on the palmar surface of the hand. A decreased triceps reflex (**B**) and weak extension of the elbow (**C**) may also be present.

6. Cervical spine radiograph findings can show narrowing of the intervertebral disc space at the site of the disc protrusion. The oblique views, which should be done in all patients, may show encroachment on the intervertebral foramen.
7. MRI is valuable for demonstrating a narrowing of intervertebral foramen and disc protrusions.
8. Electromyography (EMG) provides additional objective evidence of denervation and identifies the root or roots that are affected.

Treatment:
1. Cervical traction is an effective treatment for a protruded cervical disc, with or without mild neurologic deficits.
   a. If the patient is in bed, the head should be in a head halter, and the neck should be flexed 30 degrees (Fig. 18-9).
   b. Traction should be applied continually. More than 1.5 kg of weight is often irritating to the jaw.

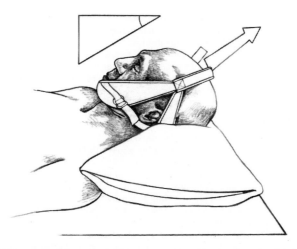

FIG. 18-9 Cervical traction in the supine position. The direction of pull is 30 degrees upward from the horizontal.

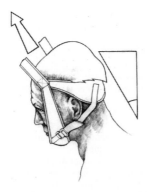

FIG. 18-10 Cervical traction in the sitting position. Note that the head is flexed 30 degrees and the direction of pull is 30 degrees from the vertical.

2. Once the patient's condition has improved, upright traction may be used intermittently. An over-the-door head-halter traction apparatus, using 5 to 7 kg of weight for 20 minutes 2 or 3 times daily (Fig. 18-10), is often effective. However, staring at a blank door does not promote compliance; we suggest modification of the over-the-door traction. (see Fig. 3-1).

3. High-dose aspirin (at least two 325-mg tablets every 4 hours) will usu-
    ally control pain and relieve inflammation. Other nonsteroidal anti-
    inflammatory drugs may be substituted.
4. For severe pain, a short course of corticosteroids (such as dexametha-
    sone in the Decadron Dose PAK) is often effective.
5. Persistent or progressive neurologic deficit indicates the need for neuro-
    surgical evaluation.

INFLAMMATION AND INFECTION

Inflammation and infection typically occur with rheumatoid arthritis or
spondylitis, hypertrophic osteoarthritis, gouty arthritis, a disc space infection, tuberculosis (TB), or Paget's disease.

▶ 1. *The most important diagnostic clue* is an insidious onset with exacer-
       bations and remissions, although an acute disc space infection
       may have a rapid onset with no remissions. The history of exacer-
       bations and remissions helps to differentiate chronic inflamma-
       tion from tumor.
   2. The patient with inflammation or infection experiences a feeling
       of general stiffness aggravated by movement and by maintenance
       of one position for a long period ("jelling effect"), such as after
       spending the night in bed; the pain may be worse in the late after-
       noon or evening, especially after an active day.
   3. Radicular symptoms are rare, but the pain may extend into the
       trapezius muscles.
   4. There may be a history of related pain in other joints.
   5. An examination shows the following:
       a. A stiffly held neck and evidence of pain on extremes of motion
           in all directions
       b. Normal reflexes, muscle strength, and sensation
   6. In the early phases, cervical spine radiographic findings may be
       normal. In the late stages, degeneration of the intervertebral discs
       and facet joints becomes apparent. In TB of the spine, there is of-
       ten a collapse of adjacent vertebrae.
   7. MRI of the cervical spine is the main diagnostic tool in inflam-
       matory disease of the spine.
   8. The ESR may be an important diagnostic clue; however, it is non-
       specific. A normal ESR does not exclude certain inflammatory
       processes, such as gouty arthritis and Paget's disease.
   9. Other valuable studies for inflammatory disease include a com-
       plete blood count (CBC), rheumatoid factor testing, antinuclear
       antibody studies, serum uric acid levels, serum calcium and serum
       alkaline phosphatase determinations, *Brucella* agglutination test-
       ing, and tuberculin skin testing.

Treatment:
1. Specific treatment for the underlying inflammatory process is
    necessary.
2. In acute disc space infection, immobilization of the cervical spine is
    mandatory. The patient should be in bed with a head-halter traction

until the infection has subsided, then placed in a halo brace or Philadelphia hard collar. In TB of the spine, apart from immobilization, appropriate antibiotic treatment is instituted. Surgical treatment is needed if there is spinal cord compression.

3. In inflammatory arthritis, physical therapy, such as diathermy and ultrasound; antiinflammatory drugs; and temporary immobilization with a soft cervical collar may relieve the pain.

STRUCTURAL BONY ABNORMALITIES

Structural bony abnormalities typically include degenerative arthritis, osteoporosis, facet asymmetry, nonunion of the odontoid, absence of bony structure, Klippel-Feil syndrome, and spinal canal stenosis (cervical spondylosis or cervical bars).

Cervical Spondylosis

Cervical spondylosis is a degenerative process involving the cervical spine that constitutes a common cause for cervical pain. The degenerative changes begin in the intervertebral space, leading to narrowing of the disc space and protrusion of the disc, with calcification and bar formation at multiple levels, most prominently at the C4 to C5, C5 to C6, and C6 to C7 levels. The clinical features are as follows:

▶ 1. *The most important diagnostic clue* of cervical spondylosis is the occurrence of chronic, nagging, centrally located cervical pain, which may radiate to the occipital areas, arms, or chest. The pain is least troublesome on rising from bed but increases with activity during the day. Recurrent episodes of neck pain, with limitation of neck movement, and bouts of upper extremity, infrascapular, or shoulder pain are characteristic.

2. The onset is usually after 50 years of age.

3. The symptoms are of a relatively long duration. (There may be a history of injury before the onset of symptoms.)

4. With spinal canal stenosis, the patient describes progressive weakness and wasting of the muscles of the arms, with a feeling of stiffness and difficulty in controlling movements of the legs.

5. Dizzy spells related to neck rotation may occur in patients in whom the degenerative changes encroach on the vertebral artery foramen.

6. Dysphagia may occur, with anterior bars compressing the esophagus.

7. Minor neck trauma may precipitate a major neurologic deficit in patients with cervical spondylosis, particularly when there is significant narrowing of the spinal canal.

8. Physical findings include the following:
   a. A cervical muscle spasm, loss of normal spinal curvature, and limitation of neck movement occur.
   b. When radiculopathy is the main feature, signs of nerve root compression are seen.

c. When there is an accompanying spinal cord involvement (spondylitic myelopathy) resulting from compression by bony bars or ischemia, the patient may show muscle atrophy, fasciculations, and decreased tendon reflexes in the upper extremities, with hyperreflexia, spasticity, and Babinski's reflex (extensor plantar responses) in the lower extremities. Myelopathy occurs more often when there is spinal canal stenosis. The differential diagnoses of spondylitic myelopathy include amyotrophic lateral sclerosis (ALS), syringomyelia, and extramedullary compression (Table 18-2).

9. Cervical spondylitic myelopathy mimics ALS, but with ALS, fasciculations and muscle atrophy are present in the tongue and legs.

10. Investigations:

   a. Radiographic testing of the cervical spine will reveal bars, narrowing of foramina, and the extent of the narrowing of the spinal canal.

   b. MRI clearly demonstrates spinal stenosis with spinal cord compression, nerve root entrapment, and osteophytes.

Treatment:

1. The treatment must at first be conservative except when progressive neurologic deficit occurs. Analgesics and muscle relaxants are given during the acute phase. A combination of aspirin (650 mg) and diazepam (5 mg) may be useful.

2. A hard cervical collar to limit neck movements may be helpful in the acute phase.

3. Surgical management (decompression of the roots and spinal cord) is indicated in patients with persistent radicular pain or increasing neurologic deficit.

MENINGEAL IRRITATION

Meningeal irritation typically occurs with hemorrhage, infection, or inflammation in the subarachnoid space.

1. The symptoms of cervical pain begin acutely or subacutely.

2. The pain is associated with a nonthrobbing occipital headache.

3. The patient complains of stiffness of the neck and a pulling sensation in the lower back with forward flexion of the neck.

4. An examination may show the following signs of meningeal irritation:

   a. An ill-appearing patient

   b. Hyperextension of the neck

   c. Guarding of the neck against forward flexion (Flexion increases the cervical pain and may produce pain between the scapulae.)

   d. No aggravation of pain with rotatory neck movements

   e. An elevated temperature

   f. Kernig's and Brudzinski's signs (see Chapter 14)

5. Patients with hemorrhage or infection in the subarachnoid space may show elevation of the peripheral white blood cell (WBC) count with a shift to the left.

6. Abnormal CSF often confirms the diagnosis. (Be sure to culture the CSF.)

Treatment:
1. Appropriate antibiotic therapy in the case of meningitis (see Chapter 14).
2. Treat subarachnoid hemorrhage appropriately. Neurosurgical consultation is indicated.

ENTRAPMENT OF THE GREATER OCCIPITAL NERVE

The C2 nerve root is wholly sensory and after exiting the intervertebral foramen, becomes the greater occipital nerve that innervates the scalp. Common causes of irritation of the greater occipital nerve (a muscle contraction or tension headache) include cervical muscle spasm from emotional stress and work-related circumstances (such as a secretary holding the head in a fixed position while working at a computer for a prolonged period), whiplash injuries, and osteoarthritis.
1. The pain radiates to the sternocleidomastoid muscles, the occiput, and over the top of the forehead. The patient may complain of a tender scalp or "painful hair."
2. Because the condition is chronic and responds poorly to treatment, the patient often is anxious or despondent.
3. An examination may show the following signs of irritation:
   a. Tense and tender paracervical and trapezius muscles
   b. A resistance to passive movement of the neck in all directions
   c. Tenderness to percussion in the high cervical area
   d. An altered sensation in the scalp

Caution: Do not be misled by nonspecific laboratory and radiographic findings. Cervical spine films in most patients over 40 years of age show some degenerative changes.

Treatment:
1. Gabapentin (Neurontin), 400 mg in the evening is often sufficient to relieve muscle spasm and pain; it may be titrated up to 2400 mg per day, but this is rarely necessary. The addition of nonsteroid anti-inflammatory drugs (we recommend indomethacin [Indocin] 25 mg 2 or 3 times a day, cost: 30 25-mg capsules $19.29) is also recommended.
2. If the aforementioned medications are not effective, cervical traction and heat and massage to the back of the neck should be added. (See page 321 for home traction.)
3. An injection of corticosteroids and anesthetics into the occipital nerve provides weeks of relief.
4. Simple measures, such as courses in stress reduction, altering the placement of the computer at regular intervals, and heat and massage to the cervical area, often make the symptoms tolerable.

BIBLIOGRAPHY

Bracken MB, Shepard MJ, Collins WF et al: A randomized controlled trial of methylprednisolone or naloxone in the treatment of acute spinal cord injury: results of the Second National Acute Spinal Cord Injury Study, *N Engl J Med* 322:1405-1411, 1990.

Shafaie FF, Wippold FJ, Gado M et al: Comparison of computed tomography myelopathy and magnetic resonance imaging in the evaluation of cervical spondylotic myelopathy and radiculopathy, *Spine* 24(17):1781-1785, 1999.

Walker MD: Acute spinal cord injury, *N Engl J Med* 324(26):1885-1887, 1991.

Wheeler JH, Peterson JA: *Back pain relief*, Champaign, Ill, 1997, Sagamore Publishing.

19

The Patient with
a Head Injury

Head trauma is the most common cause of brain damage in young adults and the leading cause of death in patients under 24 years of age. Some of this damage is avoidable if prompt management is undertaken soon after the injury. However, many physicians feel apprehensive and insecure in managing the unconscious head-injured patient. This chapter outlines the initial evaluation and treatment that should be carried out before the patient is transferred to a tertiary care center.

Remember: Evaluation and management of the patient must be carried out simultaneously.

ACUTE MANAGEMENT OF THE HEAD-INJURED PATIENT

After a head injury, the patient may arrive in the emergency department in an alert state or in a state of coma. The alert patient will need only a computed tomographic (CT) scan and careful observation, whereas the comatose patient will require urgent measures.

1. Initial management

Caution: Potentially reversible lesions may become permanent deficits secondary to hypoxia and hypotension.

   a. Stabilizing vital functions
      1) A good airway and adequate blood oxygenation must be maintained.
         a) Insert an oropharyngeal airway; suction the airway adequately to remove secretions. Insert an endotracheal tube if the patient is comatose. It is important to do this procedure rapidly and without causing any distress, since even short periods of hypoxia and hypercarbia may increase the brain edema and initiate herniation. A tracheostomy is needed urgently only in cases of severe maxillofacial and neck injuries.

    b) In the patient with respiratory distress (for whatever reason), administer oxygen in high concentration.

Note: Prompt endotracheal intubation and hyperventilation sufficient to drop partial pressure of carbon dioxide ($PaCO_2$) to less than 28 mm Hg may have contributed to a decrease in the morbidity and mortality rate after head injury.

    2) Circulatory stability must be maintained.

Note: Head trauma does not directly cause hypotension but may cause bradycardia and hypertension (Cushing's reflex).

    a) Intravenous (IV) fluids should be held to a minimum in patients with cerebral edema or possible brain herniation.
    b) The patient with low blood pressure and rapid pulse may have reduced circulating blood volume (blood loss). The source of hemorrhage may not be apparent, since the comatose patient cannot complain of pain or exhibit typical signs of bleeding (e.g., rigidity of abdominal wall with intraperitoneal hemorrhage). An IV line must be established and treatment aimed at maintaining adequate cerebral circulation by replacing blood loss and administering vasoconstrictors. A hemogram and type and crossmatch should be obtained as soon as possible. The partial pressures of oxygen (PaO_2) and the $PaCO_2$ should be carefully monitored.
2. Immediate management
    a. Once the vital functions are stabilized, there must be an ongoing determination of the level of consciousness and neurologic function (see Chapter 13) by determining the following signs:
       1) The most important criterion in the initial evaluation and follow-up of patients with head injury is the level of consciousness. The Glasgow Coma Scale (based on eye opening, best motor response, and verbal response; Table 19-1) is simple enough for repeated recording by nurses, paramedical personnel, or physicians and has been shown to provide a reliable indication of prognosis. In one study, 87% of patients with a score of more than 11 in the first 24 hours had good recovery, whereas 87% of those with scores of less than 5 remained in a vegetative state or were brain-dead.
       2) Pupillary size and reaction to light are highly useful in detecting impending herniation. With uncal herniation through the tentorial notch, the ipsilateral pupil dilates and becomes poorly reactive to light, followed by similar changes in the contralateral pupil. In a large study, 50% of patients with intact pupillary reaction made good recovery whereas 91% with nonreactive pupils (in the first 24 hours after coma) died or remained in a vegetative state.
       3) Any focal deficit, as evidenced by asymmetry of tendon reflexes or plantar responses or movements in response to painful stim-

TABLE 19-1
Glasgow Coma Scale
(Circle the Appropriate Number and Compute the Total)*

EYES OPEN	
Never	1
To pain	2
To verbal stimuli	3
Spontaneously	4
BEST VERBAL RESPONSE	
No response	1
Incomprehensible sounds	2
Inappropriate words	3
Disoriented and converses	4
Oriented and converses	5
BEST MOTOR RESPONSE	
No response	1
Extension (decerebrate rigidity)	2
Flexion abnormal (decorticate rigidity)	3
Flexion withdrawal	4
Localizes pain	5
Obeys	6
TOTAL (RANGE)	3-15

*The sum of the highest value in each category is the coma score: full mental capacity, 15; highest level of coma, 8; brain death, 3.

ulation, can help determine the level of consciousness and neurologic function.

b. An indwelling urinary catheter should be inserted to obtain a urine specimen for analysis, evaluate urinary output, and avoid overdistention of the bladder.

c. A nasogastric tube attached to suction should be inserted to prevent abdominal distention and vomiting.

d. Hyperthermia should be treated by placing the patient on a cooling blanket or by applying ice water and alcohol to the skin.

e. Seizures should be controlled with IV anticonvulsants (see Chapter 11).

f. Extreme restlessness may be treated with lorazepam (Ativan) 1 to 5 mg every 2 hours.

Caution: The most important clinical criterion in a comatose patient is the level of consciousness; it is not possible to assess the level properly if sedatives are administered to the patient. Hence, never use morphine, and give sedatives only sparingly to a patient with head injury.

g. Associated injuries should be rapidly appraised to identify intrathoracic or intraabdominal hemorrhage, fractures, or lacerations with excessive blood loss. Appropriate management of such problems must be instituted immediately.

h. It is not sufficient to assume that the unconsciousness has resulted solely from the head injury. It may be the result of shock, alcohol or drug intoxication, adrenal insufficiency, stroke, diabetic acidosis, insulin shock, or other metabolic disturbances (see Chapter 13). The relevant blood studies must be done.

i. Elevating the patient's head by 30 degrees can aid in reducing intracranial pressure.

j. As soon as the vital signs are stable, all patients with severe head injury should undergo a CT scan of the head and radiographs of the skull. (NOTE: Fractures clearly evident on one study may not be readily apparent on the other.) Radiographs of the spine, chest, abdomen, and other areas should be done depending on the clinical presentation. In a comatose patient, fractures of the extremities or pelvis can be easily missed, since the patient will not complain of pain.

Caution: Always suspect a cervical spine injury until findings of lateral cervical spine radiographs exclude it (see Chapter 18).

k. A description of the nature and mechanism of the injury from any available sources of information should be obtained. Appropriate consultations with neurosurgery, general surgery, cardiopulmonary surgery, or orthopedic surgery staff should be requested as the need for specialized care is identified. Transfer to a specialized center may be necessary.

3. Complete neurologic examination: when the patient's condition has been stabilized, a more complete neurologic examination should be performed (see Chapter 13). The examination should include the following:

a. State of consciousness.

b. Respirations. Slow, deep, or irregular respirations suggest serious intracranial abnormalities, whereas shallow, rapid respirations are more commonly associated with pathologic changes extrinsic to the nervous system, such as shock related to blood loss.

c. The degree of paresis of extremities. Early complete, flaccid paralysis occurring unilaterally suggests marked damage to the opposite cerebral hemisphere, whereas spasticity of all four extremities suggests severe brainstem or cervical spinal cord injury.

d. Peripheral cranial nerve palsies. The presence of peripheral cranial nerve palsies suggests a basilar skull fracture.

e. Spinal fluid drainage. Spinal fluid draining from the ear or nose is diagnostic of a skull fracture.

Caution: Basilar skull fractures may be missed on routing CT scans or skull radiographs.

CLASSIFICATION AND MANAGEMENT OF CRANIAL INJURY

(See Table 19-2.)

Injuries to the Scalp

1. Abrasions to the scalp should be treated by careful cleansing with soap and sterile water; the hair need not be removed. Particles embedded in the scalp should be removed with a surgical brush to avoid the tattoo effect of retained particles. The area may be left either exposed to the air or covered with a sterile, nonadherent dressing.
2. Contusions (bruises) may be treated by cold compresses.
3. Lacerations should be closed by suturing after the hair has been shaved from around the area and the area has been carefully cleansed. If a laceration extends through the galea, it is desirable to close the galea with absorbable suture *separately* from the closure of the skin.
4. Avulsions constitute a serious problem, and in all cases, the avulsed scalp should be preserved in normal saline. Microvascular surgical anastomoses of the vessels to restore circulation to the avulsed tissue is necessary.

Injuries to the Skull

1. Linear skull fractures (particularly if they occur in the base of the skull) are often difficult to identify on routine skull radiographs and may be

TABLE 19-2
Risk Groups of Patients with Head Trauma

Risk group	Clinical features
Low	Asymptomatic
	Dizziness
	Headache
	Scalp hematoma, laceration, contusion, or abrasion
	No moderate- or high-risk criteria
Moderate	Alteration in level of consciousness either at time of injury or later
	Amnesia
	Basilar skull fracture
	Drug abuse or alcohol intoxication
	Multiple trauma or facial injuries
	Possible depressed or compound skull fracture
	Posttraumatic seizure or vomiting
	Progressive headache
	Unreliable or inadequate history of injury
High	Depressed or compound skull fracture
	Focal neurologic signs
	Stupor or coma (not caused by alcohol, drugs, metabolic disorder, or seizures)

confused with vascular markings or suture lines. Skull fractures should be suspected when there is:

- a. Blood behind the eardrum or Battle's sign (black-and-blue discoloration over the mastoid) suggests a basilar skull fracture.
- b. Raccoon eyes (ecchymoses around the eyelids) suggest a frontal skull fracture.

2. Stereoscopic radiographs of the skull are the most helpful studies for evaluating linear skull fractures. Obtaining skull films in minor head trauma may not be necessary, but remember that skull fractures can occur without loss of consciousness. A patient with a skull fracture that crosses a venous sinus or a branch of a meningeal artery should be hospitalized and observed with hourly cranial checks for 24 hours (see Chapter 12).
3. A patient with a compound comminuted skull fracture should be treated with debridement and neurosurgical reconstruction.
4. A patient with depressed skull fractures should be treated with surgical elevation.

Injuries to the Dura and Leptomeninges

1. Injuries to the dura and leptomeninges are usually associated with a skull fracture.
2. An injury to the dura and leptomeninges over the paranasal sinuses or mastoid allows admission of air and infection to the intracranial contents and the escape of cerebrospinal fluid (CSF). Unless contraindicated for other reasons, patients with CSF leakage should be placed in a position with the head elevated at a 45-degree angle. This minimizes retrograde infection into the cranial cavity and encourages tamponade of the brain into the fistula tract. Prophylactic use of a broad-spectrum antibiotic in a therapeutic dose should be considered. Watch for signs of meningitis (see Chapter 14). The patient should be instructed to avoid blowing the nose. Neurosurgical consultation is advisable.
3. The following types of intracranial hemorrhage may occur in skull fractures with meningeal involvement from injury to the blood vessels:
   - a. *Extradural (epidural) hematoma:* the bleeding usually results from damage to a dural artery, most commonly the middle meningeal artery.
     1) Progressive drowsiness may follow a lucid interval, or the patient may remain unconscious from the time of the initial trauma.
     2) Progressive headache may be a symptom.
     3) A dilating pupil on the side of the hemorrhage is highly suggestive of extradural hemorrhage (resulting from herniation).
     4) A hemiparesis opposite the side of the hemorrhage may be present.
     5) A focal motor seizure in the extremities opposite the side of the hemorrhage may occur.
     6) A slowing of the pulse and respirations and an increase in blood pressure are late and ominous signs. Progressive hemiparesis occurring on the same side as the dilated pupils suggests brainstem involvement and indicates a grave prognosis.

Caution: This condition represents one of the most acute of all emergencies. Prompt neurosurgical evacuation of the clot usually results in complete functional recovery; delayed intervention results in permanent brain damage or death. If a diagnosis is suspected, immediate neurosurgical consultation is indicated. The diagnosis can be confirmed by a CT scan or magnetic resonance imaging (MRI).

   b. *Acute subdural hematoma:* the hematoma usually results from damage to the venous sinuses or to the veins communicating between the cortex and the venous sinuses. Patients may experience a variety of neurologic findings, such as seizures, progressive deepening coma, progressive headache, progressive hemiparesis, a confusional state, and signs of increased intracranial pressure.

Caution: Although the progressive deterioration in the patient with acute subdural hematoma is not usually as rapid as that in extradural hematoma, prompt neurosurgical treatment is still necessary. As with extradural hematoma, the diagnosis can be confirmed by CT or MR findings.

Injuries to the Brain

1. *Cerebral concussion* may be defined as a temporary impairment of cerebral neuronal function caused by a blow to the head. The concussion can be divided into the following categories:
   a. Mild concussion–impaired neurologic function lasting less than 5 minutes
   b. Moderate concussion–impaired neurologic function lasting more than 5 minutes but less than 3 hours, often with mild retrograde amnesia
   c. Severe concussion–impaired neurologic function lasting more than 3 hours, with retrograde and anterograde amnesia

There are no demonstrable structural abnormalities in cerebral concussion. Patients with concussion recover completely, although sometimes a postconcussional syndrome consisting of headache, dizziness, and personality changes may occur.

Treatment:

1. The patient with either a mild or moderate cerebral concussion can be managed at home if someone is ready to observe the patient's responsiveness, pupillary size, and ability to move the extremities on an hourly basis for 24 hours.
2. If the patient is hospitalized, hourly evaluation of the level of consciousness and pupillary reactions should be performed (see Chapter 12).
3. Treatment requires sports limitations. After a mild concussion, the patient should not return to the game. After a moderate concussion, the patient should play no contact sports for at least 2 weeks. After a severe concussion, the patient should play no contact sports for at least 1 month.

2. *Cerebral contusion* is an impairment of neuronal function resulting from structural damage ("bruised brain"). Focal contusions occur

under the site of impact or, more often, in the undersurface of the frontal or the anterior part of the temporal lobes, from impact against the lesser wing of the sphenoid. (The lesser wing of the sphenoid has been called the *dashboard* of the cranial cavity.) Clinical findings include focal neurologic abnormalities and loss of consciousness.

Treatment: The patient should be hospitalized with at least hourly neurologic evaluations (see Chapter 12) during the acute phase. Supportive care should be provided based on the degree of neurologic impairment.

Note: For medical, legal, and prognostic purposes, concussion and contusion may be differentiated by a CT scan or MRI and serial electroencephalograms (EEGs). In the case of a cerebral concussion, the EEGs show only temporary changes, whereas in the case of cerebral contusion, they show persistent abnormalities. A CT scan or MRI usually shows blood at the site of a cerebral contusion, but is normal with a concussion.

3. *Cerebral lacerations* are secondary to depressed skull fractures or penetrating wounds.

Treatment: Lacerations require immediate (within 6 hours) neurosurgical treatment. Emergency management should include control of the hemorrhage from the scalp at the site of the injury and application of a sterile dressing. Accompanying scalp lacerations should not be sutured until after neurosurgical reconstruction has been performed.

4. *Traumatic subarachnoid hemorrhage* should be suspected when the patient has a headache and stiff neck, with or without other neurologic signs. Subarachnoid hemorrhage may also be present in the patient with coma and a stiff neck. The diagnosis can be confirmed by the findings of a CT scan or MRI.

Treatment: Support of vital functions, elevation of the head to approximately 30 degrees, and careful observation with at least hourly neurologic evaluations (see Chapter 12) are required. An LP should be deferred for 72 hours or longer if the patient is unstable. Symptomatic improvement may be obtained by the removal of bloody CSF using repeated LPs. The CSF will be xanthochromic and under elevated pressure. The amount of fluid removed should be only the volume necessary to reduce the CSF pressure to one half of the initial reading.

5. *Traumatic intracerebral hematoma* is suggested by increased intracranial pressure, progressive focal neurologic deficits, and a deteriorating state of consciousness. The presence of blood can be readily demonstrated by a CT scan or MRI. Neurosurgical consultation is indicated.

COMMON COMPLICATIONS
Increased Intracranial Pressure

Increased intracranial pressure after head trauma is common. It may be caused by an airway obstruction with accompanying hypoxia and hypercarbia or an intracranial hematoma. Sometimes, no specific cause is demonstrable on a CT scan or an MR image. Edema of the brain after an injury may account for the increased pressure.

Treatment: Increased intracranial pressure has a deleterious effect on the outcome, and prompt treatment should be undertaken, depending on the cause. It is common practice to monitor the intracranial pressure using an epidural, subdural, or intraventricular pressure monitor. Such procedures can be done only in a neurosurgical unit. The measures used in such centers include the following:

1. Hyperventilation: Hyperventilation is an effective way of rapidly reducing intracranial pressure. The ventilatory rate should be adjusted so that the $PaCO_2$ is less than 28 mm Hg. The effect achieved on intracranial pressure is by reduced intracranial blood volume and perhaps by decreased CSF formation.

Caution: Lowering the $PaCO_2$ below 25 mm Hg may result in areas of cerebral ischemia.

2. Infusion of hyperosmolar agents, such as 20% mannitol: Use only after neurosurgical consultation, unless the patient happens to be in a state of impending herniation.
3. Corticosteroids: There is no uniformity of opinion as to the efficacy of corticosteroids in posttraumatic cerebral edema.
4. Induction of barbiturate coma: In children with posttraumatic cerebral edema (with no surgically treatable cause), the induction of a barbiturate coma is undertaken in some centers.

Posttraumatic Epilepsy
Whereas seizures may occur early in the course of a head injury, late posttraumatic epilepsy is one of the most frequent delayed complications. It occurs in approximately 5% of all patients admitted to hospitals after nonmissile head injury. The risk of epilepsy is higher when there has been intracranial hematoma, a compound depressed skull fracture, or an early seizure (in the first week after injury). The onset is most common during the first 2 years, although it has been reported even after 10 years.
Treatment: See Chapter 11.

Postconcussional Syndrome
1. After head trauma, 30% to 80% of patients have been reported to develop one or more of the following symptoms:
   a. Chronic, posttraumatic headache: a constant, dull, nonthrobbing headache often described as a tight band around the head, sometimes associated with a local area of tenderness or pain, especially if a scar is present. (Rarely, intermittent throbbing headaches may also occur.) The headache may last for several weeks to months or sometimes years.
   b. Dizziness, either intermittent or chronic (see Chapter 4).
   c. Amnesia, poor concentration, and learning difficulties in children.
   d. Emotional lability: irritability, aggressiveness, and hyperkinesis.
2. The syndrome may occur after open and closed head trauma and is thought to be a result of diffuse axonal injury. There is no consistent

correlation with the duration of unconsciousness, posttraumatic amnesia, skull fracture, or blood in the CSF.
3. Preexisting psychiatric problems (e.g., depression) and pending litigation are believed to be predisposing factors.
4. A migraine may be triggered by a minor head injury. A mild, closed head injury may trigger the onset of migraine headaches in migraine-prone patients. These must be distinguished from headaches of the postconcussion syndrome.

Treatment: Amitriptyline hydrochloride, 50 to 100 mg daily over several weeks to months, has been found to be effective, especially for the chronic posttraumatic headache. Reassure the patient and, if necessary, institute psychotherapy.

BIBLIOGRAPHY

Cantu RC: Guidelines for return to contact sports after a cerebral concussion, *Physician Sports Med* 14:75-83, 1986.

Changaris DG, McGraw CP, Richardson JD et al: Correlation of cerebral perfusion pressure and Glasgow Coma Scale to outcome, *J Trauma* 27(9):1007-1013, 1987.

Jennett B, Teasdale G: *Management of head injuries,* Philadelphia, 1981, FA Davis.

Krych D, Ashley MJ, Persel CH, Persel CS: *Working with behavior disorders: strategies for traumatic brain injury rehabilitation,* San Antonio, Texas, 1999, Psychological Corp.

Langer KG, Laatsch L, Lewis L, editors: *Psychotherapeutic interventions for adults with brain injury or stroke: a clinician's treatment resource,* Madison, Conn, 1999, Psychosocial Press.

Masters SJ, McClean PM, Arcarese MS et al: Skull x-ray examinations after head trauma: recommendations by a multidisciplinary panel and validation study, *N Engl J Med* 316(2):84-91, 1987.

Muizelaar JR, Marmarou A, Ward JD et al: Adverse effects of prolonged hyperventilation in patients with severe head injury: a randomized clinical trial, *J Neurosurg* 75(5):731-739, 1991.

Raymond MJ, editor: *Mild brain injury: a clinician's guide,* Austin, Texas, 1999, Pro-Ed.

Vogel HB: *Trauma of the head, spine and peripheral nerves.* In Earnest MP, editor: *Neurologic emergencies,* New York, 1983, Churchill Livingstone.

White RJ, Likavec MJ: The diagnosis and initial management of head injury, *N Eng J Med* 327(21):1507-1511, 1992.

WEBSITES

Brain Injury Association: www.biausa.org
Neurorehabilitation links: www.neurorehab.com/links1.html

20

Neurologic Emergencies

T he word *emergency* is used to mean those conditions which, if not treated immediately, may result in death or permanent nervous system damage. There are conditions, such as the excruciating pain of trigeminal neuralgia, that may require immediate treatment but are not included in this chapter, because lack of treatment will not result in permanent damage. What is *neurologic* is also open to discussion. Delirium tremens, the threat of suicide, and acute glaucoma are ordinarily not considered neurologic problems, although clearly they are emergencies and, if untreated, may lead to permanent nervous system damage. Table 20-1 lists neurologic conditions that we consider emergencies, along with a brief statement of why. The remainder of this chapter is devoted to an evaluation of the symptoms we consider emergencies.

COMA

See Chapter 13 for examination, differential diagnosis, and management of coma.

Immediate measures of all comatose patients include the following:
1. Determine the need for cardiopulmonary resuscitation (CPR).
2. Stabilize the patient, using the following steps:
   a. Establish and maintain a clear airway and provide ventilatory assistance, if necessary.
   b. Establish access to the circulation with an intravenous (IV) line, drawing blood samples at the same time for hematology and biochemistry tests.
   c. Maintain the blood pressure by elevating the legs and administering volume expanders (blood or plasma, normal saline, or lactated Ringer's solution).
   d. Administer:
      1) IV thiamine at least 100 mg
      2) IV glucose 1 amp D-50 (50% dextrose solution)
      3) IV naloxone (Narcan) 0.4 mg/2 min

TABLE 20-1
Neurologic Conditions Considered to be Emergencies

Process	Reason for emergency
Coma	Many causes of coma, such as a drug overdose, hypoglycemia, or an expanding cerebral mass, may cause irreversible brain damage if not treated immediately.
Transient ischemic attacks	The cause of attacks may be treatable (e.g., embolus); if untreated, permanent brain damage may occur.
Stroke	The cause of paralysis could be reversible, such as a subdural hematoma, instead of the overused diagnosis of intracerebral atherosclerosis.
Bacterial meningitis	A delayed treatment of bacterial meningitis results in irreversible brain damage or death.
Spinal cord compression	Unless pressure on the spinal cord is relieved within a few hours, permanent paralysis will result.
Status epilepticus	Prolonged seizures may result in brain damage or death.
Fracture of the spinal column	Inappropriate movement of the patient may permanently sever the spinal cord.
Thiamine deficiency	Delayed treatment of a thiamine deficiency results in an irreversible organic brain syndrome.
Temporal arteritis	Temporal arteritis may spread to intracranial arteries and cause cerebral infarction or blindness.
Severe muscle spasms	Spasms are usually caused by severe hypoglycemia or tetanus, both of which are treatable.
Myasthenia gravis	Respiratory failure in a crisis may occur suddenly and without warning.
Guillain-Barré syndrome	Respiratory failure may occur suddenly without warning in a patient who is not severely weak.

   e. Administer glucose (after blood has been drawn for a glucose determination) in the form of 25 g in a 50% glucose solution.
3. Determine the cause of the coma.

STATUS EPILEPTICUS

Convulsive status epilepticus is a medical emergency because of the respiratory compromise and subsequent hypoxic brain damage that may occur. Nonconvulsive status epilepticus should be terminated in a timely manner, but it is not as dangerous as convulsive status epilepticus because no respiratory compromise occurs. See Chapter 11 for management.

HEAD TRAUMA

See Chapter 19 for management.

FRACTURE OF THE SPINAL COLUMN AND SPINAL CORD COMPRESSION

A cervical spine fracture must be suspected after any head and neck trauma from falling, being thrown from a car, or receiving a blow to the neck. If a patient is also comatose, a cervical spine fracture must be ruled out by lateral cervical spine radiographs *before* undue manipulation of the neck occurs. If there is a neurologic deficit and plain radiographs are normal, a computed tomographic (CT) scan of the spinal column and cord or myelogram is indicated. For management, see Chapter 18.

Symptoms of spinal cord emergencies include acute paralysis of the legs and varying involvement of the trunk and upper extremities, depending on the level of the compression or injury. There is a sudden and rapidly progressive onset of sensory or motor loss, or both, of function in the trunk and extremities below the level of the lesion.

Remember: If decompression laminectomy can be performed or radiation therapy initiated (for malignancy) before all neurologic function (below the level of the lesion) has been lost, complete recovery of function is possible. High-dose IV corticosteroids initiated immediately (within 8 hours) may produce improvement. (See Chapter 17 for management.) High-dose IV methylprednisolone is the recommended treatment for traumatic myelopathy (30 mg/kg, 5.4 mg/kg/hr for 23 hours).

If pain occurs, it is often radicular from involvement of the sensory spinal nerves at the level of the spinal cord lesion; pain seldom involves the trunk or extremities below the level of the lesion.

The cause of spinal cord emergencies include the following:
1. A sudden compression of the spinal cord during trauma, usually secondary to a compression fracture or fracture-dislocation of the spine
2. Pathologic fractures of the spinal column (These are usually due to infection, neoplasia, and osteoporosis.)
3. A protruding intervertebral disc
4. Ischemia or infarction of the spinal cord from one of the following:
   a. Aortic dissection occlusive disease
   b. Progressive compression by a neoplasm, primary or metastatic, intraaxial or extraaxial
   c. Thrombosis of the anterior spinal artery
5. Spontaneous hemorrhage into the spinal cord from a vascular malformation
6. An acute or subacute infection (subdural empyema) or inflammation of the spinal cord (transverse myelitis)

Clinical Findings:
1. Clinical findings include motor weakness, hyperactive reflexes, and upgoing plantar responses in the lower extremities. The upper extrem-

ities are involved in cervical myelopathies. In acute spinal cord damage, there is often a temporary flaccid paralysis with absent deep tendon reflexes in the lower extremities from "spinal shock."

2. A sensory level is an important clue to spinal cord involvement.
   a. Begin sensory testing in an anesthetic area and work toward an area of normal sensation. (Usually a pin is used for testing.)
   b. Test for sensory level on the back, as well as on the chest and abdomen.
   c. With a high thoracic or cervical lesion, examine sensation in the arms and hands, beginning with the lower dermatome in the axilla (T2) and ending with the higher dermatome over the deltoid (C4).

3. Beevor's sign can help determine a motor level over the trunk, particularly the abdomen. Place your index finger at the level of the umbilicus and ask the patient, who is lying flat, to look at the finger. If the umbilicus moves up, the level of the lesion is at T10 or below; the normally strong upper abdominal muscles will contract, whereas the lower abdominal muscles (below the umbilicus, or T10) will not, pulling the umbilicus up toward the head.

4. Sphincter disturbance commonly occurs with spinal cord compression.

5. Spinal cord involvement localized to one half of the spinal cord will result in a Brown-Séquard syndrome.
   a. The leg on the same side will show weakness, hyperreflexia, Babinski's reflex, and loss of sensation to position and vibration.
   b. The opposite leg will show a deficit to pinprick.

6. A central cord injury of the cervical spinal cord may result in a flaccid paralysis of the muscles of the arms with absent deep tendon reflexes in the arms (caused by damage involving the anterior horn cells) and hyperactive reflexes with a Babinski reflex's in the lower extremities (caused by damage involving the corticospinal tract). This is seen in syringomyelia and intramedullary tumors.

Management:

1. In the patient with acute spinal column trauma associated with spinal cord injury, the spinal column must be kept immobile (see Chapter 17). These same principles should also be followed in cases showing acute involvement of the spinal cord from other lesions.

2. Administration of high-dose IV corticosteroids (methylprednisolone) has been shown to be beneficial if instituted within 8 hours of the acute spinal cord injury.

3. Adequate blood pressure must be maintained, since acute spinal cord damage often results in peripheral vasodilation and shock.
   a. Consider leg elevation and the administration of peripheral vasoconstrictive agents.

4. An indwelling catheter should be in place as soon as practicable to prevent overdistention of the bladder.

5. If respiratory insufficiency is present, consider the following:
   a. Suctioning and the administration of oxygen
   b. Intubation with a soft-cuff endotracheal tube or tracheostomy

6. Patients with acute spinal cord compression must be referred for urgent neurosurgical evaluation.

TRANSIENT ISCHEMIC ATTACKS (see Chapter 12)

Transient ischemic attacks (TIAs) are episodes of temporary central nervous system (CNS) dysfunction, usually lasting minutes, but always lasting less than 24 hours. Approximately 28% of patients with TIAs develop stroke within 5 years. The attacks are not necessarily ischemic, since small emboli or lacunar infarcts may resolve quickly.

Caveat: Transient dysfunction today could be a permanent dysfunction tomorrow. Many of the causes are treatable.

1. TIAs:
   a. Ischemic, including emboli from carotid disease of the heart
   b. Vascular malformation
2. Other causes of transient neurologic dysfunction:
   a. Metabolic
      1) Hypoglycemia or hyperglycemia
      2) Hypothyroidism
   b. Migraine

Treatment: Adequate treatment depends on an adequate diagnosis, and this almost invariably includes the following:

1. An immediate CT scan to rule out hemorrhage
2. Magnetic resonance imaging (MRI) of the brain to identify ischemic brain and timing of stroke
3. Doppler scan of the carotid arteries to aid in identifying carotid stenosis
4. Four-vessel cerebral angiography, which is the definitive diagnostic test for arteritis, emboli, and aneurysms, and, especially small vessel disease

Caution: Not all transient dysfunctions are "ischemic." Anticoagulation of the blood of the patient whose transient dysfunction was bleeding could be disastrous. A CT scan should be done before a decision is made to anticoagulate or initiate antiplatelet agents.

STROKE IN PROGRESSION

Stroke progression may be caused by decreased perfusion of the tissue at risk or increased edema from damaged tissue. The only way to be certain of the diagnosis of stroke in progression is to actually observe the patient's condition deteriorating over time. Since deterioration may be stuttering in temporal profile, this is difficult to judge. If the neurologic deficit is progressive, it is imperative to determine first whether bleeding is occurring, such as in hypertensive hemorrhage, subarachnoid hemorrhage secondary to aneurysm, arteriovenous malformation (AVM), or hemorrhage into a tumor. An emergent CT scan of the brain is the procedure of choice.

If there is no evidence of hemorrhage, occlusive disease (i.e., thrombosis or embolus) is the most likely cause. Within the first 24 hours, the CT scan may not show any evidence of infarct. Short-term anticoagulation may be considered (see Chapter 12) with heparin at a dosage of 800 to 1000 units IV hourly. Heparin weight-based protocol is not appropriate for stroke.

Tissue plasminogen activator (tPA) is contraindicated in an unstable deficit (see Chapter 12). Vascular interventional treatment may radically alter the outcome. An interventional radiologist, if available, may acutely lyse thrombi in the middle cerebral artery or coil an aneurysm.

STROKE

For evaluation of completed stroke, see Chapter 12.

FEVER AND CENTRAL NERVOUS SYSTEM SYMPTOMS

See Chapter 14.

Meningitis

1. Consider the possibility of bacterial meningitis in any patient with fever and even minimal mental or neurologic symptoms.
2. Whenever the diagnosis is suspected, a lumbar puncture (LP) must be performed (studies should include cultures for tuberculosis [TB], fungi, viruses).

Caution: It is far preferable to culture cerebrospinal fluid (CSF) *before* antibiotic therapy, but treatment should not be delayed if CT is not immediately available.

3. The prognosis depends on the interval between the onset of the illness and institution of therapy.

Treatment:

1. If the CSF examination is suggestive of bacterial meningitis (increased nucleated cells, particularly neutrophils, and low glucose) and after cultures have been sent, the patient must be started on IV antibiotics. The choice of antibiotics depends on the patient's age and medical history (see Chapter 14) and the results of the Gram's stain of the CSF. The antibiotic regimen can be modified when culture and sensitivity results are known.
2. Management of complications may be necessary (see Chapters 11, 13, and 14).

ENCEPHALITIS

The hallmark of encephalitis is mental status changes. It is important early in the course of the illness to recognize or suspect herpes simplex encephalitis, since it has been shown that acyclovir, instituted early, has decreased the morbidity and mortality rates remarkably. Patients with herpes simplex encephalitis classically have an acute onset of mental and behavioral symptoms, often with an amnestic syndrome, and may have lateralized findings, such as mild hemiparesis or aphasia. Seizures may be the presenting symptom. An electroencephalogram (EEG) may reveal focal slowing over the temporal lobes and (at some point during the course) periodic lateralizing epileptiform discharges (PLEDs). The CT scan or an MR image may show abnormalities of the temporal lobes.

Treatment: For herpes simplex encephalitis, begin acyclovir immediately at 10 mg/kg/day IV every 8 hours for at least 10 days.

Caveat: The disease can be so devastating and the treatment so effective that acyclovir should be started even if there is only a suspicion of the disease.

GUILLAIN-BARRÉ SYNDROME

See Chapter 15.
1. Respiratory function must be closely monitored initially with frequent (at least hourly) bedside forced vital capacity (FVC) and inspiratory force measurements. Respiratory function must be closely monitored even in patients with no apparent respiratory involvement. If the FVC falls below 20 ml/kg, tracheostomy or the insertion of a soft-cuff endotracheal tube must be seriously considered. An inspiratory force (a direct reflection of respiratory muscular strength) of less than 25 cm also indicates the probable need for tracheostomy. The frequency of monitoring of respiratory function may be reduced as the patient shows signs of clinical improvement.
2. The patient needs to be admitted to an intensive care unit (ICU) for close monitoring.
3. In addition to muscle weakness, respiratory insufficiency may be caused by the following:
   a. Aspiration pneumonia from an inability to swallow properly
   b. Pulmonary embolism from venous stasis of immobilized legs
   c. Pneumonia from decreased cough and hyperventilation
4. *Early* institution of plasmapheresis or intravenous immunoglobulin (IVIg) hastens recovery and reduces morbidity.

Caveat: Suspect this disease in any young person with a subacute onset of weakness and absent ankle reflexes.

MYASTHENIA GRAVIS

See Chapter 15.
   The patient with myasthenia gravis may have a neurologic emergency or crisis in which there is a rapidly progressive respiratory insufficiency. The crisis usually occurs in a patient with known myasthenia during added stress, such as infection, anesthesia, surgery, or medication changes; occasionally a patient with undiagnosed myasthenia gravis will have primarily respiratory failure. The crises are of the following two types:
1. *Myasthenic*—There is an increase in the severity of the disease relative to the treatment (i.e., undertreatment).

2. *Cholinergic*–There is an excess of anticholinergic activity (usually from anticholinesterase drugs) relative to the severity of the disease (i.e., overtreatment).

It is difficult to differentiate between these two types of crises at the time of presentation with imminent respiratory failure. Sometimes the evidence of excessive acetylcholine effect, such as abdominal cramps, sweating, lacrimation, bradycardia, miosis, muscle cramps, and fasciculations, may suggest that the patient is in a cholinergic crisis; however, caution is necessary, since such signs may be absent in definite cholinergic crisis or present in a myasthenic crisis.

Treatment:

1. Maintain ventilation with a soft-cuff endotracheal tube or tracheostomy. The soft-cuffed endotracheal tube may be left in place for up to a week without serious risk or distress to the patient.
2. Withdraw all medications used to treat myasthenia and all drugs with a curare-like action.
3. After 24 hours, gradually reintroduce antimyasthenic medication.
4. Plasmapheresis will result in marked improvement in patients with either cholinergic or myasthenic crises.

Remember:

1. Myasthenia is a disease characterized by muscle fatigability; artificial ventilatory support will temporarily restore respiratory strength, which will then gradually decline.
2. Respiratory failure may occur in the presence of normal arm and leg strength.

WERNICKE'S ENCEPHALOPATHY

See Chapter 8.

The signs of Wernicke's encephalopathy (resulting from a thiamine deficiency) include a patient with an acute confusional state (characterized by disorientation and an amnestic syndrome) accompanied by extraocular muscle paralysis and evidence of polyneuropathy. The classic triad is of encephalopathy, impaired extraocular movements, and ataxia. However, mental status changes alone in varying degrees may occur. Although it occurs primarily in nutritionally deficient alcoholics, it commonly occurs in other settings, such as the hospital patient receiving IV fluids without thiamine or multivitamin supplements or individuals who are on diets deficient in thiamine.

Treatment: At least 100 mg thiamine IV immediately followed by a maintenance dose of 100 mg daily is indicated.

Differential Diagnosis of Acute Paralysis of Extraocular Movement That May Have Emergency Implications

1. *Botulism:* Botulism appears as a paralysis of extraocular muscles rapidly progressing to involve swallowing problems, generalized weakness, and respiratory failure. Botulism is associated with blurred vision as a result of impaired pupillary reaction. The condition is most com-

monly associated with eating improperly home-canned acidic foods (such as green beans or salsa), and the diagnosis should be strongly suspected when several members of a family acquire symptoms.

Treatment: An antitoxin should be administered immediately. Contact the local poison control center for a supply of antitoxin. Respiratory failure should be treated with mechanical ventilatory support.

2. *Myasthenia gravis* (see Chapter 15): Paralysis of extraocular movement in ocular myasthenia may occur acutely but presents no immediate danger. There is no long-term danger if weakness is confined to those muscles. It is commonly associated with ptosis. However, if generalized myasthenia develops, respiratory failure may result.

3. *Cavernous sinus thrombosis:* Signs of cavernous sinus thrombosis include paralysis of extraocular muscles and a painful bulging red eye; it is often associated with a sinus infection. Immediate MRI and magnetic resonance angiography (MRA) are indicated, but four-vessel cerebral angiography may be necessary to establish the diagnosis. (Clinical evaluation should include auscultation of the skull and orbits for an accompanying bruit.)

Treatment: Blood and CSF cultures should be obtained; a CT scan or an MR image may reveal the source of infection of the brain and orbits. Massive doses of IV antibiotics, as if treating meningitis, should be given (see Chapter 14).

4. *Carotid-cavernous fistula:* The patient with a carotid-cavernous fistula usually has suffered a recent head injury and has extraocular palsies and a painful bulging red eye that pulsates synchronously with carotid pulsation. A bruit may be heard over the eye. Cerebral angiography will establish the diagnosis.

Treatment: Neurosurgical intervention is usually necessary for acute fistulas. An interventional neuroradiologist, if available, may treat both acute and chronic cases.

5. *Posterior communicating artery aneurysm:* The patient with a posterior communicating artery aneurysm often has third cranial (oculomotor) nerve palsy; the affected eye is turned down and out, and the pupil is dilated. The ocular palsy occurs most often when the aneurysm ruptures and the patient develops severe headache and stiff neck. Unlike the acute third cranial nerve palsy of diabetes (in which pupillary reactivity is intact), in the case of an aneurysm, the pupil is dilated and poorly reactive to light on the side of palsy. The diagnosis is established by four-vessel cerebral angiography.

Treatment: Immediate consultation by a neurosurgeon or an interventional neuroradiologist is indicated.

TEMPORAL ARTERITIS—SUDDEN LOSS OF VISION

1. In an elderly individual, new-onset headaches associated with a markedly elevated erythrocyte sedimentation rate (ESR) (usually >50 mm/first hr) suggest a diagnosis of temporal arteritis. A firm, tender temporal artery may be present.

2. Temporal arteritis is often heralded by diffuse arthralgia, myalgia, and jaw claudication. A sudden onset of monocular blindness or infarc-

tion associated with damage to other intracranial arteries is a serious complication.

3. An edematous retina with optic disc pallor may be visualized by ophthalmoscopy when a visual disturbance is present.

Treatment:

1. With headache as the only symptom, immediate treatment with prednisone 60 mg/day by mouth is recommended (see Chapter 3).
2. A temporal artery biopsy should be performed within 2 to 3 days to confirm the diagnosis. A definitive diagnosis is very comforting when long-term steroids are contemplated.

Differential Diagnosis of Sudden Visual Loss

The sudden loss of all or part of visual function is a potentially neuro-ophthalmologic emergency.

1. The type of visual loss suggests the location of the disease.
   a. Monocular visual loss suggests disease of the optic nerve or globe.
   b. Partial loss in both eyes suggests CNS disease at or behind the optic chiasm.
2. Eye pain is associated with glaucoma, infection, or optic neuritis.
3. Transient visual loss in one eye associated with paralysis of the body on the opposite side suggests emboli from the carotid artery (see Chapter 12).
4. Prodromal phenomena (zigzag lights or stars) are seen in both CNS infarction and migraine.
5. A firm globe to palpation (tonometry is much more accurate) suggests a diagnosis of glaucoma.
6. An unreactive pupil or a Marcus Gunn pupil (see Figure 10-1) suggests disease anterior to the optic chiasm.
7. With unilateral blindness, one of the following causes can often be diagnosed with the ophthalmoscope:
   a. Intraocular hemorrhage
   b. Retinal detachment
   c. Emboli
   d. Retinal infarction
   e. Infection
8. A bruit over the carotid artery raises the possibility of the artery being a source of embolus to the ophthalmic artery.
   ### Conditions requiring immediate treatment
1. Retinal artery or branch occlusion: A retinal artery or branch occlusion is a monocular defect found in the visual field corresponding to an ischemic retina with reduced or absent arterial blood flow, which is evident on ophthalmoscopic testing. Occasionally, an embolus can be visualized on ophthalmoscopy; small retinal hemorrhages and retinal edema may also be seen.

     If the blindness is transient and associated with a contralateral hemiparesis, the diagnosis of carotid artery stenosis or ulceration is strongly suggested.

Treatment: An anticoagulant (heparin) to prevent further embolization while looking for the site of origin of emboli is indicated.

2. Optic or retrobulbar neuritis: Signs of optic or retrobulbar neuritis include subacute (over hours) unilateral or bilateral visual loss with the patient complaining of eye pain with eye motion; the ophthalmologic examination may be normal, and a Marcus Gunn pupil (see Fig. 10-1) may be demonstrated. Unilateral optic neuritis is associated with multiple sclerosis (MS), whereas bilateral optic neuritis is most often associated with a toxic disturbance, such as methyl alcohol poisoning.

Treatment: Treat optic neuritis with IV corticosteroids.

Conditions requiring referral to an ophthalmologist

1. Acute glaucoma: In the case of acute glaucoma, the globe is usually hard (increased tension) with an unreactive dilated pupil and an enlarged optic cup. Assess intraocular tension by palpation or, preferably, by tonometry. Sudden blindness may occur secondary to vascular occlusion as a result of the raised intraocular pressure.

Treatment: Instill cholinergics (pilocarpine in a sufficient dose to constrict the pupil); refer the patient to an ophthalmologist to consider paracentesis of the eye.

2. Retinal detachment: A monocular visual loss in the field corresponds to the area of retinal detachment; the detachment is visible on an ophthalmoscopic examination.

Treatment: Avoid excessive head or eye movement. Refer the patient to an ophthalmologist for photocoagulation and surgery to prevent a progression of the detachment.

3. Intraocular hemorrhage: In a patient with intraocular hemorrhage, a monocular visual loss with blood is visible on ophthalmoscopic examination.

Treatment: Perform an ophthalmologic evaluation to determine the cause of bleeding and consider ocular paracentesis to reduce the pressure.

4. Intraocular infection: With an intraocular infection, there is monocular visual loss with purulent material evident on an ophthalmoscopic examination; eye pain is common.

Treatment: An ophthalmologic evaluation with paracentesis for culture and immediate antibiotic treatment similar to that used for meningitis (see Chapter 14) is indicated.

5. Retinal migraine: A transient hemianopic field defect, with retinal migraine as well as transient monocular blindness, may occur. Headache is not invariably present, especially if it is the first migraine. The ophthalmologic examination is normal. The diagnosis is suggested by a strong family history of migraine, the use of birth-control pills, or the subsequent development of a unilateral, throbbing headache.

Treatment: Acute treatment may not be necessary (see Chapter 3).

SEVERE INCAPACITATING MUSCLE SPASMS

Tetanus

1. The patient with tetanus has a fixed smile with clenched teeth (trismus). The remainder of the muscles are in constant contraction (risus sardonicus).

2. The disease appears from 1 to 54 days (within 14 days in more than half of cases) after a puncture or lacerating wound (but may appear without a demonstrable wound); it is especially common in older adults who have not been reimmunized for many years.
3. Autonomic disturbances may occur with tetanus, resulting in cardiac arrhythmias and wide fluctuations in blood pressure.

Treatment:
1. Penicillin G should be given IV at a dosage of 10 to 20 million units/day.
2. Tracheostomy should be performed in all but very mild cases. Continuous artificial ventilation is needed.
3. Analgesics should be used to relieve the pain from muscle contractions.
4. The toxin should be neutralized with human tetanus immune globulin (TIG-H) 3000 to 10,000 units intramuscularly (IM) at several sites, including the area of the presumed injury (infection).
5. Diazepam, 80 to 230 mg/day, is often effective in reducing spasms.

Hypocalcemic Tetany

1. Hypocalcemic tetany may be distinguished from tetanus by a milder degree of muscle spasm and by the presence of carpopedal spasm, Chvostek's sign (a unilateral facial muscle spasm precipitated by tapping the facial nerve near the ear), and Trousseau's sign (a carpal spasm precipitated by a brief inflation above systolic pressure of a blood pressure cuff on the arm).
2. The disease is most commonly seen in infants who drink cow's milk. It is important to recognize this disorder in infants because of the possible respiratory compromise and associated seizures.
3. Tetany in adults may be associated with hyperventilation syndrome (see Chapter 4).
4. The diagnosis is established by low serum calcium and high serum phosphate levels.

Treatment: Slow IV administration of calcium gluconate (10% solution) should be done in severe cases (up to 10 ml in children and 30 ml in adults). Oral calcium gluconate and a switch to commercially prepared formula feeding in the infant may be adequate treatment in milder cases.

BIBLIOGRAPHY

Bracken MB, Shepard MJ, Collins WF et al: A randomized controlled trial of methylprednisolone or naloxone in the treatment of acute spinal cord injury: results of the Second National Acute Spinal Cord Injury Study, *N Engl J Med* 322:1405-1411, 1990.

Cruz J: *Neurological and neurosurgical emergencies,* Philadelphia, 1998, WB Saunders.

Orland MJ, Saltman RJ, editors: *Manual of medical therapeutics,* ed 30, Philadelphia, 2001, Lippincott, Williams & Wilkins.

Samuels MA: *Manual of neurologic therapeutics,* ed 6, Philadelphia, 1999, Lippincott, Williams & Wilkins.

Wijdicks EF: *The clinical practice of critical care neurology,* Philadelphia, 1997, Lippincott-Raven.

21

Considerations in the Care of the Patient with Severe and Irreversible Nervous System Damage

Advances in medical technology have provided clinicians with the means of preserving life at the expense of a great deal of unnecessary pain and suffering by patients. The decisions with regard to neurologic patients should be governed by the same general principles as those used in other disciplines of medicine. Usually these problems have a way of providing their own solutions without the aid of complicated rules, regulations, and fancy machines. For example, cardiac resuscitation in patients with severe brain damage is rarely successful.

GENERAL PRINCIPLES

The following are a few important principles in handling patients with severe and irreversible nervous system disease:
1. Always keep the family and loved ones informed about the patient's condition. Avoid technical jargon, such as, "The cerebral angiogram showed bilateral cerebral hemisphere infarction." A preferable statement would be, "When we injected dye into the arteries of the brain, we found that no blood is reaching those parts of the brain that control movement and thought. Without blood, brain tissue dies and does not have the capability of ever recovering."
2. Designate one physician to communicate with the family. Families relate better to one physician than to a team, which can seem (to the family) to provide conflicting information.

3. Involve the patient and the family in the decision-making process. The physician has the responsibility to provide clear and simple facts that are necessary to make a decision. Often it is appropriate to give the family advice as to what action to take in a particular situation. The wishes of the patient and the family take precedence over the physician's preference.

4. Consider the quality of life *before* the current neurologic disability; for example, the patient with a clearly documented severe dementia who develops a sudden left hemiparesis may not wish for more than fluid and nutritional support.

5. Consider the quality of life *after* the neurologic disability; for example, many patients do not choose respiratory support at the end stage of amyotrophic lateral sclerosis (ALS) or muscular dystrophy (MD). A patient with ALS on a respirator faces the prospect of consciously watching his or her body wither away until he or she has no voluntary movements other than eye movements and sphincter function.

6. Carefully document all discussions and decisions in the medical record.

7. Promote the use of traditional patient and family support systems, such as clergy, close friends, and fraternal organizations, during times of severe stress.

8. Cases of suspected homicide, assault, child abuse, and the like require that the physician use special care in the decision-making process; it is always wise to seek additional (including legal) opinions.

BRAIN DEATH

Once artificial life-support systems have been instituted and irreversible coma or brain death is suspected, state or local hospital criteria for discontinuing respiratory support should be followed. These criteria often include recommendations from multiple consultants (medical and sometimes clergy and legal).

Human death is the irreversible loss of the capacity for consciousness and the capacity to breathe. The following guidelines have evolved since the late 1960s for the determination of brain death:

1. *Brain death* is defined as the irreversible cessation of all clinically ascertainable functions of the entire brain, including the brainstem (but not necessarily including the spinal cord).

2. Cessation of brain function is interpreted as both of the following:
   a. Cerebral unreceptivity and unresponsivity
   b. Absent brainstem reflexes

Note: Spinal cord activity (reflexes) and peripheral nervous system (PNS) activity may persist after brain death.

3. Minimal accepted clinical neurologic findings of brain death include the following:
   a. No spontaneous movement and no movement are elicited by painful stimuli to the face or trunk (see Chapter 13).

   b. The pupils are fully dilated or in midposition and are totally unreactive to light. (Examine the pupils under magnification with a bright light in a darkened room.)

   c. There is an absence of oculocephalic (doll's eye) and oculovestibular (caloric) responses (see Chapter 13), corneal reflex, pharyngeal reflex (the insertion and removal of a nasopharyngeal suction tube should not produce a cough or gag), and cough reflex (after suctioning or irrigation of the endotracheal tube). There should be no spontaneous blinking (eye opening) or swallowing.

   d. There are no spontaneous respirations (apnea) after the arterial carbon dioxide partial pressure ($PaCO_2$) has reached a level that provides maximal respiratory stimulus (approximately 60 mm Hg). Apnea testing should be performed with a protocol that permits pretest hyperoxygenation, exposure of the tracheobronchial tree to oxygen during the test, and monitoring of arterial $PaCO_2$ levels, which rise an average of 4 mm Hg/min during apnea.

4. Irreversibility is interpreted to mean the following:

   a. The *cause* of the coma is established, is sufficient to account for the coma, and is not a reversible condition.

Caution: The frequent reversible conditions of metabolic or drug (sedative) intoxication, hypothermia, neuromuscular blockade, and shock must be excluded.

   b. The possibility of recovery of any brain function is excluded. Demonstration of a lack of blood flow to the brain is a confirmation of irreversibility.

Caution: Conventional cerebral angiography can falsely demonstrate flow in a brain-dead patient because of the excessive injection pressure forcing dye into the intracranial vessels or the injection with the head in a dependent position, allowing contrast material to leak into the vessels.

   c. The cessation of all brain function persists for an adequate observation period (6 hours with confirmatory tests, 12 to 24 hours in the absence of confirmatory tests).

5. Confirmation of electrocerebral silence by an electroencephalogram (EEG) performed at least 6 hours after the loss of clinically ascertainable brain function is desirable when confirmatory documentation is needed to substantiate the clinical findings.

Caution: EEG tracings must be obtained using the technical guidelines established by the American Electroencephalographic Society. These guidelines have been established to ensure that tracings for electrocerebral silence are not artifactual and that all measures to maximize recording of minimal cerebral electrical activity have been performed. Usually if everything has been done by a registered EEG technologist (REEGT) and interpreted by an experienced electroencephalographer, this is assurance enough that the guidelines have been followed.

Note:

   a. Electrocerebral silence tracings may be seen in the following potentially reversible situations:
   1) Barbiturate intoxication
   2) Hypothermia
   3) A premature or full-term infant who is not brain dead
   b. Brainstem auditory-evoked responses may also be used in the diagnosis of brain death. It is known that brainstem auditory-evoked responses can be present while an EEG shows electrocerebral silence but may finally disappear when medullary function ceases.
6. Before respiratory support is discontinued, a family conference is highly desirable. Whether the patient had made a living will, the unlikelihood of recovery, the opportunity for organ donation, and permission for autopsy should be discussed.
7. Guidelines for the determination of brain death in children under 5 years of age are still in the process of development. Clinical criteria similar to those in use for patients over 5 years of age have been found to be applicable to infants and term newborns (>38 weeks' gestational age) older than 7 days of age. It has been recommended that two EEG tracings be performed in children under 1 year of age, with these tracings separated by an interval of 48 hours in patients 7 days to 2 months of age and by an interval of 24 hours in patients 2 months to 1 year of age. In patients over 1 year of age, laboratory tests are not necessary if an irreversible cause exists and clinical criteria for brain death are met.

BIBLIOGRAPHY

A definition of irreversible coma: report of ad hoc committee of the Harvard Medical School to examine the definition of brain death, *JAMA* 205:337-340, 1968.

American EEG Society: *Minimum technical standards for EEG recording in suspected cerebral death.* In Klass DW, Daly DD, editors: *Current practice of clinical electroencephalography*, New York, 1979, Raven Press.

Black PM: Brain death, *N Engl J Med* 299:338-344, 393-401, 1978.

Goldie WD, Chiappa KH, Young RR, Brooks EB: Brainstem auditory and short-latency somatosensory evoked responses in brain death, *Neurology* 31:248-256, 1981.

Guidelines for the determination of brain death in children: Task Force for the Determination of Brain Death in Children, *Arch Neurol* 44:587-588, 1987.

Guidelines for the determination of death: report of the medical consultants on the diagnosis of death to the president's commission for the study of ethical problems in medicine and biomedical and behavioral research, *JAMA* 246:2184-2186, 1981.

Kaufman HH, Beresford R, Bernat JL et al: Brain death, *Neurol Neurosurg Update Ser* 6:1-8, 1986.

Moshé SL, Alvarez LA: Diagnosis of brain death in children, *J Clin Neurophysiol* 3:239-249, 1986.

Rowland TW, Donnelly JH, Jackson AH: Apnea documentation for determination of brain death in children, *Pediatrics* 74:505-508, 1984.

Ruank JE: Initiating and withdrawing life support, *N Engl J Med* 318:25-31, 1988.

Schneider S, Ashwal S: *Determination of brain deaths in infants and children,* Mosby, St Louis, 1999.

Schwartz JA, Baxter J, Brill DR: Diagnosis of brain death in children by radio-nuclide cerebral imaging, *Pediatrics* 73:14-18, 1984.

Silverstein MD, Stocking CB, Antel JP et al: Amyotrophic lateral sclerosis and life-sustaining therapy: patient's desires for information and participation in decision making and life-sustaining therapy, *Mayo Clin Proc* 66:906-913, 1991.

Sundram JC: Informed consent for major medical treatment of mentally disabled people, *N Engl J Med* 318:1368-1373, 1988.

Task force for the determination of brain death in children: Guidelines for the determination of brain death in children, *Ann Neurol* 22:616-617, 1987.

Youngner SJ, Bartlett ET: Human death and high technology: the failure of the whole-brain formulations, *Ann Intern Med* 99:252-258, 1983.

APPENDIX A

Head Circumference Charts* and Denver Developmental Test†

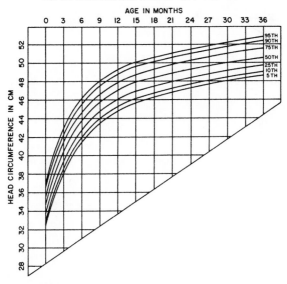

Boys head circumference by age percentiles : ages birth - 36 months

AGE IN MONTHS

HEAD CIRCUMFERENCE IN CM

*Growth charts courtesy of National Center for Health Statistics: NSCH Growth Charts, 1976. Monthly Vital Statistics Report, Volume 3, Supplement (HRA) 76-1120 Health Resources Administration, Rockville, Maryland. Used by permission.
†From William K. Frankenburg, MD, and Josiah B. Dodds, PhD, University of Colorado Medical Center. Used by permission.

Girls head circumference by age percentiles : ages birth – 36 months

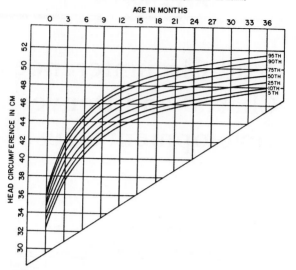

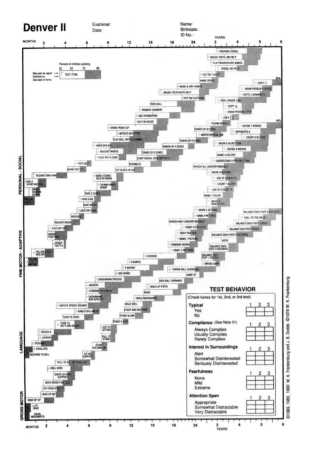

DIRECTIONS FOR ADMINISTRATION

1. Try to get child to smile by smiling, talking or waving. Do not touch him/her.
2. Child must stare at hand several seconds.
3. Parent may help guide toothbrush and put toothpaste on brush.
4. Child does not have to be able to tie shoes or button/zip in the back.
5. Move yarn slowly in an arc from one side to the other, about 8" above child's face.
6. Pass if child grasps rattle when it is touched to the backs or tips of fingers.
7. Pass if child tries to see where yarn went. Yarn should be dropped quickly from sight from tester's hand without arm movement.
8. Child must transfer cube from hand to hand without help of body, mouth, or table.
9. Pass if child picks up raisin with any part of thumb and finger.
10. Line can vary only 30 degrees or less from tester's line.
11. Make a fist with thumb pointing upward and wiggle only the thumb. Pass if child imitates and does not move any fingers other than the thumb.

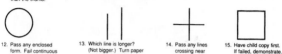

12. Pass any enclosed form. Fail continuous round motions.
13. Which line is longer? (Not bigger.) Turn paper upside down and repeat. (pass 3 of 3 or 5 of 6)
14. Pass any lines crossing near midpoint.
15. Have child copy first. If failed, demonstrate.

When giving items 12, 14. and 15, do not name the forms. Do not demonstrate 12 and 14.

16. When scoring, each pair (2 arms, 2 legs, etc.) counts as one part.
17. Place one cube in cup and shake gently near child's ear, but out of sight. Repeat for other ear.
18. Point to picture and have child name it. (No credit is given for sounds only.)
    If less than 4 pictures are named correctly, have child point to picture as each is named by tester.

19. Using doll, tell child: Show me the nose, eyes, ears, mouth, hands, feet, tummy, hair. Pass 6 of 8.
20. Using pictures, ask child: Which one flies?... says meow?... talks?... barks?... gallops? Pass 2 of 5, 4 of 5.
21. Ask child: What do you do when you are cold?... tired?... hungry? Pass 2 of 3, 3 of 3.
22. Ask child: What do you do with a cup? What is a chair used for? What is a pencil used for?
    Action words must be included in answers.
23. Pass if child correctly places <u>and</u> says how many blocks are on paper. (1, 5).
24. Tell child: Put block **on** table; **under** table; **in front of** me, **behind** me. Pass 4 of 4.
    (Do not help child by pointing, moving head or eyes.)
25. Ask child: What is a ball?... lake?... desk?... house?... banana?... curtain?... fence?... ceiling? Pass if defined in terms of use, shape, what it is made of, or general category (such as banana is fruit, not just yellow). Pass 5 of 8, 7 of 8.
26. Ask child: If a horse is big, a mouse is __? If fire is hot, ice is __? If the sun shines during the day, the moon shines during the __? Pass 2 of 3.
27. Child may use wall or rail only, not person. May not crawl.
28. Child must throw ball overhand 3 feet to within arm's reach of tester.
29. Child must perform standing broad jump over width of test sheet (8 1/2 inches).
30. Tell child to walk forward, heel within 1 inch of toe. Tester may demonstrate.
    Child must walk 4 consecutive steps.
31. In the second year, half of normal children are non-compliant.

OBSERVATIONS:

B

The Symptom-Oriented Neurologic Examination

This appendix is written to assist with the mastery of the neurologic examination. Each phase of the examination is divided into three parts: step-by-step directions on how to proceed, common problems the beginner faces, and common abnormalities.

The first eight sections make up the "routine examination." With a cooperative patient an experienced examiner can perform the examination in less than 15 minutes. However, with each patient the examiner must individually modify it according to the chief complaint, age, degree of cooperation, and other individual factors. The neurologic examination is never the same, even for patients with the same age and complaint.

The most important part of the neurologic evaluation is the history taking. It is during the interview that the examiner forms hypotheses concerning the nature of the complaints. The examiner then tailors the examination to gather objective data to verify these hypotheses. This appendix focuses only on the form in which the history should be recorded. The *art* of gathering this history is a by-product of astuteness in listening, experience, and individual communication style.

It is important to emphasize that there are many correct ways to do a neurologic examination. What is presented here is certainly not the only "right" examination but simply one that has worked for the authors over many years. The astute physician will ultimately adopt those techniques that work best for him or her.

PATIENT RECORD

Introduction

The general principles of interviewing and examining the patient with a neurologic complaint are no different from those of interviewing and examining the patient with any medical illness—only the emphasis is different. In every patient encounter, the physician must form *hypotheses* as to the cause of the patient's distress. These hypotheses are strengthened or discarded according to the facts that emerge during the interview and examination. This section is a general framework for recording the illness of a patient with a neurologic complaint. Obviously, such a framework emphasizes a neurologic review of systems and the neurologic examination. The purpose of preparing such a record is to communicate information concerning the patient's illness in an organized, succinct, and legible manner.

The uniqueness of each patient encounter cannot be overemphasized. Thus it is impossible to present a "cookbook" that outlines precisely how to proceed. For example, it is useless to spend much time taking a history and review of systems from a patient with a severe memory deficit. Information in such circumstances is best gathered from other sources. If the physician performs a "routine" neurologic examination on every patient, important data will be routinely missed. For example, palpation of the temporal arteries and a careful search for early papilledema are important in the elderly patient with the complaint of headache, but tests usually reserved for the patient complaining of low back pain (such as straight leg raising, abdominal reflexes, cremasteric reflexes, and internal hamstring reflexes) will yield little useful information. The problem-oriented approach to neurologic examination necessitates individualization (Table B-1).

The following is a "template" that can be given to a transcriptionist or entered in a computer. This satisfies a level 1 Centers for Medicare & Medicaid Services outpatient consult. If default information is used, this necessitates that the review of systems, physical examination, and neurological examination be done exactly the same on every patient and the default script changed accordingly. "If it isn't written down, you didn't do it."

Comments on the Outline of the Medical Record of the Patient with a Neurologic Complaint

Demographic data:
Date of visit:
Site:
Patient name:
Birth date:
Age:
Patient phone number:
Address:
SS#:
Referring doctor:
Chief complaint: (Why you are seeing the patient)
Present illness: (Include pertinent positives and negatives)
Past history: (Operations, accidents, medical illnesses)
Medication allergies:
Medications:
Family history:

TABLE B-1
Steps in Arriving at a Neurologic Diagnosis

Process	Concepts	Skill	Knowledge
History	Anatomic and pathologic concept of the disorder *[A]*	Interrogative skill	Basic neuroscience and neuropathology
Physical signs	Anatomic and functional localization *[B];* confirm or refute *[A]*	Clinical examination	Interpretation of physical signs to localize and to assess dysfunction
Differential diagnosis investigations	Confirm or refute *[A]* or *[B]*	Discriminative	Knowledge of sensitivity and predictability of tests
Final diagnosis			

Marital status, employment status, education, habits, hobbies:
Review of systems:

Constitutional:	No weight loss, recent infections, heat or cold intolerance or malaise.
HEENT:	No headache, head trauma, visual changes, speech or swallowing, abnormalities.
Neck back and spine:	No trauma or pain.
Skin:	No rash, scars or birthmarks.
Respiratory:	No coughing, wheezing, or shortness of breath.
Cardiovascular:	No chest pain or palpitation.
GI and/or GU:	Normal bowel and bladder function; normal appetite.
Musculoskeletal:	No leg cramps, muscle weakness or joint pain.
Mental status/psychiatric:	No sleep disturbance or forgetfulness.

Physical Examination
Constitutional:

Height: **Weight:**

General appearance:	Healthy, well groomed, appearance, appropriate for age.
Extremities:	No deformities or skin changes.

Peripheral vasculature:	No edema, varicosities, or abnormal pulses; no carotid bruits.
HEENT:	No scars, abnormal coloration, pharyngeal inflammation, or nasal discharge.
Cardiac:	No murmurs and rubs; normal rhythm.
Chest:	Normal breath sounds on auscultation; no chest deformities.
Neck and spine:	Normal range of motion and alignment; no tenderness to percussion.

Neurologic Examination

| Mental status: | Oriented to time, place and person; intact recent and remote memory; normal attention span, concentration, and language; normal spontaneous speech, fund of knowledge, and vocabulary. **Mini-Mental Status Examination (MMSE) (see p. 422) Clock drawing** |

Cranial nerves (CN):

CN I:	Smells in each nostril.
CN II:	Visual fields are normal to confrontation. The disk margins are sharp and normal in color. There are normal retinal vein pulsations and visual acuity.
CN III, IV, VI:	Extraocular movements are full and without nystagmus or ptosis. Pupils are equal, round, and reactive to light.
CN V:	The corneal reflex is normal and symmetric. There is normal facial sensation to light touch.
CN VII:	Facial movements are symmetric.
CN VIII:	Auditory acuity is normal as judged by the ability to hear rubbed fingers.
CN IX, X:	Palatal movements and pharyngeal reflex are normal; phonation is normal.
CN XI:	Sternocleidomastoid and trapezius muscle are of normal strength.
CN XII:	The tongue is at the midline with no atrophy or fasciculations.
Coordination:	A finger-to-nose test was done accurately with no action tremor. Rapid alternating movements were normal.
Muscle stretch reflexes:	Reflexes are normal and symmetric in the upper and lower extremities. Plantar responses are flexor.
Motor:	There are no fasciculations or alternation in tone: bulk is normal: There is no weakness.

Station and gait:	There was a normal gait that showed no abnormalities. Walking on the heels, toes, and sides of feet was done without difficulty. A tandem walk was normal. No abnormal movements were noted. A Romberg's test was negative.
Sensation:	Sensation was intact to light touch, pinprick, vibration, and position.

Discussion:
  Localization
  Dx
Tests ordered:
  None
Therapy:

Discussion. The differential diagnosis of neurologic problems begins with an assessment of the anatomic location of the pathology. For example, "The patient has a peripheral polyneuropathy because of the bilateral distal loss of sensation and tendon reflexes." When localizing a disease process, it is often helpful to go through the following checklist mentally:

1. Does the problem involve the central or the peripheral nervous system?
2. If it involves the peripheral nervous system, is muscle or nerve primarily involved?
3. If it involves the central nervous system (CNS), is the lesion above or below the foramen magnum?
4. If the lesion is above the foramen magnum, is it above the tentorium cerebelli (anterior or middle cerebral fossae) or below (posterior fossa)?
5. If the lesion is above the tentorium, is it in the right or left hemisphere? Is it gray matter or white matter disease?
6. Are multiple systems involved?

This should be followed by a discussion of the pathophysiologic process involved. For example, the sudden onset of symptoms suggests vascular occlusion; a slow progression, a positive family history, and multiple system involvement suggest a degenerative process. Discuss the possible diagnoses and the reasons for considering them and for excluding other conditions. For example, in a patient with a peripheral neuropathy, because the patient has had insulin dependent diabetes mellitus for 8 years and the neuropathy is primarily sensory, the most probable diagnosis is diabetic peripheral polyneuropathy. However, because of the history of a gastrectomy 12 years ago and possible recent exposure to lead, subacute combined degeneration of the spinal cord (combined system disease) and lead intoxication must also be considered as possible diagnoses.

Differential diagnosis. This should be a list, in order of probability, of all diseases that reasonably account for the clinical picture. The diagnosis you think the patient has is listed first. Specific diseases should be listed, not generalities such as "some kind of degenerative disease." The differential diagnosis serves as a guide to proper evaluation because appropriate tests will be chosen to confirm or exclude each condition listed.

Pertinent diagnostic tests. In the example of the patient with a peripheral neuropathy, indicated tests would include an electromyogram (EMG), nerve conduction velocity studies (NCV), a glucose tolerance test (GTT), serum vitamin B_{12} levels, a red blood cell smear for morphologic evaluation, and urinary screening for heavy metals. "Routine" studies (e.g., complete blood count [CBC], urinalysis, serum chemistry panel, electrocardiography [ECG], chest radiographs) need not be reiterated, unless specific tests are critical in confirming or excluding one of the differential diagnoses. Table B-2 lists commonly ordered diagnostic tests.

COMMON TOOLS FOUND IN THE MEDICAL BAG OF A NEUROLOGIST

The medical bag of the neurologist might contain many of the following items:

1. Ophthalmoscope: this instrument should have a bright light source (good batteries, quartz-halogen bulb), a light aperture that can be adjusted to provide various sizes and colors of light beams, multiple lenses calibrated in a range of diopters, and an otoscope head (with a removable ear speculum) for examining small or irregular pupils under magnification.
2. Reflex hammer: there are at least 20 varieties available; the Queen's Square hammer is the one we favor because the flexible long handle greatly simplifies elicitation of reflex activity.
3. Blood pressure cuff: the aneroid style with the hand-held gauge is preferable because it facilitates measuring postural hypotension.
4. Stethoscope: this is also useful in detecting cranial and spinal bruits.
5. Flashlight: a bright, pinpoint light source is preferable. Disposable pocket flashlights generally provide inadequate light.
6. Visual acuity test card: this hand-held card tests nearsightedness. If the patient wears corrective lenses (glasses or contact lenses), they should be worn during this test.
7. Red target on a wire (larger than a dime): this is used to detect visual field defects. A red-headed hat pin may also be used.
8. Opticokinetic tape: testing for opticokinetic nystagmus may be useful. An easily constructed homemade cloth tape consisting of alternating 2-inch-wide light and dark stripes is all that is necessary.
9. Tape measure: a tape measure is required for measuring head circumference and muscle atrophy.
10. Pin: a pin can be used for testing pain sensation. Other sharp objects are inadequate; injection needles are too sharp and diaper pins do not permit quantitation. CAUTION: human immunodeficiency virus (HIV) (the virus of acquired immune deficiency syndrome [AIDS]), and hepatitis B and C can be spread with contaminated pins; therefore it is mandatory that a new pin be used for each patient.
11. Key: because of the serrated edge, a key is the optimal instrument that should be used for plantar stimulation to elicit Babinski's reflex. Sharp or very smooth objects are ineffective.

TABLE B-2
Diagnostic Tests in Neurologic Disorders

Test	Anatomic/ physiologic basis	Most useful in
Electroencephalogram (EEG)	Spontaneous electrical activity of cerebral cortical neurons	Seizure disorders Metabolic encephalopathy Tumors Infectious encephalopathy Dementia Brain death determination
Visual evoked potentials (VEPs)	Arrival of electrical signals at the visual cortex through the visual pathways, when the retina is stimulated	Multiple sclerosis Disorders of optic nerve Lesions of optic tract, radiations, or occipital cortex
Brainstem auditory evoked potentials (BAEPs)	Passage of electrical signals through auditory nerve, auditory nuclei, lateral leminiscus, and inferior colliculus to auditory cortex	Acoustic neurilemmoma (neuroma) Brainstem tumor Brainstem infarct Multiple sclerosis
Somatosensory evoked potentials (SSEPs)	Passage of electrical signals through peripheral nerves to central somatosensory pathways (including dorsal columns, medial lemnisci, thalamus, thalamo-cortical pathways) and arrival at sensory cortex	Multiple sclerosis Spinal cord tumors Myelopathy
Nerve conduction studies	Conduction of electrical signals through myelinated nerve fibers (motor or sensory)	Peripheral neuropathy Nerve trauma Nerve compression (e.g., carpal tunnel syndrome)

Continued

TABLE B-2
Diagnostic Tests in Neurologic Disorders—cont'd

Test	Anatomic/physiologic basis	Most useful in
Needle electromyography (EMG)	Electrical activity of muscle during rest and voluntary contraction	Denervating disease (e.g., amyotrophic lateral sclerosis [ALS]) Muscular dystrophy Polymyositis
Repetitive nerve stimulation test (Jolly test)	Neuromuscular transmission	Myasthenia gravis Lambert-Eaton (myasthenic) syndrome
Muscle biopsy	Morphology and histochemistry of muscle fibers	Muscular dystrophy Polymyositis Metabolic disorders
Nerve biopsy	Morphology of axons and myelin	Peripheral neuropathy
Cerebrospinal fluid (CSF) study	CSF pressure, biochemistry, cell count, serology, microbiology	Meningitis Encephalitis Subarachnoid hemorrhage Multiple sclerosis Central nervous system (CNS) syphilis
Myelogram	Outline of spinal canal and its contents via radiopaque contrast in subarachnoid CSF space may be combined with computed tomography (CT)	Cervical or lumbar disc herniations Spinal cord tumors
Magnetic resonance imaging (MRI)	Different responses of protons in various tissues and compartment of nervous system to high-intensity magnetic fields	Multiple sclerosis Tumors (especially in posterior fossa) Spinal cord lesions Infarcts Malformations
Computed tomography (CT)	Different x-ray absorption coefficients of various tissues and compartments within nervous system	Hemorrhage Infarct Tumor Hydrocephalus Dementia Head trauma

12. Tuning forks (128 Hz and 256 Hz): use a 128-Hz tuning fork for measuring vibratory sense; use the higher-frequency (256 Hz) tuning fork to test auditory acuity.

13. Assorted small objects: these objects (penny, dime, sandpaper, silk, key, safety pin, etc.) can be used for testing astereognosis.

14. Syringe with soft plastic catheter: a syringe can be used for caloric testing with ice water.

15. Red piece of plastic or glass: these can be used for analysis of diplopia (the red-glass test).

16. Cotton-tipped swabs: a wisp from the end is useful for testing the corneal reflex; swabs can also be used to elicit the pharyngeal reflex.

17. Tongue depressor: a tongue depressor may be necessary for depressing the tongue when eliciting the pharyngeal reflex. When broken, it may also be used for eliciting cutaneous reflexes.

18. *Aids to the examination of the peripheral nervous system* (Her Majesty's Stationery Office, London): this compact reference provides a detailed description for the testing for peripheral nerve and muscle dysfunction.

EXAMINATION OF THE CRANIAL NERVES
Optic Nerve (Cranial Nerve II)
1. **Examining the optic fundus with the ophthalmoscope.**
   a. The room should not be totally darkened, since pupillary constriction will occur from shining the bright ophthalmoscope light into the patient's eye and the patient will not be able to see a fixation point. However, dimming the room lights may diminish glares and reflections from the cornea and iris that can be distracting and interfere with the examination of the retina.
   b. Instruct the patient to look at an object more than 5 feet away.
   c. In general, both the examiner and the patient should remove their eyeglasses (although contact lenses (except some very darkly tinted lenses) may be left in place.
   d. Ophthalmoscope lights should be as bright as possible, and the size of the light should be adjusted to match the size of the pupil. If the light is larger than the pupil, the fundus will be difficult to see because of light reflected from the iris.
   e. The examiner should use the right eye to examine the patient's right fundus and the left eye to examine the patient's left fundus.
   f. Systematically examine the fundus (Fig. B-1).

Common problems:
1. Pupils are too small: in selected cases in which information is vital, a drop of 1% tropicamide (Mydriacyl) or 2.5% neosynephrine may be used to dilate the pupils temporarily. An experienced examiner rarely needs to do this.

Caution: This should not be done in patients who have a history of glaucoma or have abnormally firm globes. Check pupillary reactions before using dilating agents. When pupillary size and reactivity may be of criti-

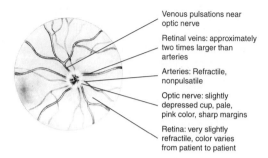

Venous pulsations near
optic nerve

Retinal veins: approximately
two times larger than
arteries

Arteries: Refractile,
nonpulsatile

Optic nerve: slightly
depressed cup, pale,
pink color, sharp margins

Retina: very slightly
refractile, color varies
from patient to patient

FIG. B-1 Funduscopic examination.

cal diagnostic significance (such as in head trauma, subarachnoid hemorrhage, or intercerebral hemorrhage), dilating agents should *not* be used.

2. Cataracts: unless very severe, the fundus still can be visualized. Dilation of the pupils may help.
3. Lens is absent (usually after a cataract operation): the fundus will appear small, but the usual features are still visible. Try using the +10D (+10 diopters) lens on the ophthalmoscope to visualize the retina.
4. Patient is uncooperative: the experienced examiner is quick and efficient; in rare cases sedation or restraints may be necessary. In children the examination of the fundus can be upsetting and should be performed at the conclusion of the neurologic examination, often with the infant or child sitting in the mother's lap.
5. There is difficulty locating the retina: beginners who have trouble locating the retina while looking through the ophthalmoscope can try identifying the red reflex through the zero diopter (0D lens) of the ophthalmoscope from a distance away from the eye and then move in closer.

Normal variations:

1. Congenital medullation of nerve fibers: White areas that fan out from the optic disc following the normal course of the retinal nerve fibers are of no pathologic significance but may be confused with papilledema.
2. Tigroid retina: The retina tends to be pale orange in light-skinned individuals and darkly pigmented in dark-skinned individuals; the tigroid retina resembles retinitis pigmentosa but has no pathologic significance.
3. Drusen: Whitish cobblestone-like projections near the optic disc may be mistaken for early papilledema.

Important abnormalities:

1. Papilledema (Fig. B-2): elevation of the optic nerve head is caused by any process that impedes venous return from the retina (such as increased intracranial pressure or right-sided heart failure) or any process that inflames the optic nerve (such as papillitis). Early signs of

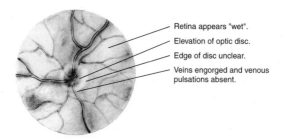

Retina appears "wet".
Elevation of optic disc.
Edge of disc unclear.
Veins engorged and venous pulsations absent.

FIG. B-2 Papilledema.

papilledema are slight blurring and elevation of the optic nerve, loss of venous pulsations (note that venous pulsations may be absent in 30% of normals), engorgement of the veins, an increased venous to arterial size (diameter) ratio, and a "wet" reflective appearance of the retina. Elevation of the optic nerve is measured by focusing from a high positive lens (such as +8D) to a less positive lens (such as +1D), until the surface of the optic nerve is in focus. Then, go back to the high positive lens and focus on the retina in the same manner. The difference in the power of the lenses necessary to focus on the retina and the optic nerve is the number of diopters of papilledema. For example, if the nerve is in focus at +4D and the retina is in focus at +1D, there are 3 diopters of papilledema.

Papillitis can be differentiated from papilledema by the early, rapid loss of visual acuity, which is not characteristic of papilledema.

2. **Examining visual fields.** If a visual field defect is *not* suspected, examine both eyes simultaneously (Fig. B-3).
   a. The examiner and the patient are seated approximately 2 feet apart. The patient is instructed to look at the examiner's nose. The examiner's fingers are midway between himself or herself and the patient and at the outer limit of vision.
   b. The examiner wiggles one finger and asks the patient to point to the one that moved. Both fingers are then wiggled simultaneously. Normally the patient will perceive all movements correctly.
   c. The process is repeated on the other diagonal.
   d. The visual field examination is concluded by the examiner placing his or her right hand over the patient's right eye. The examiner then closes his or her own left eye and instructs the patient to "look at the pupil in my right eye." The examiner brings the left finger toward the patient's nasal field on the diagonal while instructing the patient to "tell me when you can first see my finger." Normally both the patient and the examiner should see the finger at approximately the same time. The other eye is then tested similarly.

A

B

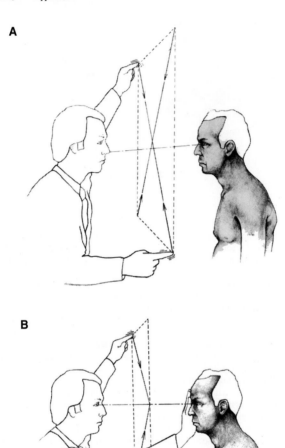

FIG. B-3 **A** and **B**, Visual field testing.

C

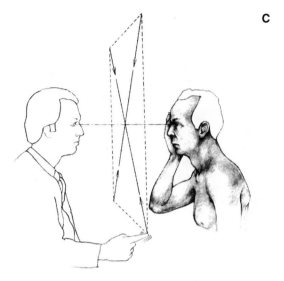

FIG. B-3, cont'd C, Visual field testing.

Important abnormalities:
1. With the phenomenon of "extinction" or "neglect," the patient correctly perceives finger movement individually but not simultaneously, suggesting a contralateral parietal lobe lesion.

If a defect is suspected or suggested by the screening procedure, each eye must be tested separately (Fig. B-3).

The patient should cover one eye (a patch may be necessary). The examiner then closes one of his or her own eyes (on the same side as the closed eye of the patient), and the patient and examiner look into each other's pupils. The examiner then brings his or her finger on the diagonal toward the midline until it is perceived by the patient. In effect, the examiner is comparing his or her visual field with that of the patient. The test is more accurate if the examiner uses a small red object, such as a 5-mm ball on a hat pin, as a target (Fig. B-4).

3. **Checking visual acuity (Fig. B-5).**
   a. Place the pocket Snellen chart approximately 14 inches (36 cm) from the eye.
   b. The room should be well lighted, the patient should wear any corrective lenses (eyeglasses or contact lenses), and one eye should be covered.
   c. The numbers on the chart that accompany the smallest type the patient can read indicate the patient's visual acuity. For example,

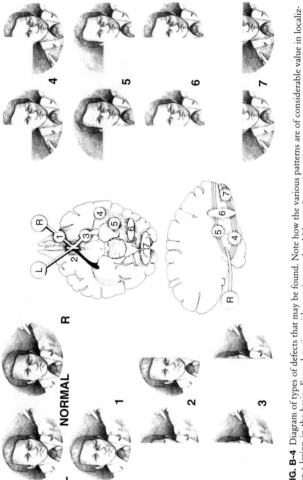

FIG. B-4 Diagram of types of defects that may be found. Note how the various patterns are of considerable value in localizing a lesion in the brain. Formal testing with a perimeter should be performed in all patients in whom a defect is demonstrated. Note that all visual input from the left side of the patient's environment ultimately goes to the right occipital lobe and all visual input above the horizontal goes below the calcarine fissure.

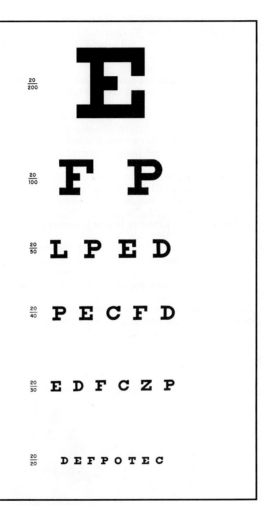

FIG. B-5 Snellen chart for testing visual acuity.

20/50 means that the patient can see at 20 feet what the normal individual can see at 50 feet.

Oculomotor (III), Trochlear (IV), and Abducens (VI)

Cranial nerves III, IV, and VI control movement of the eyes and are tested together. The third cranial nerve also controls pupillary size and eyelid elevation.

1. Testing ocular movement
   a. Place one hand on the patient's head to prevent the natural tendency to turn the head as the eyes follow an object. Instruct the patient to follow the examiner's finger as it moves laterally in the horizontal plane. Continue the lateral movement until the outer edge of the iris (limbus) of the *adducting* eye (eye moving medially) just touches the punctum (the red area at the medial corner of the eye). Then test lateral movement in the opposite direction (Fig. B-6, *A*).
   b. Test vertical movement by having the patient look upward at the examiner's finger (Fig. B-6, *B*). Then quickly bring the finger down (observing how quickly the lids follow) for downward gaze. In Fig. B-6, *C*, there is "lid lag" suggestive of thyroid disease.
   c. Finally, ask the patient to look at his or her nose and observe for constriction of the pupils.
2. Testing pupillary reaction to direct light: the swinging flashlight test should be performed using a bright, pinpoint source of light to determine both direct and consensual pupillary reaction. This test is used to detect the Marcus Gunn pupil (Figs. B-7, *A* and B-7, *B*).

Common abnormalities:
1. Marcus Gunn pupil: when the sequence for testing the pupillary reaction to direct light (swinging flashlight test) is used, a pupil that

A

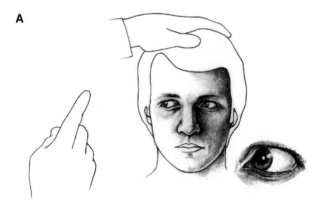

FIG. B-6 A, Horizontal eye movement.

apparently dilates to direct light may be observed. This phenomenon ("afferent pupillary defect") occurs with a lesion in the optic nerve anterior to the optic chiasm in which the consensual pupillary reflex is preserved, whereas the direct reflex is impaired (i.e., the pupil dilates because there is less stimulus for pupillary constriction from light shown directly into the abnormal eye, whereas maximal pupillary constriction occurs from the consensual reflex when light is shown in the normal eye) (Fig. B-7, *C*).

2. Nystagmus: nystagmus is a rhythmic, involuntary abnormal eye movement that may be present at rest or induced by eye movement and persists after eye movement has ceased. Nystagmus can be described as slow deviation of the eye in one direction with quick jerking eye movements in the opposite direction. By convention, nystagmus is named for its quick component. The following types may be noted:

   a. "End point" nystagmus (also called *physiologic nystagmus*) results when the normal patient gazes too far laterally. Therefore the examiner should have the patient gaze laterally only to the point where the edge of the iris or limbus of the adducting eye meets the lacrimal punctum.

   b. Asymmetrical lateral nystagmus (absent or reduced in one direction of gaze compared to the opposite direction of gaze) suggests either CNS or end organ dysfunction.

B

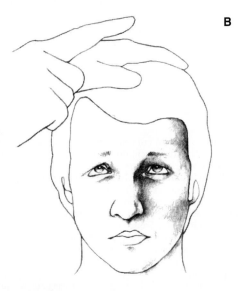

FIG. B-6, cont'd **B,** Vertical eye movement.

Continued

C

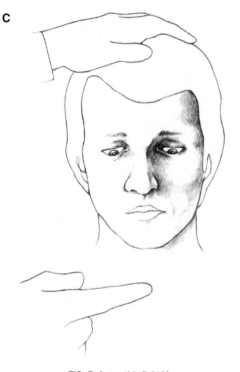

FIG. B-6, cont'd C, Lid lag.

c. Nystagmus with the fast component upward (upbeat nystagmus) or with the fast component downward (downbeat nystagmus), often most easily elicited on upward or downward gaze, usually indicates CNS disease, often at the level of the brainstem.

d. Nystagmus associated with dysconjugate eye movements or nystagmus in only one eye (monocular nystagmus), such as internuclear ophthalmoplegia (see page 378) in multiple sclerosis (MS), would be indicative of CNS disease.

e. Congenital nystagmus is pendular lateral nystagmus that disappears with convergence and has a lateral movement even on upward gaze. It is usually associated with congenital bilateral visual impairment (blindness).

f. Drug-induced or CNS nystagmus: if nystagmus is equal in both directions of gaze, suspect toxic or metabolic disorder; rarely brainstem dysfunction may produce similar nystagmus.

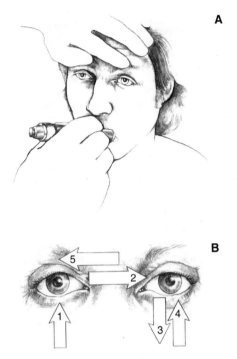

FIG. B-7 The swinging flashlight test. Instruct the patient to keep the eyelids open while a light is flashed in the eyes. (The examiner may need to hold the eyelids open, **A.**) The sequence of light movement is depicted by numbered arrows in **B.** Swing the light from below up to the first eye, shining the light directly into the pupil. The pupil in the tested eye should immediately constrict, as should the pupil in the opposite eye. Then quickly swing the light to the opposite eye; there should be no change in the size of either pupil. Swing the light down from the second eye; both pupils should dilate promptly; then swing the light back up to the second eye (pupils should constrict) and quickly back to the first eye (no change in pupillary size).

Continued

3. Third nerve palsy: (Fig. B-8, *A*) the oculomotor nerve (third cranial nerve) innervates all extraocular muscles (including the levator of the upper eyelid) except the lateral rectus and the superior oblique. Thus with a complete third nerve palsy, the eye is abducted and deviated slightly downward, the upper eyelid droops, and the pupil is dilated and unreactive to light. Because the autonomic pupillary constrictor fibers are in the periphery of this nerve, when diabetic vascular disease affects the third nerve (by producing infarction), the pupil is frequently

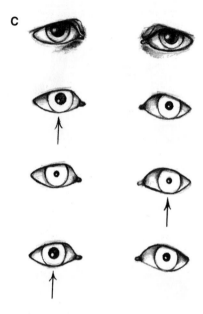

FIG. B-7, cont'd C, Marcus Gunn pupil.

spared. In contrast, when the third nerve is damaged by cerebral herniation resulting from a temporal lobe mass causing the nerve to be compressed against the tentorium, or compression by a posterior communicating artery aneurysm, the peripheral pupillary fibers are affected first and the pupil frequently dilates before paralysis of the extraocular muscles occurs.

4. Sixth nerve palsy: (Fig. B-8, *B*) the abducens nerve (sixth cranial nerve) innervates the lateral rectus muscle. Therefore with sixth nerve palsy, the eye is in an adducted position and does not move laterally beyond the midline. The pupil is not affected. A sixth nerve palsy may be a false localizing sign and is frequently seen with raised intracranial pressure.

5. Internuclear ophthalmoplegia (INO): (Fig. B-8, *C*) this abnormality superficially resembles a medial rectus palsy except that the ability to converge and look at a near object is spared. When the patient attempts to look laterally, the *abducting* eye moves laterally and develops nystagmus, whereas the *adducting* eye does not move past the midline. The abnormality is caused by a lesion of the medial longitudinal fasciculus in the central part of the pons and is often associated with MS.

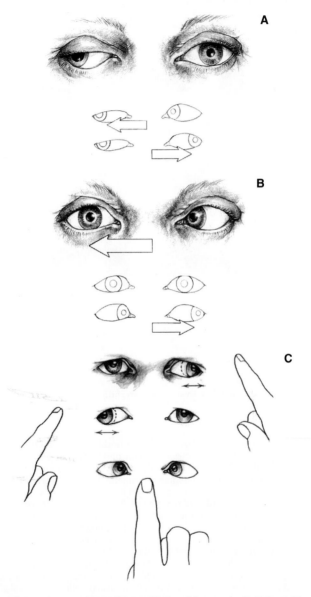

FIG. B-8 Ocular nerve abnormalities. **A,** Third cranial nerve palsy. **B,** Sixth cranial nerve palsy. **C,** Internuclear ophthalmoplegia.

Continued

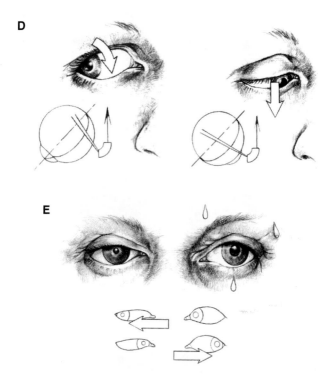

FIG. B-8, cont'd D, Fourth cranial nerve palsy. E, Horner's syndrome.

6. Fourth nerve palsy: (Fig. B-8, *D*) the trochlear nerve (fourth cranial nerve) innervates the superior oblique muscle that rotates the top of the globe toward the nose in the abducted position and turns the globe downward in the adducted position. The muscle normally functions to keep the visual image upright by rotating the eye slightly during minor sideward head movements. Patients with fourth nerve palsy will complain of a vertical diplopia, especially when looking downward at relatively near objects (e.g., walking down stairs). Patients may develop a slight head tilt to prevent this diplopia. Isolated fourth nerve palsy is often caused by diabetes or head trauma.

7. Horner's syndrome: (Fig. B-8, *E*) Horner's syndrome is caused by damage to the sympathetic nerve supply to the eye and not by damage to cranial nerves III, IV, or VI. The pupil is small (miotic), there is a slight drooping of the eyelid (ptosis), and sweating on that side of the face is impaired (anhidrosis). Damage may occur anywhere in the course of

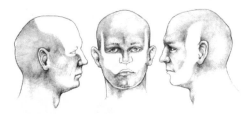

FIG. B-9 Trigeminal nerve. The divisions are ophthalmic, maxillary, and mandibular.

the sympathetic pathway from the hypothalamus to the eye globe; some of the more common lesion sites are the cervical spinal cord, apex of the lungs (affecting the sympathetic chain), and along the carotid artery (atherosclerotic damage at the carotid bifurcation).
8. Argyll Robertson pupil: an Argyll Robertson pupil is an irregular small pupil that does not react to direct light but constricts on accommodation; it is classically described with neurosyphilis.

Trigeminal Nerve (V)
The fifth cranial nerve provides sensation for the face and cornea (Fig. B-9).
1. Elicit the corneal reflex in both eyes (Fig. B-10).

Caution: False results will be obtained if the examiner elicits a blink to threat or if the sclera, rather than cornea, is touched.

2. Testing facial sensation: if the patient has an abnormal corneal reflex (an asymmetric or absent blink) or if the patient complains of pain, numbness, paresthesias, or other sensory disturbances about the face, check each division of the trigeminal nerve bilaterally with a wisp of cotton (light touch) and a pin (pain). (For technique, see the following section on sensory testing.)
Common abnormalities:
1. If the patient has fifth cranial nerve dysfunction, the eye on that side will not blink to direct touch but will blink when the opposite cornea is touched, and the patient will report a difference in sensation between the eyes.
2. If the patient has facial nerve (seventh cranial nerve) paralysis, the eye on that side will not blink regardless of which cornea is touched, although the patient will report sensation is the same in each eye. A partial facial nerve paralysis may be evident as a slower blink on the affected side compared to the normal side.

Caveat: The trigeminal nerve also innervates the muscles of mastication, and if affected, the jaw will deviate toward the side of the lesion during jaw opening.

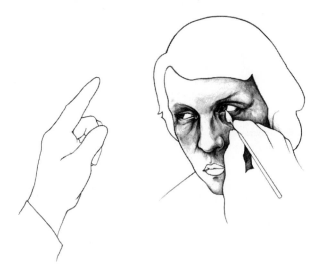

FIG. B-10 Corneal reflex. Tease a wisp of cotton from the end of a clean cotton-tipped applicator. Tell the patient what will be done before the test. Ask the patient to look laterally and lightly touch the cornea, approaching laterally from the side opposite the gaze. (This avoids a threat reflex.) Be certain to touch the cornea and not just the sclera. Normally, a rapid involuntary blink will occur and both eyes blink simultaneously. Finally, ask the patient if the wisp of cotton feels the same in both corneas.

Facial Nerve (VII)

1. Observation for facial asymmetries (Fig. B-11, *A*): on close inspection, many normal patients have slight asymmetries of the nasolabial folds and height of the palpebral fissures (size of the eyelid opening). However, excessive flattening of one nasolabial fold or excessive opening of one palpebral fissure is abnormal.
2. Observation of facial movement (Fig. B-11, *B*)
   a. Instruct the patient to grimace ("show me your teeth" usually communicates this movement) and wrinkle the forehead (Fig. B-11, *C*), observing for any asymmetry.
   b. To resolve doubt concerning weakness, instruct the patient to close the eyelids tightly; attempt to open them as illustrated in Fig. B-11, *D*. When the eyelids are tightly closed, the eyelashes are not visible. If the eyelashes are seen, there may be partial facial nerve palsy. The examiner can also instruct the patient to puff out his or her cheeks while the examiner taps on them; a tap on the weak side more easily expels air (Fig. B-11, *E*).

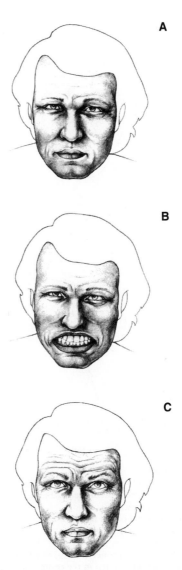

FIG. B-11 A, Observation for facial asymmetry. **B,** Observation for facial movement (grimace and wrinkle forehead). **C,** Wrinkling the forehead.

Continued

D

E

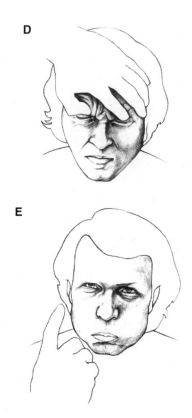

FIG. B-11, cont'd D, Forcibly opening eyes. **E,** Blowing out cheeks.

Common problems:
1. Absent teeth may create the impression of facial paralysis.
2. Asymmetry of movement is a more reliable sign of abnormality than asymmetry of appearance.
3. A patient with bilateral partial facial palsy may appear normal but will not be able to voluntarily show teeth.

Common abnormalities:
1. A patient with upper motor neuron weakness (lesion above the brainstem facial nucleus, most often in the contralateral motor cortex) will be able to wrinkle the forehead (and partially close the eyelids) but will have paresis of the remainder of the face (Fig. B-12). These patients may have preserved facial movements with emotion.

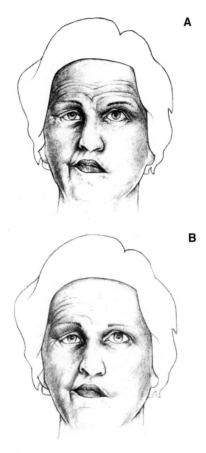

FIG. B-12 A, Upper motor neuron facial weakness. **B,** Lower motor neuron facial weakness.

2. A patient with a lower motor neuron facial weakness (lesion in the brainstem facial nucleus or along the facial nerve) will have weakness of all the facial muscles (including the forehead) on the same side as the lesion.

Auditory Nerve (VIII)

1. Testing of auditory acuity bilaterally: auditory acuity may be tested by lightly rubbing the fingers together several inches from the patient's ears (Fig. B-13, *A*).

A

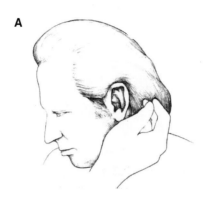

FIG. B-13 A, Testing auditory acuity.

2. Confirming a deficit in auditory acuity: if a hearing deficit is demonstrated, the Weber's and Rinne tests should be performed.
   a. Rinne test (Fig. B-13, *B*): lightly tap a 256-Hz tuning fork and place it firmly against the mastoid process. Ask the patient to indicate when it is no longer heard. Then place it in front of the external auditory meatus and note the period of time during which it is heard. A normal individual will have a positive Rinne test in which the tuning fork is heard twice as long by air conduction as by bone conduction.
   b. Weber's test (Fig. B-13, *C*): tap a 256-Hz tuning fork lightly, place the base of the fork on the forehead, and ask, "Is the buzzing equally loud in both ears?" The normal patient will answer, "The buzzing is the same in both ears."

Common problems:
1. Diminished auditory acuity is misdiagnosed because of wax or other foreign matter in the ear.
2. A high or low frequency loss is missed because specific frequencies are not tested.

Common abnormalities:
1. Conductive hearing loss (usually otosclerosis): bone conduction is greater than air conduction (Rinne test), and the tuning fork on the forehead lateralizes to the affected ear (Weber's test).
2. Sensorineural loss: air conduction is greater than bone conduction (Rinne test), and the tuning fork on the forehead lateralizes to the *normal* ear (Weber's test)

Glossopharyngeal Nerve (IX) and Vagus Nerve (X)

1. Observation of soft palate. Instruct the patient to open the mouth; the arches of the soft palate should be symmetric.

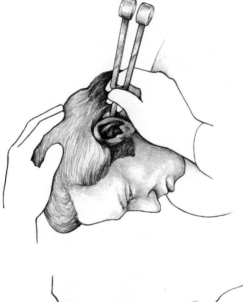

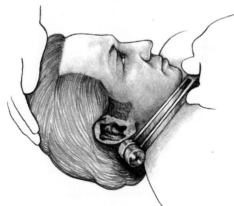

FIG. B-13, cont'd B, Rinne test.

Continued

B

C

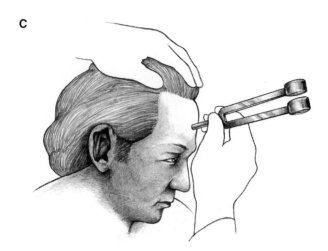

FIG. B-13, cont'd C, Weber's test.

2. Observation of palate movement. Instruct the patient to say "ah" and observe symmetric elevation of the soft palate.
3. Eliciting the pharyngeal reflex (Fig. B-14). Touch both sides of the soft palate with a cotton-tipped applicator and observe the symmetric elevation of the soft palate. Ask the patient if the sensation is the same on both sides.
4. Listen to voice quality.

Common problems:
1. If the tongue interferes with adequate visualization of the palate, depress it with a flashlight on a wooden tongue depressor.
2. Some normal individuals may have bilateral slight or absent pharyngeal reflexes; sensation, however, remains normal. It is not necessary to make the patient gag. Stimulation with a tongue depressor rather than a cotton applicator is not necessary.

Common abnormalities:
1. A unilateral vagal nerve (X) paresis results in failure of the palate to move either voluntarily or to sensory stimulation. The arch will be asymmetric, and the uvula will deviate toward the normal side (Fig. B-15).
2. Patients with bilateral vagal paralysis will have little or no palatal movement and, in addition, will exhibit considerable difficulty in swallowing, but the uvula will be midline.
3. With palatal weakness, the voice has a nasal quality (from air escaping into the nose), whereas with vocal cord paresis the voice is hoarse.

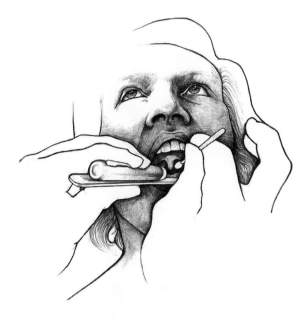

FIG. B-14 Pharyngeal reflex.

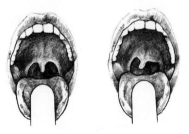

FIG. B-15 Palatal deviation caused by unilateral vagal nerve paralysis.

Spinal Accessory Nerve (XI)

1. Testing the strength of sternocleidomastoid and trapezius muscles
   a. Instruct the patient to turn the head to one side and keep it there. Attempt to overcome this resistance by pushing at the angle of the jaw (Fig. B-16, *A*).
   b. Instruct the patient to shrug the shoulders. Place both hands on the shoulders and attempt to push them down (Fig. B-16, *B*).

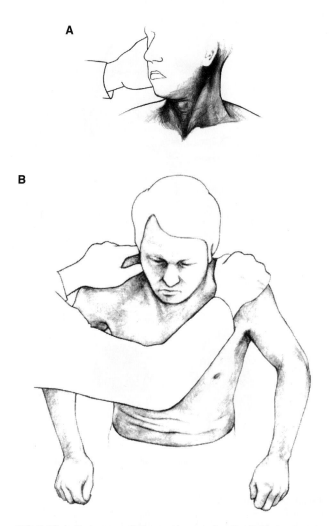

FIG. B-16 A, Testing sternocleidomastoid muscle function. **B,** Testing trapezius muscle function.

c. Instruct the patient to extend the shoulders by placing the hands forward on the wall when standing. Observe for winging of the scapula with shoulder extension.

Common problems:

1. The examiner forgets that the left sternocleidomastoid muscle turns the head to the right.
2. Neck pain or limitation of motion interferes with proper testing of muscle strength.

Common abnormalities:

1. Weakness of these muscles is rare except when the lower motor neuron portion is injured. Cerebral lesions usually cause only minimal weakness.
2. Weakness of the trapezius muscle may lead to drooping and winging of the scapula.

Hypoglossal Nerve (XII)

1. Testing tongue movement. Instruct the patient to stick out the tongue; observe carefully for deviation, symmetry, and abnormal movements (Fig. B-17, *A*).

Common problem:

1. A patient with a facial nerve paralysis may give the illusion of having a deviated tongue. The illusion is proved false when the crease in the middle of the tongue lines up with the tip of the nose.

Common abnormalities:

1. A cerebral lesion (upper motor neuron) causes slight or no deviation of the tongue.
2. A lesion of the hypoglossal nucleus, or the twelfth cranial nerve, causes the tongue to deviate toward the side of the lesion and, with time, ipsilateral atrophy. Atrophy gives the tongue a wrinkled appearance (Fig. B-17, *B*).
3. A tongue may be normally "wiggly." Fibrillations are best seen at the lateral edge of a tongue when it is lying in the mouth. Retract the inside of the cheek with a tongue blade and shine a flashlight onto the lateral edge of the tongue.

STATION AND GAIT

In an area with 20 feet of straight walking space (with the patient barefooted and in hospital gown), the patient is instructed to perform a series of tasks to assess station and gait (Table B-3 and Fig. B-18). By doing the station and gait testing in this manner, a skillful examiner can obtain in 1 minute a glimpse of mental status (how well the patient comprehends instructions), upper motor neuron function (posturing of arms and by gait), lower motor neuron function (muscle atrophy and weakness), muscle disease (proximal weakness), basal ganglia (abnormal posture movement), cerebellum (balance and tandem walk), and the sensory system (poor balance with eyes closed [the Romberg test]). Station and gait testing serves as a "screening neurologic examination." A patient who can perform all the maneuvers normally will rarely have a significant neurologic

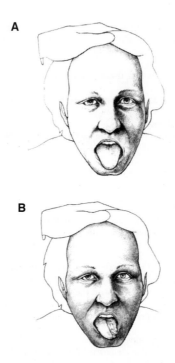

FIG. B-17 A, Tongue protrusion. **B,** Tongue deviation.

abnormality. Abnormalities noted can be more specifically tested in the remainder of the neurologic examination. For example, if station and gait testing suggests cerebellar abnormality, more specific cerebellar tests should be performed.

Common problems:

1. The examiner forgets to perform the station and gait testing (one of the most valuable parts of the neurologic examination) because the examination is conducted only with the patient lying in bed.
2. The examiner does not adequately protect the ataxic patient, who may fall and be injured.
3. The examiner fixates on the patient's legs and forgets to look at the arms for associated abnormal postures (dystonic) or lessened arm swing.
4. Modesty must be preserved with appropriate clothing to allow the patient to walk with the arms free. Clothing should not be too long as to cover the feet.

TABLE B-3
Procedure for Station and Gait Testing

Instructions	Things to note
Walk the distance normally.	Asymmetric arm swing, abnormal arm and hand postures, and instability of the trunk should be noted.
Rapidly turn around and walk on tiptoe.	Extra steps while turning around and inability to rise completely on the tips of the toes should be noted.
Rapidly turn and walk on heels.	Foot drop should be noted.
Turn and walk with heels touching toes (tandem walk).	Instability characteristic of midline cerebellar lesions should be noted.
Turn and "walk on outsides of feet like a bowlegged cowboy does" (walking on lateral aspects of feet).	This maneuver specifically brings out hemiplegic posturing of an arm from subtle or old upper motor neuron damage.
Do a deep knee bend (preferably with hands on hips; if there is an obvious balance problem, patient may hold onto an object, such as a chair).	Loss of balance indicates cerebellar difficulties; inability to rise indicates proximal weakness.
Stand with feet together, eyes closed, and arms outstretched with palms facing ceiling and fingers spread apart.	Increased swaying with eyes closed indicates either posterior column disease or a peripheral neuropathy; with subtle hemiparesis the affected arm will pronate, whereas in more obvious hemiparesis the arm will pronate and then drift downward and outward.

5. Uninformed examiners incorrectly interpret the Romberg test as a cerebellar sign.

EVALUATION OF TENDON (MUSCLE STRETCH) REFLEXES AND PLANTAR STIMULATION
Muscle Stretch Reflexes
Technique for eliciting tendon reflexes
1. A muscle stretch (or tendon) reflex is the brief contraction of a muscle in response to a sudden stretch. The reflex therefore depends on the following factors:
   a. Whether the tendon is struck.
   b. How hard the tendon is struck.
   c. How quickly the tendon is struck.

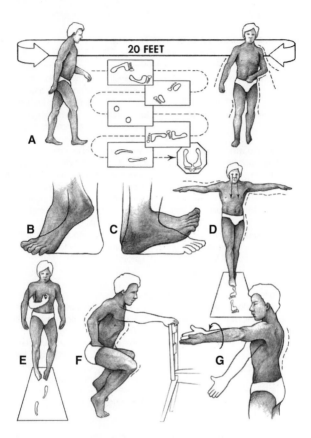

FIG. B-18 Station and gait testing.

2. Reflex hammers:
   a. A hammer with a soft rubber head and flexible handle will aid the examiner in delivering a quick tap.
   b. A hammer with a long handle will aid in more accurate grading of reflexes and tapping the tendons in inconvenient positions.
   c. We prefer a Queen's Square style of hammer that is available in two sizes–a small one for children and a large one for adults.
3. Grading reflexes: reflexes are normal, hypoactive, absent, hyperactive, or clonic. Muscle stretch reflexes may be graded as follows: 0, absent; +, present but diminished; ++, normal; +++, increased but not

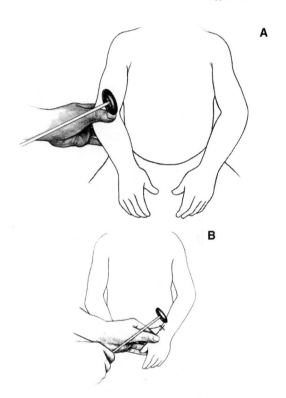

FIG. B-19 A, Biceps reflex. B, Brachioradialis reflex.

Continued

necessarily to a pathologic degree; $+++$, markedly hyperactive often with associated clonus.

4. Muscle contraction may be observed or felt.

Specific "routine" reflexes

1. Biceps reflex (C5 and C6 spinal roots: musculocutaneous nerve) (Fig. B-19, *A*): the arms must be slightly flexed, relaxed, and symmetrically resting on the patient's thighs. The examiner lightly presses the biceps tendon with the thumb and taps the thumb with the hammer. Elbow flexion will be observed, and contraction of the biceps tendon against the thumb will be felt.

2. Brachioradialis reflex (C5 and C6 spinal roots; radial nerve) (Fig. B-19, *B*): with the arms positioned and relaxed as in eliciting the biceps reflex, a tap is delivered above the styloid process at the distal end of

C

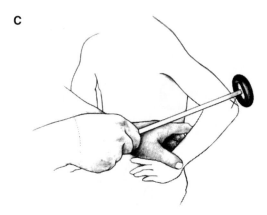

FIG. B-19, cont'd C, Triceps reflex.

the radius. Elbow flexion and slight outward rotation of the forearm will be observed.

3. Triceps reflex (C6, C7, and C8 spinal roots; radial nerve) (Fig. B-19, *C*): with the patient's arms resting on the hips, the examiner identifies (by palpation) the triceps tendon just above the bony prominence of the elbow (olecranon), and then delivers a tap to this tendon. Contraction of the triceps muscle will be observed along with elbow extension.

4. Patellar (knee) reflex (L2, L3, and L4 spinal roots; femoral nerve) (Fig. B-20, *A*): the patient should be sitting with the knees slightly beyond the edge of the table and the legs relaxed, dangling, and not touching the floor. The patellar tendon should be palpated before it is tapped (this is especially important in obese patients or patients with a bony deformity). Tapping the patellar tendon results in knee extension. In some patients with hypoactive reflexes or in whom the tendon is difficult to localize, placing the thumb on the tendon and tapping the thumb may elicit the reflex. In addition to eliciting the patellar reflex, the examiner should observe for contraction of the ipsilateral or contralateral adductor muscle or contralateral quadriceps (such abnormal reflex spread is seen with hyperactive reflexes) and excessive swinging of the leg back and forth. (This "pendular" reflex is an indication of hypotonia.)

5. Achilles (ankle) reflex (S1 spinal root; tibial nerve) (Fig. B-20, *B*): with the patient in the same position as for the patellar reflex, the examiner places his or her hand under the patient's foot and slightly extends the foot. The patient is instructed to apply light pressure to the palm of the examiner's hand while the examiner strikes the Achilles tendon. The foot should move downward against the examiner's hand.

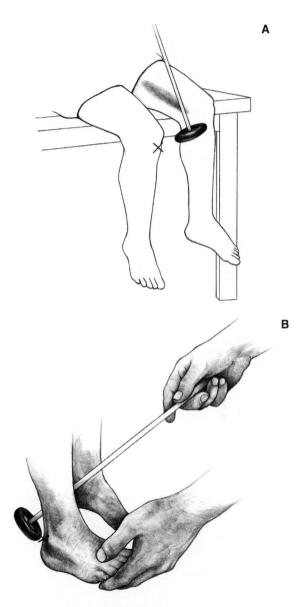

FIG. B-20 A, Patellar reflex. **B,** Achilles reflex.

Common problems:
1. The patient is not appropriately undressed.
2. A reflex hammer with an aged, hard rubber head is used.
3. The patient is not relaxed or is improperly positioned.
4. An inexperienced examiner reports a reflex as present when it is really absent. (Usually the inexperienced examiner does this out of anxiety that the reflex was missed because his technique was defective and that a more experienced examiner will find the reflex present.) REMEMBER: There is some normal variability in reflex activity such that two quite experienced examiners may find slightly different degrees of reflex activity.
5. Reflexes should be present in normal elderly patients; however, peripheral nerve dysfunction from a variety of causes is very common in elderly patients who thus have absent reflexes on the basis of pathologic findings.

Common abnormalities:
1. Hyperactive reflexes: tense patients tend to have brisk reflexes, and there is a wide range of what is considered "normal." Pathologic hyperactive reflexes tend to have a "spread" of reflex activity (e.g., muscles distal from the one whose tendon is being tapped also contract [a crossed adductor response when tapping the adductor tendon on one side] or finger flexion when the biceps tendon is tapped). The presence of a pectoral reflex is also pathologic. Hyperactive reflexes suggest an upper motor neuron lesion.
2. Clonus may be elicited by rapidly dorsiflexing the ankle; a rhythmic alternating dorsiflexion (extension) and plantar flexion of the ankle ensue and may last seconds to minutes (Fig. B-21). Clonus indicates an upper motor neuron lesion, although patients who tense their calf muscles because of anxiety may have unsustained clonus.
3. Absent reflexes suggest damage to any part of the reflex arc: muscle spindle or sensory or motor nerves. An absent Achilles (ankle) reflex has a different sound (a "thud") than that elicited with a normally active reflex.

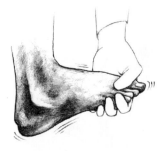

FIG. B-21 Ankle clonus.

4. A slowed relaxation phase of the Achilles reflex suggests hypothyroidism.
5. The most common abnormality observed is *reflex asymmetry*, rather than absent or hyperactive reflexes. Asymmetries are best appreciated by using the lightest tap possible that will still elicit the reflex. Many examiners strike the tendons with too much force. The advantage of the Queen's Square hammer is that, rather than striking the patellar tendon, it can be dropped by gravity at equal distances from the right and left. Using the minimal distance necessary to elicit a knee jerk will usually make any asymmetry more obvious.

Plantar Responses
Technique for eliciting the plantar response
1. The plantar response is a complex cutaneous reflex; the type of response elicited depends on the type of stimulation used (we recommend a key), how quickly the stimulus is delivered, and the position of the patient. The key is used to stimulate the lateral aspect of the plantar surface of the foot beginning at the heel and moving up to the ball of the foot, staying lateral to the great toe (Fig. B-22 and Table B-4).
2. Because the abnormal plantar response is such an important sign of nervous system disease, the best approach to recording the results, if in doubt, is to record exactly the observed movements.

Common problems:
1. Too sharp a stimulus is used and a withdrawal reflex is elicited.
2. Too light a stimulus is used, and no response occurs.
3. The response may change from time to time depending on the time of day, medication, and the patient's position (sitting or lying). Since the character of the plantar reflex may change with position, stimulation should be done with the patient in both the lying and sitting positions in a situation where the response is critical.
4. The examiner brings the stimulus over the base of the big toe, causing mechanical flexion of the big toe.

MUSCLE APPEARANCE, STRENGTH, RANGE OF MOTION, AND INVOLUNTARY MOVEMENTS
1. Plan the evaluation of muscles on the basis of the history, station and gait testing, reflex examination, and coordination.

Remember, reflex examination and station and gait testing involve the following:
   a. Distal strength (the ability to walk on tiptoes and heels).
   b. Proximal strength (the ability to perform deep knee bends while holding arms outstretched and the ability to rise from sitting position).
   c. Abnormal postures and movement.
   d. Abnormal muscle bulk by observation.
   e. Abnormal tone (hyperactive reflexes suggest hypertonia; pendular reflexes suggest hypotonia).

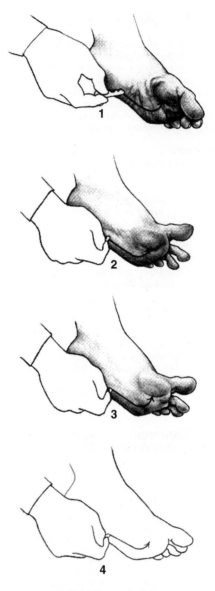

FIG. B-22 Plantar stimulation.

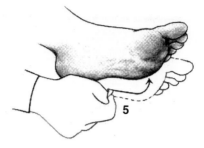

FIG. B-22, cont'd

TABLE B-4
Responses to Plantar Stimulation

Name	Observation	Interpretation
Normal response (flexor plantar response)	First movement of great toe is flexion.	Normal
Classic Babinski's reflex (classic extensor plantar response)	Extension of great toe with extension and fanning of other toes occur.	Most often seen in upper motor neuron lesions (below the foramen magnum)
Babinski's reflex (extensor plantar response)	First movement of great toe is extension (there may be subsequent flexion of great toes); other toes either show no movement or flexion.	Seen in upper motor neuron lesions (especially above the foramen magnum)
Mute plantar response	Nothing happens.	Seen in severe sensory loss or paralysis of foot
Withdrawal	Patient pulls foot away.	Often seen in toxic-metabolic peripheral neuropathies
Asymmetric response	Mute plantar response on one side and flexor plantar response on other side occur.	Is indication of need to look for other signs of neurologic disease

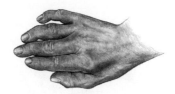

FIG. B-23 Hand atrophy.

    f. Abnormal coordination (may be a sign of weakness as well as cerebellar disease).

Therefore if the station and gait testing and reflex examination are normal and the patient does not complain of weakness, cramps, stiffness or a change in muscle bulk, detailed muscle testing may not be necessary.

2. Common abnormalities seen on an inspection.

    a. Muscle atrophy is often best appreciated by looking at the muscle (first dorsal interosseous) between the thumb and first finger. Normally, the superficial contour in this area should be convex; with atrophy it is flat or concave. The thenar and hypothenar areas should also have a convex surface; with atrophy they become flat (Fig. B-23).

    b. If atrophy is present in the thighs, upper arms, or forearms, the degree of wasting should be documented by measurement. For example, if atrophy of the gastrocnemii is suspected, measure from a convenient landmark (e.g., the lateral malleolus to the midpoint of the muscle) and then measure the girth of the legs bilaterally at these points (Fig. B-24).

    c. Muscle hypertrophy is rare and is most commonly seen in the gastrocnemii of boys with Duchenne's muscular dystrophy.

    d. Fasciculations are seen as brief (less than 1 second), troughlike dimpling of the skin over the muscle. They are easiest to see in large muscles with the use of cross-lighting. Several light taps with a percussion hammer may precipitate a flurry of fasciculations, but clinical conclusions from fasciculations elicited in this manner should be made with caution (Fig. B-25).

3. Testing muscle strength.

    a. For suspected muscle weakness, first have the patient contract the muscle and allow the full normal movement of the body part to take place. Then instruct the patient to hold that posture while you attempt to return the body part to a more neutral position (Fig. B -26). For example, to test the bicep muscle, tell the patient to "make a muscle like Popeye." (You might even demonstrate the movement to the patient.) Then grasp the forearm near the elbow and tell the patient, "don't let me extend your arm," while applying force to extend the arm.

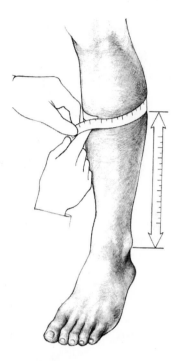

FIG. B-24 Measurement of leg girth.

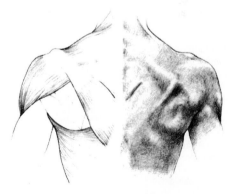

FIG. B-25 Fasciculations in back muscles.

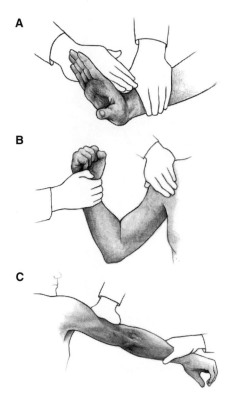

FIG. B-26 Muscle strength testing.

Most muscles in the body can be tested in a similar manner; we recommend that examiners keep a copy of *Aids to the examination of the peripheral nervous system* for quick reference in case detailed muscle testing is required.

   b. Formal grading of muscle strength: the following classification of strength is most commonly used (derived by the British Medical Research Council and termed the *MRC scale*):

5	Normal, full strength.
4	Movement against resistance that can be overcome.
3	Movement is possible against gravity (e.g., the patient can flex the supinated arm until the hand touches the shoulder, Fig. B-27).
2	Movement is possible only when the force of gravity is eliminated (e.g., with the shoulder abducted, the patient can flex and extend the arm on the horizontal plane, Fig. B-27).

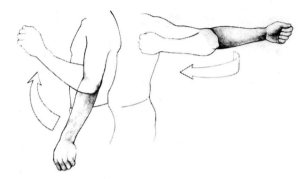

FIG. B-27 Medical Research Council (MRC) muscle testing.

| 1 | Contraction of muscle is seen or palpated but no movement takes place. |
| 0 | No muscle contraction is apparent. |

Caveat: As many as 60% of the myofibers in a given muscle may be destroyed without producing a clinically detectable weakness. The majority of weak patients will fall into the "4" category, which is subjective; therefore the grading system is not perfect.

    c. Functional grading of muscle strength: in patients whose weakness may be either improving or deteriorating, it is important to test and document their strength frequently. Pick a task that a patient can perform, but just barely. Suggestions include (Fig. B-28) the following:
       1) Rise from a chair with the arms crossed.
       2) Raise the arms above the head.
       3) Extend the leg from a sitting position.
       4) Hop on one foot.
4. Testing range of movement.
    a. If muscles are not periodically stretched, they lose their elasticity and become pathologically shortened in what is termed a *contracture.* Thus a patient with a hemiplegia may not be able to fully extend the elbow, not because of weakness but because the length of the biceps makes it impossible to do so.
    b. The range of motion may also be limited by pain, muscle spasm, or a joint deformity.
5. Abnormal muscle tone: instruct the patient to relax an arm "like a rag doll." The examiner then flexes and extends the forearm. The following abnormalities may be noted:
    a. An increased resistance to passive movement that is greater at the start of the movement and becomes less as the movement is

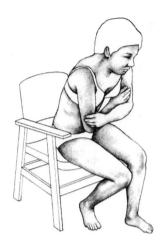

FIG. B-28 Rising from a chair.

completed is known as the *clasp knife phenomenon* and may be seen in severe upper motor neuron lesions.

   b. Increased resistance throughout the range of movement is known as *lead pipe rigidity* and may be seen in the parkinsonian syndrome.

   c. A severely floppy extremity is hypotonic, which is seen in severe peripheral nerve lesions and cerebellar disease. Acute upper motor neuron lesions cause an initial hypotonia before hypertonia.

6. Abnormal posture and movement.

   a. Chorea and athetosis are abnormal movements that really are repetitive assumptions of inappropriate postures. Call the movement *athetosis* if it is proximal and writhing and *chorea* if it is jerky in nature, distal and irregularly irregular in rhythm.

   b. Tremor is an involuntary, rhythmic oscillatory movement of a body part proximal or distal, as seen in familial (senile) tremor, benign essential tremor, parkinsonian syndrome, and thyrotoxicosis. It may also be seen only with action, as in cerebellar or cerebellar outflow lesions. It may be present both at rest and with action, as in midbrain disease (rubral tremor).

   c. Myoclonus is a spontaneous, irregular, rapid contraction of a part of a muscle causing movement across a joint. It is caused by the simultaneous contraction of agonists and antagonists and may occur focally, multifocally, or generalized. When axial musculature is involved, sudden falls in which the patient seems thrown to the ground can occur.

   d. Asterixis is elicited by having the patient dorsiflex the wrists. Brief lapses in tone make the patient appear to be waving "bye-bye" (Fig. B-29).

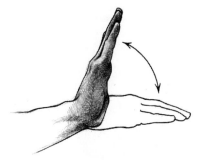

FIG. B-29 Asterixis.

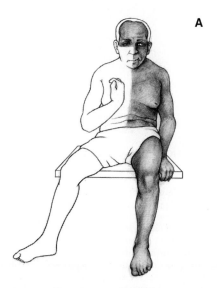

A

FIG. B-30 A, Hemiplegic posture.

Continued

e. Common abnormal postures include the hemiplegic posture (flexion of elbow and wrist, adduction of the shoulder, extension of the
leg and feet) (Fig. B-30, *A*) and the parkinsonian posture (forward
flexion of the body, shoulders internally rotated, arms at side with
palms facing backward) (Fig. B-30, *B*).

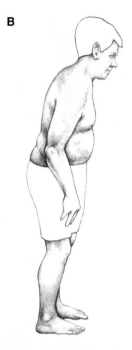

FIG. B-30, cont'd B, Parkinsonian posture.

7. If the patient complains of muscle stiffness or has a long thin "hatchet" face, test for the presence of myotonia (Figs. B-31 to B-33).
8. If the patient complains of easy fatigability, suspect myasthenia gravis and attempt to demonstrate fatigability (Fig. B-34).
   a. Have the patient sustain an upward gaze for at least 2 minutes; in patients with myasthenia gravis, one or both lids may droop.
   b. Have the patient perform some repetitive act relative to the complaint of weakness. For example, have the patient do repeated deep knee bends if the complaint is leg weakness. Have the patient repeatedly squeeze a manometer cuff if the complaint is weakness of grip. Myasthenics often gradually lose muscle power when performing such repetitive acts. The voice may lose volume during rapid loud counting.
9. Common peripheral nerve lesions.
   a. Radial nerve (Fig. B-35, *A*) damage produces weakness of dorsiflexion of the wrist and extension of the elbow. The lesion often is the result of compression of the nerve at the spiral groove of the humerus.

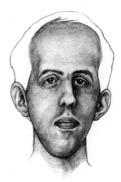

FIG. B-31 Hatchet face of myotonic dystrophy.

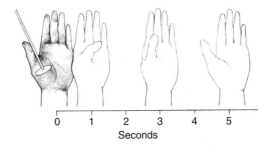

FIG. B-32 Demonstration of myotonia. Percuss the thenar eminence; if myotonia is present, the thumb will make a quick, involuntary opposing movement and then slowly relax. Have the patient make a hard fist and then suddenly open it; if myotonia is present, opening the fist will be slow and laborious.

b. Median nerve damage results in weakness of opposition of the thumb and the little finger if the lesion is at the wrist (carpal tunnel syndrome). More proximal lesions in the arm result in a weakness of pronation of the forearm and flexion of the radial three fingers (middle, ring, and little fingers) (Fig. B-35, *B*).

c. Ulnar nerve injury results in the weakness of abduction and adduction of the fingers, flexions of the ring and little fingers, and ulnar flexion of the wrist. The lesion is most often the result of compression of the nerve in the ulnar groove of the elbow (Fig. B-35, *C*).

d. Peroneal nerve damage results in weakness of extension (dorsiflexion) and eversion of the foot. The most common site for injury is at the fibular head.

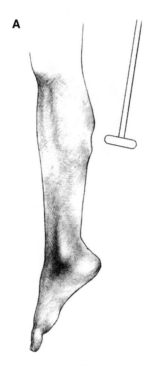

FIG. B-33 Demonstration of myoedema and myotonia. With the patient prone, percuss the gastrocnemius muscles with a reflex hammer. **A,** If myotonia is present, a persistent depression at the point of percussion will appear.

TESTING OF CEREBELLAR FUNCTION

1. Finger-nose-finger test: the examiner places his or her finger in front of the patient's nose at nearly the patient's arm length. The patient is then instructed to "touch my finger and then your nose, and back and forth."
2. Rapid alternating movements: the examiner demonstrates to the patient alternately slapping the palm and dorsal surface of the hand on the thigh and then requests that the patient do the same with each hand.
3. Heel-to-toe walking (tandem gait): The examiner instructs the patient to walk a line, heel to toe (this is usually done as a part of station and gait testing).
4. Heel-to-shin test: Instruct the patient in the lying position to run the heel of one leg smoothly up and down the shin of the other leg (Fig. B-36).

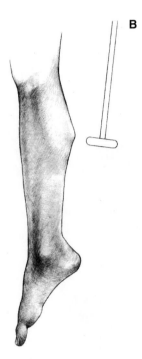

FIG. B-33, cont'd B, If myoedema is present, a lump will appear.

Common problems:
1. If the patient performs the finger-to-nose test too rapidly, the increase in tremor that occurs as the target is approached may be difficult for the examiner to appreciate.
2. The examiner's finger must be held at arm's length to increase excursion of the patient's arm and enhance the tremor.
3. The coordination may be difficult or impossible to test in a weak or paralyzed arm.
4. An abnormal tone (such as the rigidity of Parkinson's disease or with spasticity) may significantly interfere with the performance of rapid alternating movements.
5. The inexperienced examiner may not recognize that a patient with severe midline cerebellar disease can have relatively normal rapid alternating movements and a finger-to-nose test.
6. Other movement disorders, such as benign essential tremor, may make the finger-to-nose test difficult to interpret.

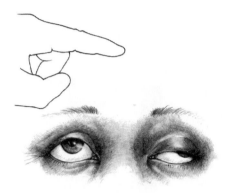

FIG. B-34 Myasthenia gravis.

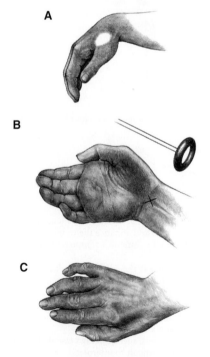

A

B

C

FIG. B-35 A, Radial nerve. B, Median nerve. C, Ulnar nerve.

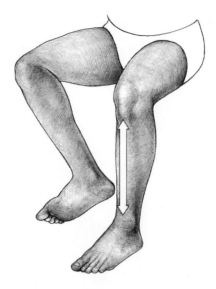

FIG. B-36 Heel-to-shin test.

Common abnormalities:
1. Dysfunction of a cerebellar hemisphere will cause an ipsilateral tremor notable during the finger-to-nose test. The tremor worsens as the target is approached and is not present in the resting hand or arm (Fig. B-37).
2. Dysfunction of a cerebellar hemisphere will cause an ipsilateral decrease in the ability to perform rapid alternating movements quickly and rhythmically.
3. Midline cerebellar dysfunction will cause balance difficulties during heel-to-toe walking. Truncal ataxia may also be present in the sitting position.

Other signs of cerebellar dysfunction:
1. Hypotonia may be manifested by a pendular knee reflex (Fig. B-38).
2. Speech melody may be disturbed, and speech may become "explosive" and ataxic. This is particularly noticeable when pronouncing "tongue-twister" phrases such as "Methodist Episcopal."
3. In acute cerebellar disease, the patient's voice may be hypophonic (low volume) or even mute temporarily.
4. When a patient is flexing the arm against resistance and the examiner suddenly lets go, the patient may be unable to avoid striking his or her face. This is known as *rebound*. The examiner should use his or her arm to protect the patient (Fig. B-39).
5. Titubation: in the sitting position, or when standing with the feet together and the eyes open, the patient wobbles unsteadily. This is a sign, along with abnormal tandem gait, of midline cerebellar dysfunction.

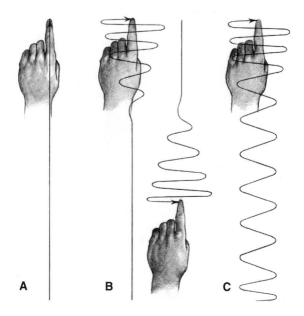

FIG. B-37 Tremor.

SENSORY AND AUTONOMIC EXAMINATION

Examination of Peripheral Sensation

The evaluation of sensation is subjective, and therefore the examiner must be certain that the patient correctly interprets the procedure. Sensory testing is the least reliable portion of the neurologic examination, and diagnosis should rarely, if ever, be made on the basis of the patient's reporting alone.

1. Testing the sensation of pain (Fig. B-40, *A*).
   a. Gently grasp the shaft of a pin (not a safety pin, ECG calipers, etc.) and test an area presumed to be normal (e.g., the neck). The pin should slide through the thumb and forefinger as skin contact is made. Ask the patient, "Does this feel sharp?"
   b. To evaluate lower extremity sensation, repeat the procedure on the dorsum of the foot and ask, "Does this feel the same?" If the patient says, "No, it's not so sharp on my foot," then ask the patient to quantitate the difference between the two if possible. The same procedure can be repeated on the dorsum of the hand to test upper extremity sensation.

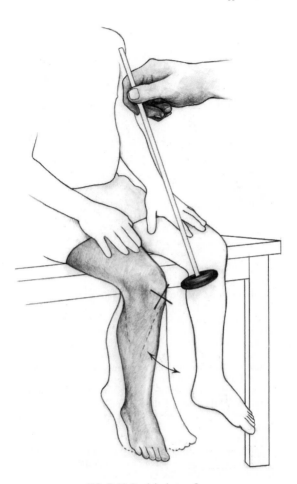

FIG. B-38 Pendular knee reflex.

Note: Always use a fresh pin for each patient to avoid the spread of infections such as hepatitis or HIV.

2. Testing light touch. Instruct the patient to keep the eyes closed and respond whenever touched. Take a wisp of cotton or facial tissue and touch the patient on random areas of the skin. Ask the patient to point to the part being touched.

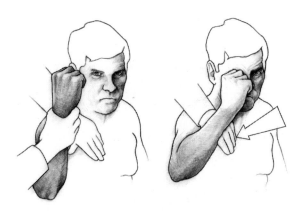

FIG. B-39 Rebound.

3. Testing vibratory sense (Fig. B-40, *B*).
   a. Establish rapport with the patient by placing the shaft of a lightly vibrating 128-Hz tuning fork on the distal finger of the patient's hand and ask, "Do you feel the buzzing?" Then ask the patient to "Tell me when the buzzing stops." When the patient says "stop," place the shaft of the fork on the knuckle of your hand. Normally, the examiner would also detect no vibration.
   b. To test vibratory sensation in the lower extremities, lightly tap the fork and place the shaft on the patient's big toe, again asking the patient to tell you when the buzzing stops. When the patient says "stop," place the shaft of the fork on the knuckle of your own hand. Normally, only a very slight vibration will still be felt by the examiner.
4. Testing position sense in the big toes.
   a. Establish rapport with the patient by grasping the patient's big toe *by the sides* and, with the patient observing the foot, say, "When I move the toe in this direction (demonstrating) I mean up, and when I move it in this direction (demonstrating) I mean down." It is helpful to fix the proximal joints with the examiner's opposite hand (Fig. B-40, *C*).
   b. With the patient's eyes closed, instruct the patient, "Tell me when I move your toe and whether I move it up or down." Move the toe unpredictably (e.g., up twice, down once). Normally, a patient will be able to detect movements of about 5 mm or less.
5. Testing for cortical sensation (Fig. B-40, *D*).
   a. Ascertain that primary sensory modalities (pain and vibratory sensation) are intact in the hands; if sensation is not intact, this test is not valid.

A

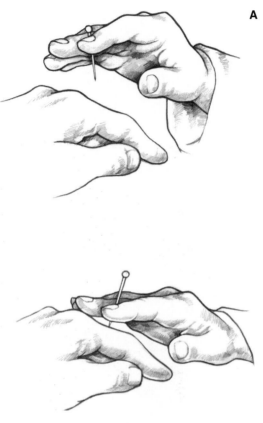

FIG. B-40 A, Testing for pain sensation.   *Continued*

b. To establish rapport with the patient, while the patient watches, draw a number or letter on the patient's palm (using the dull point of an object such as a key) and ask, "What number did I draw?" It is preferable to test the dominant hand first (unless a known neurologic defect exists on that side of the body), and the number should be written so that it is right side up to the patient. Then have the patient look away or close the eyes and repeat the procedure.

c. Then have the patient identify an object placed in his or her hand with the eyes closed. The object can be identified verbally—by naming it—or, in aphasic patients, picking the object correctly from an array of multiple objects.

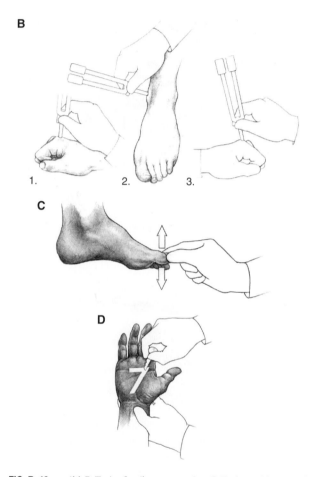

FIG. B-40, cont'd B, Testing for vibratory sensation. C, Testing position sensation in the toes. D, Testing cortical sensation.

Common problems:
1. The patient and examiner do not communicate adequately. The sensory examination is of limited value in patients with low intelligence, altered consciousness, aphasia, and psychiatric disturbances.
2. The examiner tests an area of sensory disturbance with a pin asking only, "Is this sharp or dull?" and does not compare with a normal area; many less severe sensory disturbances are thus undiagnosed.

E

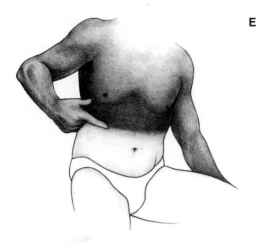

FIG B-40, cont'd E, Sensory self-examination.

3. The patient may think the response is what the examiner wants to hear; this is not necessarily malingering but is simply a human foible of attempting to please an authority figure.
4. Posterior column disease or a cortical sensory loss cannot be demonstrated if the patient has a peripheral nerve disturbance that affects all sensory modalities.

Common abnormalities:

1. Patients with peripheral neuropathies (especially those secondary to diabetes, alcohol, or deficiency states) will have a symmetric sensory loss in the feet in the distribution of the socks. Often the phenomenon of summation will be present; this is tested as follows:
   a. Normally, during repeatedly pricking of a skin area with a pin, the patient, if asked, "Does this become sharper?" will indicate that the pricks seem to be about of equal intensity.
   b. In an area of sensory abnormality, the examiner watching the patient's face will notice a sudden grimace after a dozen or so pricks if summation is present, and the patient will report that the intensity of the pin prick suddenly becomes unbearably sharp.
2. Intelligent, cooperative patients can often outline sensory disturbances better than the examiner. The patient should be instructed to place a finger in an area of disturbed sensation and move it until an area of normal sensitivity is found (Fig. B-40, *E*).
3. If a cortical sensory loss is suspected from the patient's inability to recognize numbers or letters written in the palms of the hand, other tests of cortical sensation should be used.
   a. With the eyes closed, the patient should be able to discriminate between various sizes of coins and identify a common object such as a key.

   b. With the patient's eyes closed, the examiner touches one arm, the other arm, and then both arms simultaneously. If the patient perceives the individual stimuli but consistently neglects one stimulus during simultaneous touching, the phenomenon of extinction is present.

   c. Other tests of cortical sensation include tactile localization (with eyes closed, a normal patient can accurately localize the examiner's touch) and two-point discrimination (with eyes closed, the normal patient can distinguish two sharp points separated by 5 mm on the fingertips) and extinction to double simultaneous touch of both hands.

AUTONOMIC NERVOUS SYSTEM

1. Examine the patient's blood pressure and heart rate in the supine and erect positions. Determine whether postural hypotension and compensatory tachycardia are present.
2. Instruct the patient to take a deep breath and bear down as if having a bowel movement (the Valsalva maneuver). The normal slowing of the heart associated with this maneuver can often best be appreciated with ECG monitoring.
3. Demonstrate the normal triple response (of Lewis) by scratching the patient's skin with a broken throat stick; normally, a white line will initially appear on the skin, followed by a red line, then reddening around the red line (flare), and finally slight elevation of the line (wheal).
4. Place the patient's hand in warm water for 10 or more minutes. The normal response is for the fingertips to become wrinkled.
5. Assess the pupillary size and response (which are controlled by both sympathetic and parasympathetic innervation).

Common abnormalities:

1. Diabetic peripheral polyneuropathies usually cause orthostatic hypotension, loss of finger wrinkling response, and loss of the flare in the triple response.
2. A small pupil may be caused by sympathetic denervation of the eye (Horner's syndrome). In a darkened room, the normal pupil will dilate, whereas the sympathetically denervated pupil will not change in size. Failure of the pupil to dilate to the instillation of a solution of 1% hydroxyamphetamine (Paredrine) suggests a lesion involving the peripheral sympathetic fibers (lesion of the third order sympathetic neuron).
3. A large pupil that does not constrict to bright light is the result of parasympathetic denervation as occurs with third cranial nerve palsy.

PATIENTS WITH ABNORMALITIES OF MENTATION

1. Deciding whether a formal evaluation of mentation is necessary. A mini-mental status examination (MMSE) should be done once at the time of the patient's first presentation. Further cognitive testing would be necessary if this is abnormal.

a. Consider the chief complaint and the clinical hypotheses formed during the history-taking; if a CNS mass lesion, diffuse CNS dysfunction, or focal CNS damage is under consideration, formal testing of mental status is necessary.

b. Consider certain information obtained in the history as "red flags." For example, patients with a history of ethanol abuse should be formally tested because the conversation and appearance of a patient with Korsakoff's psychosis may be superficially normal.

c. A formal mental status examination is mandatory when friends or family report mental deterioration or when there is a history of deterioration of occupational performance.

2. If a CNS dysfunction is suspected and formal mental status testing is anticipated, the following observations should be recorded:

a. The patient's mood is sad, elated, withdrawn, tearful, or bland

b. The appropriateness of behavior

c. The ability to relate the history relative to the complaint in a concise and logical manner

d. The ability to follow directions

e. Unusual behavior that might indicate the patient is experiencing hallucinations, such as suddenly looking at or listening to sensory stimuli which are not there

f. The presence or absence of perseverations; this may consist of the patient continuing a motor movement such as rapid alternating movements for an inappropriate length of time (Another example of perseveration would be the inability to change easily from one topic of conversation to another.)

g. The presence or absence of motor impersistence, which consists of the patient's inability to sustain a given motor test such as keeping the eyes closed (often noted during the sensory examination) or keeping the tongue protruded

3. Before starting the questioning, reassure the patient with a statement such as, "I'm now going to ask you some questions which may sound foolish but it is just part of the routine examination."

a. Mini-Mental Status Examination (Box B-2).

b. Standard mental status examination.

1) Memory

a) Immediate recall: the examiner slowly and distinctly pronounces a series of random numbers and has the patient repeat them in order. Start with a series of three numbers and continue with longer series until the patient successfully repeats a series of seven numbers, or fails twice. (If the patient fails to repeat six digits forward two times, but was able to repeat a series of five digits, record the success as five digits forward.) Then, have patient repeat the series backward. Normally, subjects repeat backward two digits less than they repeat forward.

b) Recent memory: tell the patient three unrelated nouns (e.g., "fox," "car," "blue") and have the patient repeat them. Indicate that the patient will be asked to repeat these words in

---

BOX B-2
Mini-Mental Status Examination

The Mini-Mental Status Examination (MMSE) is a brief, 30-point scale that screens cognition in the following areas:
- Orientation (time: date, year, month, season; and place: location, floor, city, county, state)
- Registration (repeating three words)
- Attention and calculations (spelling *world* backward or subtracting serials sevens)
- Recall (recalling the three words from the registration section)
- Language (naming two common objects, repeating a simple phrase such as, "No ifs, ands, or buts," following a three-stage command, following a written command, and writing a sentence)
- Construction (copying intersecting pentagons)

---

approximately 3 minutes. Then distract the patient with a few other questions before asking him or her to repeat the words. In addition, in obtaining the patient's history, questions regarding the last few hours (if the examiner can confirm the facts) are also indicative of recent memory ability.

   c) Remote memory: testing of remote memory can be incorporated with obtaining family and social histories. Information such as the patient's age, date of birth, and order of siblings, marriage date, and number and names of children is appropriate. The examiner may also use readily available historical facts. Ask for information that the patient should have known before the onset of the illness; occupational and recreational facts are much more reliable than such questions as naming presidents or other political figures. Questions concerning a favorite television show, a favorite sport, or wars a veteran may have lived through or participated in are useful.

2) The ability to follow instructions can usually be assessed during the physical and neurologic examination.

3) General information: rather than asking questions that are indicative of education and reminiscent of school examinations, it is as meaningful, and less threatening, to ask about the patient's occupation or hobbies. The patient should discuss either with interest and reasonable knowledge. Another useful line of questioning may concern a favorite television show and the plot from a recent episode. This combines recent memory with the ability to tell a story and may give insight into the patient's character as well.

4) Mathematical ability (calculation): ask simple, everyday problems of calculation such as "A newsman collected 25 cents from each of six customers. What is the total amount he or she col-

lected?" or "If five apples cost a quarter, how much does one apple cost?"

Caveat: Serial-sevens (subtracting 7 from 100 and continuing to subtract 7 from each number obtained) is not a simple calculation problem. It involves not only calculation but also recent memory and the ability to concentrate. Remember that under stress even normal persons may have difficulty performing serial-sevens, and poorly educated normal persons may not be able to perform this task. A person with above average IQ can subtract serial sevens from 100 and end at 2 in 20 seconds.

5) Judgment and abstract thinking are difficult to assess but may be the earliest functions to be impaired. Evidence of poor judgment often can be obtained by a history of occupational performance and daily activities. Commonsense questions can be used such as: "If you traveled to an unfamiliar city to visit a friend, what would you do to find him?" Or, "If you got into your car one morning to go to work and it didn't start, what would you do?" Another useful test involves similarities and differences. Ask the patient how two items are alike (what properties different objects have in common). For example, "What do a river and a lake have in common?" Other useful pairs of items to ask about include an orange and a banana, a dog and a lion, and a coat and a dress; the best answers would be conceptual ones such as fruit, animals, or clothing, whereas concrete answers may be given, such as both are edible, have four legs, or have sleeves. Patients with dementia often can give differences, but not similarities.

Note: Interpretation of proverbs such as "People who live in glass houses shouldn't throw stones" or "A golden hammer breaks an iron door" is often used by physicians as a test of judgment but may be difficult even for normal persons, especially if they are from a different cultural background.

Common problems in assessing mental status:
1) The examiner records in the chart "oriented ×3"; this is significant only if that is *all* the patient can do, but a patient may have a very serious impairment and still be "oriented ×3."
2) The examiner fails to take into account the patient's educational level or ethnic background.
3) The examiner fails to appreciate that the patient is depressed or hallucinating and therefore is unable to respond correctly.
4) The examiner asks the questions under stressful circumstances (e.g., in the presence of other physicians or patients).
5) Aphasic patients are mistaken as being demented.
6) The examiner fails to appreciate the difference between the patient who never, from birth, had the ability to perform well on a mental status examination and the patient who has *lost* the capacity to perform well on the examination. Dementia is a deterioration of whatever

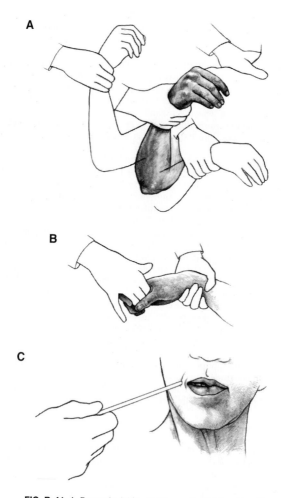

FIG. B-41 **A,** Paratonic rigidity. **B,** Grasp reflex. **C,** Rooting reflex.

previous mental capacity the individual had, even if the previous level was subnormal.
4. Abnormal reflexes seen in patients with generalized CNS disease.
  a. Paratonic rigidity (Gegenhalten) (Fig. B-41, *A*): The examiner requests the patient to relax an arm "like a rag doll." The examiner then moves the arm quickly and unexpectedly back and forth and

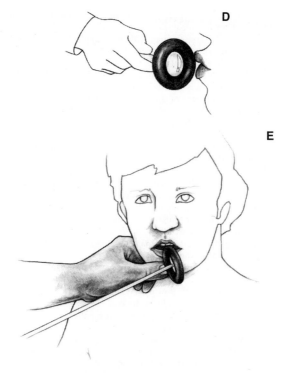

FIG. B-41 cont'd D, Snout reflex. E, Jaw reflex.

from side to side. The result is positive when it seems as if the patient is not relaxing the arm. (The inexperienced examiner may become impatient because of a mistaken perception that the patient is uncooperative.)

b. Grasp reflex (Fig. B-41, *B*): when the examiner strokes the patient's palm from the hypothenar eminence to the thumb and forefinger, the patient squeezes the examiner's fingers (a normal response in infants).

c. Rooting reflex (Fig. B-41, *C*): lightly stroking away from the corner of the patient's lips causes a movement of the lips or movement of the mouth toward the stimulus (a normal response in infants).

d. Snout reflex (Fig. B-41, *D*): a light tap on the patient's closed lips with a reflex hammer will cause the lips to pucker.

e. Jaw reflex (Fig. B-41, *E*): with the patient's mouth slightly open, the examiner lightly taps a thumb placed on the patient's chin, resulting in momentary closing of the jaws. This is a tendon reflex that normally is difficult to elicit; an easily elicited reflex indicates bilateral corticobulbar tract abnormalities.

  f. Eliciting reflexes associated with generalized CNS dysfunction results in the following problems:

    1) All of the abnormal reflexes are rarely present in the same patient; the reliability of each reflex as an indication of CNS dysfunction largely depends on the skill and experience of the examiner.

    2) The significance of the abnormal reflex must be viewed in the context of the patient's history and examination (e.g., some normal patients who are very nervous may have an easily elicitable jaw reflex).

5. Important disorders of higher cortical function caused by focal lesions.

  a. Aphasia: the disturbance of comprehension and production of language.

  b. Apraxia: a difficulty in performing a motor sequence in the absence of any significant weakness, sensory loss, incoordination, or difficulty understanding the task.

  c. Agnosia: a failure to interpret sensory information despite the lack of primary sensory deficit.

  d. Following is a short examination of higher cortical functions for aphasia, apraxia, and agnosia:

    1) Listen for abnormalities of spontaneous speech: word output, rhythm, effort, syntax, and paraphasias.

    2) Evaluate speech flow by having the patient name the days of the week and months of the year.

    3) Evaluate repetition by having the patient repeat a sentence (e.g., "The weather is nice outside today.").

    4) Assess reading ability and comprehension of written material by having the patient read several sentences or a paragraph aloud (a page from a magazine is useful) and discuss what was read.

    5) Evaluate the patient's naming ability by asking him or her to name several objects pointed out by the examiner (e.g., coins, pen, comb, button).

    6) Determine whether singing is performed better than ordinary speech by having the patient sing a familiar melody such as "Happy Birthday" either without or with prompting.

    7) Evaluate the ability of the patient to understand and follow one-, two-, and three-step oral instructions (e.g., "Stand up," "Go to the door," "Take the glass, fill it with water, and put the glass on the table in the corner of the room.").

    8) Assess the ability of the patient to follow written instructions ("Stand up," "Sit down," "Take the glass and fill it with water.").

    9) Evaluate the writing ability by having the patient write several sentences spontaneously (e.g., ask the patient to write a description of the weather); then have the patient copy several short sentences written by the examiner.

    10) Evaluate spatial abilities by having the patient draw a house, a clock, and a cube.

11) Evaluate the patient for evidence of agnosia and right-left disorientation by giving the patient complex body instructions (e.g., "Put your right thumb on your nose and your left thumb on your right ear.").

12) Evaluate the patient for evidence of apraxia by instructing the patient to perform a variety of motor tasks spontaneously and following the examiner's demonstration (e.g., "Stick out your tongue," "Stand up," "Pretend to use a hammer," "Show me how you comb your hair," "Show me how to pound a nail into a board.").

Common problems:

1. Many patients have elements of several aphasic syndromes caused by the involvement of several focal brain areas involved in language function.

2. The aphasic patient is mistakenly considered to be demented; the aphasic patient has difficulty only in communication, but other cognitive functions are intact.

3. The speech abnormality of Wernicke's aphasia is confused with the "word salad" characteristic of schizophrenia.

4. Mutism is mistaken for aphasia.

Common abnormalities:

1. Broca's aphasia (anterior, motor, or expressive aphasia).
   a. The cardinal difficulty is that quantity of speech is reduced ("nonfluent" aphasia).
   b. Conversational speech requires extra effort.
   c. Prepositions, articles, and conjunctions are often omitted (telegraphic speech).
   d. The patient is aware of the deficit and often is embarrassed and frustrated.
   e. The patient's comprehension is intact, but repetition is poor.
   f. Emotional speech, including profanity, is often preserved.
   g. Naming of objects may be intact or impaired.

2. Wernicke's aphasia (posterior, sensory, or receptive aphasia).
   a. The cardinal difficulty is understanding the examiner's words.
   b. The total quantity of speech is normal or increased ("fluent" aphasia).
   c. Meaningless, nonsense, or inappropriate words are substituted for correct words (paraphasias, such as "desk" for table or "phone" for stone); this is often referred to as *jargon speech.*
   d. The patient has difficulty repeating words and sentences.
   e. The patient's speech intonation and rhythm are intact (normal speech melody).
   f. The patient is often unaware of the deficit.
   g. The patient writes letters that are well formed, but the content is abnormal with normal words mixed with unintelligible words.

3. Conduction aphasia.
   a. The patient's cardinal difficulty is with repetition.
   b. The patient's comprehension is normal (in contrast to Wernicke's aphasia).

    c. The patient uses paraphasias excessively, but with excellent articulation (in contrast to Broca's aphasia).

    d. The patient has difficulty in naming objects.

    e. The patient can often sing better than speak.

4. Apraxia.

    a. Ideomotor apraxia: the patient has difficulty with simple motor tasks but improves on repetition, particularly after the examiner demonstrates the task.

    b. Ideational apraxia: the patient can perform simple motor tasks and individual steps of a complex motor task but has difficulty performing the correct sequence of steps or complex motor tasks.

    c. Constructional apraxia: the patient has difficulty drawing or copying two-dimensional or three-dimensional objects or arranging or building puzzles.

5. Alexia without agraphia.

    a. The patient can write but cannot read what has just been written.

    b. This condition is usually associated with a right homonymous hemianopia.

    c. This is secondary to a lesion involving the left occipital cortex and the splenium of the corpus callosum.

PATIENT SUSPECTED OF HAVING A NONORGANIC PROCESS

1. Suspect that a patient may have a nonorganic ("functional") lesion under the following circumstances:

    a. The motor or sensory deficit is not accompanied by objective abnormalities (e.g., reflex changes).

    b. The pattern of motor or sensory deficit violates known anatomic principles.

    c. The patient shows no concern over the deficit and may even seem pleased about being disabled.

    d. The deficit potentially could result in considerable financial or psychologic gain for the patient.

    e. The patient has a history of multiple hospitalizations or complaints without objective pathologic findings.

    f. The patient dresses inappropriately for the occasion (e.g., a female excessively groomed in a provocative negligee, presenting with a hemiparesis).

2. Procedures that may help in identifying a nonorganic complaint.

    a. If one leg is paralyzed (Fig. B-42):

        1) With the patient supine, the examiner places both palms beneath the heels of the patient (Fig. B-42, *A*). The patient is asked to lift the paralyzed leg. Then when asked to lift the nonparalyzed leg, the patient will unconsciously increase the pressure on the examiner's palm beneath the supposedly paralyzed leg. (Fig. B-42, *B*).

        2) The patient is then asked to press down with both heels (Fig. B-42, *C*). If the pressure to the examiner's palm is not equal to

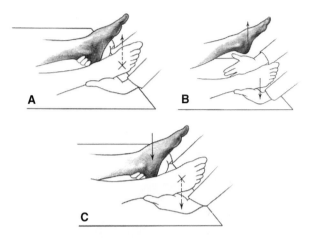

FIG. B-42 Testing for pseudoparalysis caused by conversion reaction.

that applied when the patient lifted the nonparalyzed leg, a conversion reaction can be suspected. This is called the *Hoover's sign.*
b. If the patient complains of sensory disturbance in one hand: have the patient clasp together inverted hands (Fig. B-43, *A*) and bring the arms upward; this places the right hand on the left side of the body (and vice versa) and distorts a person's sense of which hand is which; thus quickly reexamining the patient's sensibility to pinprick or a cotton wisp will give different results if the sensory disturbance is due to a conversion reaction (Fig. B-43, *B*).
c. When the hand of a comatose patient is lifted above the face and then dropped, it will strike the face (Fig. B-44, *A*); the hand of the patient with a nonorganic abnormality will veer to the side to avoid striking the face (Fig. B-44, *B*).
d. The patient with hemiparesis will have weakness in turning the head away from the paralyzed side caused by paresis of the sternocleidomastoid muscle (Fig. B-45). The patient with a nonorganic hemiparesis will often have normal strength turning to the opposite side but weakness turning to the same side.
e. The patient with a nonorganic positive straight leg raising test will complain of pain in the supine position (Fig. B-46, *A*), but not when the leg is straightened by the examiner to the same angle in the sitting position, even though the geometry is the same in both positions (Fig. B-46, *B*).
f. If a patient complains of weakness on one side of the body, test the strength on both sides simultaneously. It is difficult to "give way" with one muscle group while maintaining normal strength on the opposite side (Fig. B-47).

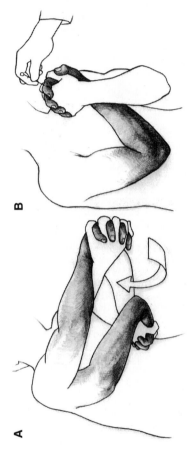

FIG. B-43 Testing for sensory disturbance in conversion reaction.

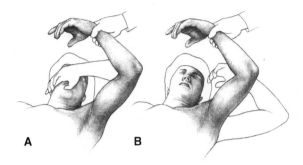

FIG. B-44 Demonstrating pseudocoma caused by conversion reaction.

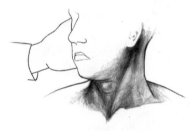

FIG. B-45 Testing for hemiparesis by evaluating weakness in head turning.

g. If the patient complains of an area of anesthesia, instruct the patient to close the eyes and answer "yes" if feeling the pinprick or "no" if not. (Obviously the only appropriate answer is silence when the supposedly anesthetic area is touched.)

h. A patient with an organic hemisensory deficit in the face can still feel the vibrations of a tuning fork placed on either side of the face owing to the conductive properties of bone; a patient with a nonorganic lesion will often report no vibratory feeling at all on the affected side (Fig. B-48). This test also works on the sternum.

i. If the patient complains of total blindness in one eye, the lesion must be anterior to the optic chiasm, and a Marcus-Gunn pupil or another pupillary abnormality must be present.

j. If the patient complains of a visual field defect, plot the defect on a tangent screen at two different distances; with an organic lesion, the field defect should increase as the distance from the patient to the chart increases.

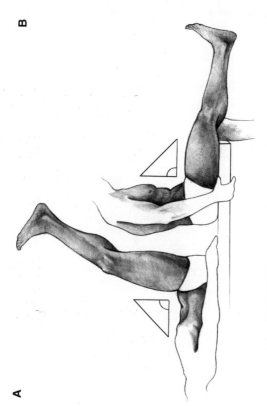

FIG. B-46 Nonorganic positive straight leg raising test.

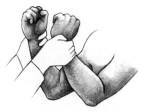

FIG. B-47 Simultaneous bilateral testing of muscle strength to demonstrate weakness caused by conversion reaction.

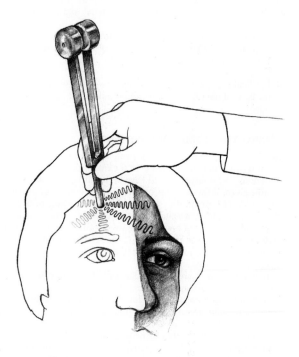

FIG. B-48 Testing for nonorganic hemisensory deficit on the face.

k. A patient with bilateral blindness will not blink when the examiner's hand is suddenly thrust at the patient's face in a threatening manner; the patient with nonorganic blindness often will blink.

l. The patient with nonorganic total blindness will not be able to suppress the nystagmus induced by an opticokinetic tape.

Common problems:

1. The examiner does not appreciate that many patients with organic lesions elaborate on symptoms and appear to have a psychiatric disturbance.

2. The examiner hastily makes a diagnosis on subjective findings and submits the patient to dangerous and expensive tests.

3. The examiner becomes angry with the patient with nonorganic complaints and fails to appreciate that the patient is in distress and needs sympathy and understanding, along with referral to a psychiatrist or psychologist.

4. The examiner feels insecure in his or her knowledge of psychiatry and neurology and considers a psychiatric diagnosis only after organic causes are ruled out.

Caveat: Psychiatric diagnoses, like neurologic diagnoses, should be made only on the basis of objective evidence and should never be made simply by exclusion.

EXAMINING THE COMATOSE PATIENT

1. Before examining the comatose patient, make certain that respirations and circulation are adequate. In the emergency department, an intravenous (IV) infusion should have been started and glucose and thiamine given. If there is a history of trauma, a fracture of the cervical spine must be excluded by radiographic studies. The general physical examination may give clues as to the causes of coma: jaundice of hepatic failure, bleeding ear or Battle's sign of trauma, petechiae of infections, or neoplastic and bleeding disorders. Check for characteristic breath odor (alcohol or diabetic ketoacidosis).

2. Obtain blood pressure and pulse.

   a. An elevated blood pressure is commonly found in patients with intracranial hemorrhage or cerebral edema.

   b. Increasing blood pressure and slowing of the pulse can be associated with medullary compression from cerebral herniation caused by increased intracranial pressure.

   c. Low blood pressure is often associated with toxic-metabolic coma.

   d. A rapid pulse may indicate severely depleted blood volume.

3. Observe the character of the breathing pattern (Fig. B-49).

4. Record rectal temperature.

   a. Temperature is usually normal or decreased in metabolic coma.

   b. Temperature is often increased in structural CNS coma, meningitis, and heat stroke.

Caveat: Infants and the elderly may not have elevated temperatures with infection.

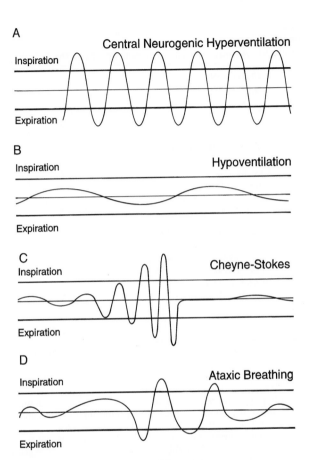

FIG. B-49 Common abnormal breathing patterns include: **A,** Central neurogenic hyperventilation (deep, rapid, regular). **B,** Hypoventilation (shallow, slow, regular). **C,** Cheyne-Stokes (apneic spells followed by respiration that gradually increase in rate and depth and then gradually decrease in rate and depth until apnea again occurs). **D,** Ataxic breathing (respirations totally unpredictable as to depth, rate, or rhythm; this is the only respiratory pattern diagnostic of a CNS lesion).

5. If the patient is spontaneously moving, note whether the movements are symmetric or asymmetric. Asymmetric movements are suggestive of a structural CNS lesion.
6. Determine the level of consciousness according to the Glasgow Coma Scale (Table B-5).

TABLE B-5
Glasgow Coma Scale
(Circle the Appropriate Number and Compute the Total)*

EYES OPEN	
Never	1
To pain	2
To verbal stimuli	3
Spontaneously	4
BEST VERBAL RESPONSE	
No response	1
Incomprehensible sounds	2
Inappropriate words	3
Disoriented and converses	4
Oriented and converses	5
BEST MOTOR RESPONSE	
No response	1
Extension (decerebrate rigidity)	2
Flexion abnormal (decorticate rigidity)	3
Flexion withdrawal	4
Localizes pain	5
Obeys	6
TOTAL (RANGE)	**3-15**

*The sum of the highest value in each category is the coma score: full mental capacity, 15; highest level of coma, 8; brain death, 3.

7. The type of movement in response to painful stimulation can suggest the site of the lesion. To produce the painful stimulation, stand behind the patient and apply pressure to the styloid process.
   a. Symmetric decerebrate posturing (Fig. B-50, *A*) or decorticate posturing (Fig. B-50, *B*) is suggestive of metabolic coma or of central rostral-caudal brain herniation.
   b. Asymmetric posturing (Fig. B-50, *C*) is suggestive of coma from a structural CNS lesion.
8. Check for neck suppleness by placing one hand under the occiput and attempting to flex the patient's neck.

Caveat: Do not manipulate the neck if cervical fracture is a possibility.

Common observations:
   a. Normal response: the chin should easily touch the chest.
   b. Stiff neck: with subarachnoid hemorrhage or meningitis, the examiner often can raise the upper part of the body without inducing neck flexion.

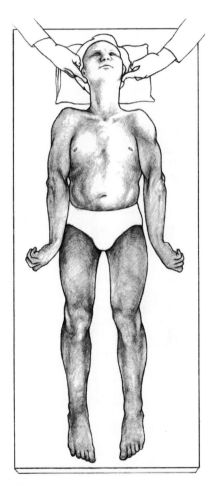

FIG. B-50 A, Symmetric decerebrate posturing in response to painful stimulation.

Continued

A

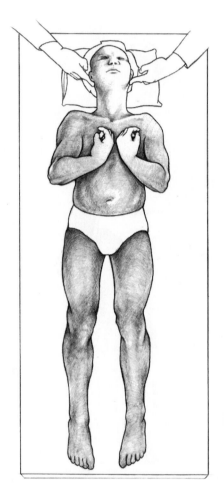

B

FIG. B-50, cont'd B, Symmetric decorticate posturing in response to painful stimulation.

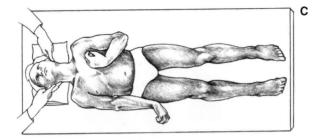

FIG. B-50, cont'd **C,** Asymmetric posturing in response to painful stimulation.

9. Check for muscle tone.
   a. Lift both arms together above the chest and let them fall simultaneously. The hypotonic arm will fall faster.
   b. Lift both lower extremities at the knees so that both knees and hips are flexed. When released, the hypotonic leg will externally rotate and extend faster.
   c. The resistance to passive movement should be tested separately in each limb.
10. Evaluation of cranial nerves and brainstem integrity.
    a. Examine the optic fundus (see the section on examination of the cranial nerves in this appendix). Papilledema is usually associated with structural CNS lesions but can also occur with metabolic abnormalities that cause cerebral edema.
    b. Observe pupils for size, symmetry, and reaction to light (see the section on examination of the cranial nerves).

Note: Use a bright, pinpoint source of light; when there is doubt about whether the pupils are reactive, observing the pupil through the magnification lens of the otoscope may be helpful.

    c. Common abnormalities:
       1) Pinch the skin at the neck and observe if pupils dilate bilaterally. If so, the brainstem is largely intact (ciliospinal reflex).
       2) Pinpoint pupils are suggestive of pontine hemorrhage, narcotic overdose, or cholinergic drugs.
       3) Unilaterally dilated and fixed or poorly reactive pupils are suggestive of intracerebral hemorrhage causing damage to cranial nerve III.
       4) Bilaterally large and poorly reactive pupils are suggestive of anoxia or anticholinergic or adrenergic drugs.
       5) Asymmetric pupils are suggestive of coma from a structural CNS lesion. (Symmetric pupils suggest metabolic coma.)
    d. Oculocephalic (doll's eye) reflex. Holding the eyelids open, passively rotate the patient's head rapidly to each side (Fig. B-51, *A*).

A

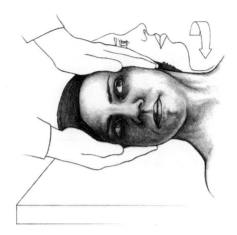

B

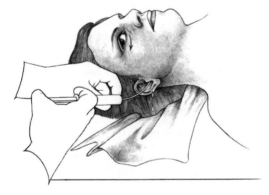

FIG. B-51 **A,** Oculocephalic reflex. **B,** Oculovestibular reflexes.

In the comatose patient with an intact brainstem, the eyes deviate away from the direction of the rotation, then return to the neutral "straight ahead" position. Awake patients have no oculocephalic reflex.

Caveat: This should never be done in comatose patients with head trauma until a neck fracture has been ruled out.

Common observations:
1) No response (eyes turn with head) occurs in both severe metabolic and CNS structural coma.

2) Dysconjugate movement of the eyes is seen in coma from CNS structural lesion damaging the brainstem.
3) A response indicates that the brainstem is intact from cranial nerves III to VIII and that the coma is probably caused by a metabolic abnormality.

e. Oculovestibular (caloric) reflex (Fig. B-51, *B*) (performed if there is suspicion of a neck fracture or if the oculocephalic reflex is equivocal): check to see that the tympanic membrane is intact and that the external auditory canal is not blocked by wax or blood; inject at least 10 ml of ice water through a small polyethylene catheter into the external auditory canal and then immediately elevate the head to approximately 30 degrees from the horizontal.

Caveat: If a neck fracture is suspected, do not move the head or neck. Instead, tilt the table to elevate the head.

Common observations:
1) In a comatose patient with an intact brainstem from cranial nerves III to VIII, there is conjugate deviation of the eyes toward the cooled ear and no nystagmus occurs.
2) No response suggests either severe metabolic or a structural CNS lesion, whereas dysconjugate eye movement indicates a structural lesion damaging the brainstem.

f. Corneal reflex.
Common observations:
1) No response is seen in patients with deep coma from any cause.
2) A symmetric response indicates the brainstem between cranial nerves V and VII is intact.
3) An asymmetric response is seen in structural CNS coma.

g. Evaluation of facial symmetry (cranial nerve VII): with facial asymmetry, as the patient breathes a paralyzed cheek will exhibit more movement than the nonparalyzed cheek. This is seen in coma from structural CNS lesions.

h. Evaluation of the pharyngeal reflex (refer to testing of cranial nerve X in this appendix).
Common observations:
1) No response is seen in patients in deep coma from any cause.
2) Asymmetric response indicates structural CNS coma.

11. Evaluation of muscle stretch reflexes and plantar response (Fig. B-52).
Common problems:
a. An acutely paralyzed limb may exhibit either absent or hypoactive reflexes even if the paralysis is caused by an upper motor neuron lesion.
b. Occasionally patients may have asymmetric posturing, movement, or reflexes when the cause of the coma is metabolic; this is especially true if there is an old injury to the CNS system.
Common observations:
1) Symmetric reflexes (hyperactive, hypoactive, or absent) are seen primarily in metabolic coma.

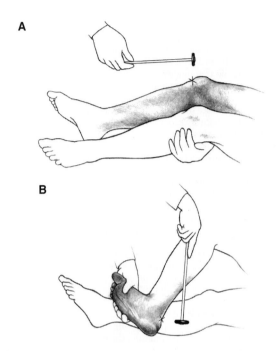

FIG. B-52 A, Eliciting patellar reflexes in a comatose patient. Place an arm under both knees so that the knees are slightly flexed and then strike the patellar tendon with a reflex hammer. Pay close attention to reflex asymmetries and crossed adductor responses. **B,** In the comatose patient, the Achilles reflex is elicited by crossing the legs and slightly dorsiflexing the foot before tapping the Achilles tendon.

2) Asymmetric reflexes are seen most often in structural CNS coma.

NEUROVASCULAR EXAMINATION

1. Determine the blood pressure.
   a. The blood pressure cuff should be of suitable size. (A normal-size blood pressure cuff on an obese patient may give a falsely high reading.)
   b. Brachial blood pressure is measured in both arms, usually both in supine and erect positions.
      1) An asymmetric blood pressure of more than 10 mm Hg suggests occlusive disease in the proximal artery, usually the subclavian artery.

2) A blood pressure change of 30 mm Hg or more in systolic pressure in assuming the erect from the supine position suggests peripheral autonomic dysfunction; a lack of compensatory tachycardia substantiates autonomic dysfunction.

Common problems:

1. Blood pressure changes must be correlated with the patient's symptoms.
2. Especially in the elderly, blood pressure changes may vary; orthostatic hypotension is usually more prominent in the morning because of dehydration.
3. The patient must be protected from falling.
4. The examiner should perform the measurements (rather than relying on nurses or technicians) to correlate the symptoms with the measurements.
5. An accurate handheld manometer is more convenient to use than a mercury manometer.
6. An appropriate manometer cuff should be used relative to arm size.

2. Examine the blood vessels: Palpate the superficial temporal, radial, femoral, and dorsalis pedis arteries to evaluate collateral circulation and find evidence of atherosclerosis or emboli.

Common abnormalities:

1. A reduced or absent pulse in superficial temporal artery is seen in occlusion of the common carotid artery.
2. Tenderness and beading of the superficial temporal artery suggests temporal arteritis.
3. An irregular pulse suggests the possibility of emboli originating in the heart.

Caveat: Palpation of the carotid artery may cause bradycardia and has the potential of dislodging a clot. An occluded artery may appear to have a relatively normal pulsation, and therefore palpation is of limited value.

3. Auscultation.
   a. Carotid artery bruits are best heard at the bifurcation.
   b. Subclavian artery bruits are best detected in the supraclavicular fossa.
   c. Intracranial bruits are best heard over the orbits.

Note: Bruits are best heard by using the bell of the stethoscope.

Common problems:

1. Transmitted heart murmurs may be mistaken for bruits.
2. Too firm pressure from the stethoscope bell may create an artificial bruit.
3. Fluttering of the eyelids can be mistaken for a bruit.
4. The loudness of the bruit does not correlate with the degree of stenosis or pathologic condition.

TABLE B-6
Funduscopic Vascular Findings

Lesion	Findings
Subarachnoid hemorrhage	Subhyaloid hemorrhage (between retina and vitreous)
Hollenhorst plaques	Yellow refractile cholesterol emboli in retinal arterioles
Fibrin-platelet emboli	White emboli in retinal arterioles
Septic emboli	Small retinal hemorrhages with a central white spot (Roth's spots)
Central retinal artery occlusion	Pale retina, attenuated arterioles, and red macula
Diabetic retinopathy	Microaneurysms, hard exudates, neovascularization, vitreous hemorrhage, retinal detachment
Hypertensive retinopathy	Copper- or silver-wiring appearance of narrowed arterioles, flame hemorrhages, cotton-wool exudates, and (in later stages) papilledema

Common abnormalities:
1. Carotid or subclavian bruits suggest arterial stenosis.
2. Orbital bruits suggest intracranial arteriovenous malformation or carotid-cavernous fistula.
4. Retinal examination. Funduscopic vascular findings are presented in Table B-6.

Index

Page numbers followed by b indicate boxes; f, figures; t, tables.

445